Clinical Reasoning and Decision-Making in Psychiatry

In *Clinical Reasoning and Decision-Making in Psychiatry*, Drs. Joseph Goldberg and Stephen Stahl, two well-respected psychiatrists with expertise in mood disorders and psychopharmacology, clarify the thinking that goes into the provision of personalized medicine. They cogently illustrate the many dilemmas psychiatrists face in their everyday practices: how to weigh clinical observations with the scientific literature guiding expert treatment without losing sight of individual patients' histories, objectives, and preferences. Clinical vignettes bring to life the shared physician/patient decision-making that is key to successful personalized treatment. The reader comes away knowing what a seasoned clinician would do under the complex situations that often appear in practice but are not always discussed in treatment guidelines. This is a must-read for new or experienced clinicians who seek to improve their practices by collaborating with and meeting the needs of their individual patients.

David J. Miklowitz, Ph.D.
Distinguished Professor of Psychiatry and Behavior Sciences,
UCLA School of Medicine, Los Angeles, CA

Clinical decision-making is an art that depends on effective translation of prior scientific evidence and experience to the care of an individual patient. This volume is designed to help both experienced clinicians and those earlier in their careers navigate that process. The authors bring to this challenging task the valuable perspectives of researchers with a deep knowledge of the clinical studies that underlie our diagnostic formulations and those that yield the medications and other treatments that are available for use. They couple this knowledge with extensive clinical experience in addressing the treatment of patients. Their goal is to develop a model that views clinical decisions about diagnosis or treatment as a test of a hypothesis that will be confirmed or rejected based on an observable outcome for the patient. Following that model will reward clinicians and their patients.

Nina R. Schooler, Ph.D.
Professor of Psychiatry and Behavioral Sciences, SUNY Downstate Health Sciences Center,
Brooklyn, NY

This terrific book is an indispensable resource for mental health clinicians. Drs. Goldberg and Stahl, both luminaries in the field, provide nuanced, practical, and person-centered recommendations for addressing the needs of patients, especially those with diagnostic complexity or treatment resistance. The authors engage readers in useful consideration of common clinical concerns such as optimal use of diagnostic categories, off-label treatment options, and management of complex clinical dilemmas. Humorous tips, informative vignettes, and easy-to-reference summaries bring the material to life. Readers will appreciate the authors' encyclopedic knowledge of psychopharmacology, sage clinical wisdom, and thoughtful approach to shared decision-making. If you want to take better care of your psychiatric patients, this book is for you.

Holly A. Swartz, M.D.
Professor of Psychiatry, University of Pittsburgh, Pittsburgh, PA
Editor-in-Chief, *American Journal of Psychotherapy*

Psychiatry, at best, is both a science and an art. Lacking formal tools like x-rays and pathology tests in the main, generating a valid diagnosis and then determining the optimal treatment requires both domains to be brought into play by the psychiatrist. Some learn criteria lists and weight guidelines documents, a process that risks a "painting by numbers" approach. Some "hear the music" and meld (or iterate) left-brain and right-brain thinking to operate to a pattern analytic approach. Malcolm Gladwell has argued that any skill requires ten thousand hours to obtain expertise. This book by two skilled clinicians and educators can be guaranteed to reduce that period, being jam-packed with clinical wisdom. Their focus on a non-patriarchal shared decision-making model is illuminating. Will Rogers once astutely observed that "Common sense ain't that common." This book is redolent with common sense and at a level rarely observed in medicine let alone psychiatry.

Gordon Parker
Scientia Professor of Psychiatry, University of New South Wales, Sydney

This is a comprehensive and indispensable resource for mental health professionals seeking to master two essential psychiatric skill sets. They delve deep and offer a profound exploration of the intricate processes that guide clinical decision-making in this field. Drs. Goldberg and Stahl provide a well-balanced blend of theoretical insights and practical wisdom. Readers will benefit from guidance on navigating the nuanced landscape of psychiatric diagnoses, refining relevant skills, and formulating evidence-based treatment plans. The authors emphasize the importance of considering both the biological and psychosocial aspects of mental health, ensuring a holistic approach to patient care. With its clear, accessible language and evidence-based approach, *Clinical Reasoning and Decision-Making in Psychiatry* is an essential companion for psychiatric clinicians, residents, and all students, offering a robust foundation for delivering compassionate and effective care in the field of psychiatry.

Professor Allan H. Young
Director, Centre for Affective Disorders and Academic Director,
Psychological Medicine and Older Adults Clinical Academic Group,
Institute of Psychiatry, Psychology and Neuroscience, King's College London

Psychiatrists perform one of the most difficult tasks in medicine. In our training we must acquire knowledge and understanding of all the determinants of behavior and how to address symptomatic behavior. As clinicians we have one tool in which to assess and determine how to treat our patients, our minds. Drs. Goldberg and Stahl provide a conceptual guide as to how to address and order the information that we attain in our clinical interactions. They apply this guide to initial patient assessments where we develop diagnoses and therapeutic treatment plans and then to all the complex elements that affect our work throughout a course of patient treatment. This is not a volume that tells us what to do. Instead, it teaches how to engage in essential clinical thinking and hypothesis formation in all areas of practice. This volume provides the critical foundation as to how to be a modern psychiatrist.

Sidney Weissman, M.D.
Clinical Professor of Psychiatry and Behavioral Science, Northwestern University/Feinberg
School of Medicine, Chicago, IL Emeritus Faculty, Chicago Psychoanalytic Institute, Chicago, IL
Past President, American Association of Directors of Psychiatric Residency Training

A psychiatrist has to master a great deal of information – signs, symptoms, diagnoses, treatments, and much more. However, information is not enough. The clinical process involves how to think, not only what to think about. This volume, by two expert clinical psychopharmacologists, shifts attention to this broader clinical process: coping with diagnostic ambiguity, determining the appropriate level of care, when and how to start, stop, change, or end a course of treatment, how to construct a strategic plan that recognizes that treatment often doesn't work, how to evaluate whether it is working (including a primer on what a clinician can learn from research statistical methods), and finally, most important, how to include the patient in every step along the way. This book belongs on the shelf of every psychiatrist who has mastered the basics and is ready to become a seasoned expert, a consultant to others and, most of all, to his or her own work.

Robert Michels, M.D.
Walsh McDermott University Professor of Medicine and University Professor of Psychiatry,
Weill Medical College, Cornell University, Ithaca, NY

Clinical Reasoning and Decision-Making in Psychiatry

Joseph F. Goldberg
Icahn School of Medicine at Mount Sinai, New York

Stephen M. Stahl
University of California, San Diego

CAMBRIDGE
UNIVERSITY PRESS

CAMBRIDGE
UNIVERSITY PRESS

Shaftesbury Road, Cambridge CB2 8EA, United Kingdom

One Liberty Plaza, 20th Floor, New York, NY 10006, USA

477 Williamstown Road, Port Melbourne, VIC 3207, Australia

314–321, 3rd Floor, Plot 3, Splendor Forum, Jasola District Centre, New Delhi – 110025, India

103 Penang Road, #05–06/07, Visioncrest Commercial, Singapore 238467

Cambridge University Press is part of Cambridge University Press & Assessment, a department of the University of Cambridge.

We share the University's mission to contribute to society through the pursuit of education, learning and research at the highest international levels of excellence.

www.cambridge.org
Information on this title: www.cambridge.org/9781009181556

DOI: 10.1017/9781009181549

First published 2024

Printed in Mexico by Litográfica Ingramex, S.A. de C.V.

A catalogue record for this publication is available from the British Library

Library of Congress Cataloging-in-Publication Data
Names: Goldberg, Joseph F., 1963– author. | Stahl, Stephen M. 1951– author.
Title: Clinical reasoning and decision-making in psychiatry / Joseph F. Goldberg, Stephen M. Stahl.
Description: Cambridge, United Kingdom ; New York, NY : Cambridge University Press, 2024. | Includes bibliographical references. |
Identifiers: LCCN 2023045640 (print) | LCCN 2023045641 (ebook) | ISBN 9781009181556 (paperback) | ISBN 9781009181549 (ebook)
Subjects: MESH: Mental Disorders – diagnosis | Clinical Decision-Making – methods | Mental Disorders – therapy | Psychiatry – methods
Classification: LCC RC469 (print) | LCC RC469 (ebook) | NLM WM 141 | DDC 616.89/075–dc23/eng/20231215
LC record available at https://lccn.loc.gov/2023045640
LC ebook record available at https://lccn.loc.gov/2023045641

ISBN 978-1-009-18155-6 Paperback

Contents

Foreword

This book aspires to explain, promote, and facilitate the implementation of patient-centered psychopharmacological or psychotherapeutic treatments, thereby minimizing the growing trend toward recipe-driven mental health treatment. This seminal contribution is particularly timely for three reasons: inadequate evidence, inadequate training, and inadequate opportunity in practice to deliver personalized care. These three challenges have led to guideline-mandated rather than guideline-informed care, which is both dangerous and ineffective. The development of artificial intelligence could exacerbate this situation if not managed with caution and deliberation (as noted by the authors at various points throughout this book).

Our evidence base for treatment effectiveness largely relies on randomized controlled trials that exclude the complex, comorbid, severe, and chronic patients whom we see in routine practice – thus making "evidence-based medicine" more aspirational than we'd like to believe. Consequently, once we decide what *might be* (not what *is*) wrong and what *might be* (not what *is*) a good treatment, we need plans for diagnostic revisions and for what and when a second treatment step might be indicated should the first fail.

Second, training in the mental health specialties, especially in the practice of psychopharmacology, focuses on identifying the diagnosis, differential diagnoses, and learning the available treatment options based on the above-noted limited evidence – for example, which kinds of pharmacological mechanisms should be combined based on what clinical findings? Similarly, there is an emphasis on treatment algorithms, and using techniques in "manual-based therapies" in a more recipe-like fashion than initially intended. This focus on "what is wrong" and "what to do" (sometimes called strategic decisions) fails to address the "how" and "when" to deliver which treatment(s) to which patients (sometimes called tactical decisions). Even if we get the strategic decisions right (diagnosis and treatment choice), if we fail to personalize the dose, duration, or timing (tactical failures), the treatment will underperform or fail.

Third, current practice management, emphasizing "production" and "volume" rather than "value"-based medicine, may hamper thoughtful patient-centered clinical decision-making given time limitations.

Drs. Goldberg and Stahl address each of these challenges to patient-centered decision-making by examining the strategic and tactical decision-making processes entailed in diagnosing and treating mental health patients (e.g., defining the goals, when they are expected, anticipating problems, and deciding when and how to proceed if the initial steps fail, etc.). They make explicit the kinds of thinking that underlie clinical decisions. For example, they promote and illustrate the idea of formulating clinical problems as testable hypotheses that then form the basis for shared decision-making with patients. This helps the reader frame clinical decisions as deductive reasoning processes based on pro–con analyses when there is often no single "right" course of action. The reader will learn how to weight the relative importance of both clinicians' and patients' goals and priorities in constructing patient-specific treatment plans or decision trees. This approach helps clinicians devise iterative treatment strategies tailored to individual patients (rather than large diagnostic groups) based on patient-specific historical and current clinical characteristics.

Clinicians who incorporate these techniques will find themselves a step closer toward practicing personalized medicine. Some of these tactical and strategic decisions are things seasoned veterans sometimes do intuitively, or sometimes not at all. Readers at all levels of expertise will welcome the way Drs. Goldberg and Stahl illustrate processes of sophisticated clinical reasoning in ways that can only enhance their confidence in how to assess, formulate, and render care for patients across the spectrum of psychiatric disorders.

The authors make generous use of engaging clinical vignettes that illustrate how to apply these techniques to deliver personalized care despite the evidence limitations. Thinking through the clinical evidence provided by the patients, their circumstances, and their histories, as well the research evidence and its applicability in each case, helps readers to thoughtfully bridge the gap between what we know, what we think we know, and what we need to do on a case-by-case basis.

This book will help mental health practitioners as well as trainees from all backgrounds and levels of expertise become more systematic and analytic about the choices they make and the ways they can deliver on those choices, with a focus on patients first. The approach outlined in the pages ahead will very likely make our patient care safer, more collaborative, more personalized, and more effective.

Augustus John Rush, MD
Professor Emeritus, Duke-National University of Singapore;
Adjunct Professor of Psychiatry and Behavioral Sciences,
Duke Medical School,
Durham NC;
CEO Curbstone Consultant LLC

Preface

When faced with multiple options for how to solve a clinical problem, how do clinicians decide which is the best, or which hierarchically to pursue first, then second, and then third? How do they mentally construct an algorithm, formally or informally, both pharmacologically and psychosocially, about how to follow a sequenced pattern of interventions? How do they choose when to make unilateral decisions versus collaboratively engaging patients (or third parties) in the decision-making process? Treatment decisions by clinicians hinge fundamentally on thorough diagnostic and clinical assessments – one must know exactly what one is treating before deciding how best to deliver the most appropriate intervention – but then comes the challenge of decision-making. What factors go into the mental calculus for devising a treatment plan? Ideally, one considers evidence-based information about the efficacy of one intervention versus another. (That is, is there a robust database of randomized trials supporting a particular intervention? And how impactful is one intervention relative to another?) One also weighs the pros and cons of various candidate treatment options (including efficacy versus tolerability and acceptability of a proposed treatment) and the degree to which viable alternative options exist. One takes into account patient preferences but also the confronting or dispelling of inaccurate biases and wrongly sourced information. Add in factors such as cost, dosing complexity, formulary availability, and co-prescribed medications that bring their own drug interactions, and the net sum becomes a complex equation with multiple unknowns.

The purpose of this book is to provide mental health clinicians from all backgrounds with a systematic strategy for clinical decision-making – spanning pharmacotherapy, psychotherapy, treatment settings, and team-based approaches – and gaining a broadened ability to recognize and make explicit the many factors that go into the process of choosing from among plausible interventions. Whether they consciously realize it or not, clinicians often form implicit hypotheses about what they think might work best for a given patient and then test those hypotheses, often in a sequential fashion. They also, consciously or otherwise, blend their own experiences with learned knowledge (either from firsthand reading of the literature, attending research presentations, pharmaceutical marketing materials, or sheer scuttlebutt), and then implement some self-generated algorithm that merges "evidence-based prescribing" with "prescribing-based evidence."

One of our goals in writing this book has been to help practitioners make this tacit process more explicit and deliberate. Doing so has numerous advantages: contingency-planning lends a more cohesive longitudinal structure to a global treatment plan ("if X doesn't work we'll try Y; if Y fails then Z is the next most logical option"); it conveys a sense of purposefulness and strategy by devising a comprehensive, iterative operation that takes into account the results of previous undertakings (e.g., choosing a third step will depend on what exactly happens after the first two steps have been attempted); and it engages the patient as an active partner in the shared decision-making process.

Seldom is there one and only one appropriate intervention for any given mental health condition – though there are exceptions: for example, nothing has ever been shown to be more efficacious than electroconvulsive therapy for treatment-resistant depression, nor has any treatment ever been shown to be superior to clozapine for refractory schizophrenia. Some interventions are well studied in treatment-resistant depression while others are not. Decision-making conundrums arise when a clinician does not discuss options, makes no mention of back-up plans, or draws no distinctions between well-studied versus poorly studied treatment options for a given situation. Deliberate decision-making means contrasting purposeful with arbitrary treatment options. There is no a priori reason to expect greater success from a third or fourth serotonergic antidepressant for depression after several adequate trials of drugs with similar mechanisms have failed. Nor should one expect that a newly available drug will likely help a refractory population if it has not formally been studied in that setting. Clinicians working in the trenches may feel desperate to think of any viable next option without necessarily taking into account whether or not there is a compelling evidence base or rationale for guiding a next iterative treatment option.

In severely ill patients, should one routinely prioritize efficacy over tolerability (and rely on motivational interviewing skills to persuade a reluctant patient to accept a more impactful but onerous treatment option)? When should clinicians accept defeat (or claim partial victory) in the setting of residual symptoms that cannot readily be leveraged despite multiple efforts? There are undeniable instances in which the goals of treatment shift from disease modification to disease management, and reorienting the patient toward strategies for coping with a chronic condition.

Iterative treatment studies, such as the Sequenced Treatment Alternatives to Relieve Depression (STAR*D) trial, teach us that, at least in the case of depression, most of the time there is no definitive next step, from among an array of reasonable options, after an inadequate response to an initial intervention. (In fact, in that setting, practitioners really have only a limited number of meaningful opportunities to effect some improvement before descending into the often inescapable abyss of treatment refractoriness.) Clinical trials of second-generation antipsychotic medications for schizophrenia or bipolar mania also tend to show overlapping confidence intervals that imply little evidence for meaningfully greater efficacy of one therapy over another (apart from clozapine) – collectively making decisions about iterative treatment dependent on an array of interacting nuanced factors such as drug tolerability, utility for comorbid conditions, cost, compatibility with co-therapies, possible synergies, and – not least of all – patients' own preferences.

Rote decision trees or algorithms (such as practice guidelines) provide some sequential roadmap for identifying iterative treatment options, but a fundamental problem of such approaches is their failure to take into account the outcomes of prior trials, coupled with the unique clinical characteristics of a given patient that might inform which next option may be better suited to one patient versus another. No two patients are the same. A bipolar disorder patient with psychotic mania who is morbidly obese and has steatohepatitis and coronary heart disease may be better served by the most metabolically neutral option, while a chronically depressed patient with severe comorbid anxiety may not improve without accepting an option for which weight gain or sedation can reasonably be avoided.

Our hope is that readers of this book will become more mindful about how they make treatment decisions, and minimize the element of arbitrariness (or worse, having no clear rationale) in the process of formulating a treatment plan imbued with contingency steps and iterative strategies depending on the outcomes of prior undertakings. Wise clinicians often frame their recommendations within a conditional context – as when they forecast the likelihood of an outcome followed by a plan for next steps (e.g., "here are the best options to pursue if the first recommendation fails"). Forecasting a plan of successive steps in itself often helps to engender hope.

Direct experience is perhaps the best teacher of all, and we have tried to bring to bear our collective understanding of ways to utilize, comprehend, and interpret the literature, as well as deploy a scientific method to evaluate clinical problems and devise systematic ways to outline strategic management plans. As we are fond of telling patients, the one thing we can promise is a rationale. In real-world practice, haphazard treatment plans unfortunately often abound (and sometimes might only loosely be called "plans"). Our hope is that readers of this book will find that it provides a kind of modus operandi for undertaking a systematic approach to the mechanics of clinical assessment and decision-making at all levels of psychiatric care.

We do not intend for this book to be a "how to" manual or a technical guide for implementing a cookbook-style recipe-based approach to patient care. This is not meant to be a handbook or reference resource for looking up facts, algorithms, or instructions. Instead, think of this book as more of a preceptorship on paper (or its electronic format counterpart). As educators, our goal in the way we have designed and presented the material ahead is to prompt clinicians about *how to think*, rather than *what to think*, when they evaluate patients and make treatment decisions. This is a fundamental point. Rather than pointing to which drug to use for which diagnosis, our intention is to equip readers with knowledge about how to evaluate the ever-evolving database of clinical trials and craft patient-specific treatments by adopting a more artisanal than rote approach.

We wish to convey our gratitude to the many patients and their family members, and colleagues, whose own experiences have given us the opportunity to observe and learn about the process of decision-making from diverse perspectives. We hope that in the pages ahead readers at all levels of expertise will discover useful ideas, engaging cases, and thought-provoking strategies to undertake the process of clinical reasoning and decision-making with optimal deliberation, purposefulness, and confidence.

Joseph F. Goldberg, M.D., M.S.

Stephen M. Stahl, M.D., Ph.D., D.Sc. (Hon.)

1 Making Sense of the Senseless: How to Gather and Organize Pertinent Information

LEARNING OBJECTIVES

- ☐ Recognize the pertinent positive and negative features that comprise an organized psychiatric clinical history
- ☐ Identify cohesion versus disparities between signs and symptoms
- ☐ Understand the RIME model for developing sophisticated clinical assessments as a precursor to devising clinical formulations and pursuing therapeutic decision-making

A IT'S ALL ABOUT THE NARRATIVE

Patient histories are, fundamentally, stories. As such, their details either hang together in a logical and cohesive fashion or they appear fragmented and mystifying. The challenge for clinicians is to frame the story in a coherent narrative. Purposeful data-gathering allows one to triage information and discern the relevant from the nonrelevant, follow threads that point to a unified phenomenon, formulate testable hypotheses about likely psychopathological processes, and match appropriate treatments to a coherent symptom picture for a given patient. Appropriate treatment options can enter into the picture only after enough pertinent information has been distilled and organized into a cogent summary of symptoms and clinical problems that might otherwise seem disparate and arbitrarily strung together. Clinical reasoning and decision-making hinge on obtaining high-quality data. A cogent summary includes elements such as:

- Affirming that symptom presentations fit within known epidemiological parameters; for instance, it is awfully rare to see new-onset psychosis or mania arise de novo in older adults (suggesting that either an earlier history was concealed, denied, or missed; or that truly new psychiatric symptoms are high-probability secondary manifestations of an underlying medical or toxic-metabolic condition)
- Appreciating the match between symptoms and functioning (e.g., complaints of "anxiety" or "depressed mood" *alone* may not sufficiently account for pervasively impaired functioning, such as chronic unemployment or a persistent inability to live independently in the community)

- Appreciating behavioral, cognitive, or emotional *departures from a baseline* versus the static persistence of problems that show little deviation over time (i.e., distinguishing states versus traits)
- Recognizing symptoms that belong together within a known pattern or constellation (for example, complaints of "inattention" that also involve a formal thought disorder may point more to schizophrenia, while those involving vegetative signs may reflect depression, and those involving behavioral apraxias may suggest dementia; or strange ideas that are fixed and resistant to challenge or scrutiny point more toward psychosis, while those that seem odd to the patient himself may more likely reflect obsessional thoughts)
- Formulating a hierarchical explanation about how symptoms are best accounted for under an overarching conceptualization. Occam's razor favors the simplest and most parsimonious explanation for a phenomenon, as when a single syndrome or cause accounts for multiple signs and symptoms. Parsimony also aligns with the modern nosological principle that symptoms potentially associated with one disorder are not better accounted for by another (e.g., impulsive aggression that results more proximally from alcohol intoxication than "underlying" bipolar disorder)

B ORGANIZING A COHERENT HISTORY: START FROM THE BEGINNING

The core foundation of excellent psychiatric treatment starts with obtaining a coherent history, preferably as a longitudinal narrative that follows a chronological timeline, with an emphasis on parsing relevant pertinent "positives" and "negatives" from that narrative. A simple organizing principle is to have patients present their concerns from a chronological perspective, in order for the clinician to develop a clear narrative. "When was the very first time you recall having any problems involving your mental health?" provides a good starting point, followed by "When was the first time you sought any kind of treatment for those problems?" A chronologically organized narrative gives some sense not only about the backdrop and longevity of a psychiatric disorder but, moreover, clues about the degree of distress and disruption caused by symptoms, the potential duration of untreated illness, and symptom severity as reflected by the kinds of interventions that previously occurred. A clinical timeline that starts with years of psychotherapy differs from one that begins with an involuntary psychiatric hospitalization or a suicide attempt; low-grade symptoms that persist for extended periods unnoticed by others, or cause no outward functional impairment, imply a different level of severity and debilitation, and possible prognosis, from those linked with more obvious outward signs of disability.

For persistent problems, one always wonders why the patient is seeking help *now* and not a week or month or two ago.

Careful clinical assessments are not a race to formulate a diagnostic impression as fast as possible; quite the contrary, when facing symptoms that might overlap across two or more constellations (such as anxiety, psychosis, or inattention), the time spent reasoning through a thoughtful differential diagnosis often pays its eventual dividends in perpetuity. Box 1.1 summarizes a number of basic principles for framing a patient's history within a meaningful clinical context.

Box 1.1

Key considerations for contextualizing the history of present illness

- Clarify sudden versus gradual onset of symptoms, and changes to a "stable" equilibrium state of affairs
- Identify how (and whether) symptom complaints represent a clear departure from (versus exacerbation of) someone's usual state
- Why now? Particularly for more longstanding complaints, what factors have prompted help-seeking behavior now as opposed to any time previously?
- Is the decision to seek treatment the patient's, or someone else's? (That is, are the patient's problems more bothersome to themselves or to someone around them?)

Subjective symptoms should correspond to outward signs that together reflect a distinct core underlying problem. Wise clinicians can anticipate problems almost intuitively when they truly recognize the signature pattern of a particular ailment – such as the anosognostic detachment from reality in psychosis, or the flat vacancy and absence of emotion in negative symptoms versus the presence of sadness and "feelingful" despair in depression, coupled with a sheer absence of hedonic capacity. The art of psychiatric evaluation means more than applying DSM-5 (the fifth edition of Diagnostic and Statistical Manual of Mental Disorders; American Psychiatric Association, 2013) criteria to arrive at a most likely diagnosis – or, for that matter, simply making "just" a diagnosis from checklist criteria. It involves sifting relevant from extraneous information in order to render plausible explanations for symptoms, drug effects, or the environmental contexts in which symptom profiles arise. It is more the clinician's than the patient's job to order their narrative, and to understand the context in which symptoms arise.

Tip

Negative/deficit symptoms, such as flat affect, entail the *absence* of emotion; depression involves the amplified *presence* of sadness and despair.

In fact, when we elicit a chief complaint by asking the proverbial open-ended question, "Tell me what brings you here," an enormous amount of data comes forth in the moments that follow. The "sifting" clinician learns the following by not (yet) interrupting the patient's verbiage:

- Can the patient tell a coherent narrative? Do they present logical threads that can be followed without the need to interrupt for clarification?
- Does the patient lose their train of thought? If flow of thinking is not linear and coherent, what are the possible explanations? Is a formal thought disorder present? Is the patient intoxicated? Is a delirium, dementia, or other major cognitive disorder present? Could they be malingering?
- Does the patient display intact social cognition? That is, do they check in with the clinician to see if they are being understood? Or are they oblivious to their effect on the listener?
- Is the patient reasonable? Entitled? Demanding? Aggressive or threatening? Cognizant of the impact of their words and actions on other people?
- Do they display insight into the nature of their condition and an appreciation for the risks, benefits, alternatives, and consequences of proposed treatment options?
- Do "pertinent positives" occur contemporaneously in ways that point to a cohesive clinical entity? Or are symptoms disjointed and fail to add up to a recognizable syndrome?

C ARE DIAGNOSTIC CRITERIA MET?

Meeting the operational definition of a syndrome is often a bugaboo for both clinicians and researchers. The crux of such approaches to diagnosis involves the concept that diagnoses equate to the number, severity, and persistence of signs and symptoms that comprise the criteria for recognizing a clinical entity as unique. Does fleeting psychosis fall under the heading of trauma-related phenomena or micropsychosis during times of stress in someone with borderline personality disorder, rather than a more full-fledged psychotic disorder? Could a thyroid-stimulating hormone level of 5.1 mU/L really be enough to account for current mood symptoms? Clinical investigators can agonize at length over a given patient's history in order to determine whether or not formal diagnostic criteria for a particular clinical entity are or are not met, in a rigid and binary fashion.

Clinical investigators undergo formal training in how to administer semi-structured clinical interviews, which they then rely on to form operational definitions of a suspected diagnosis. In clinical trials, diagnosticians must gain inter-rater reliability (meaning, they must demonstrate a minimally acceptable level of consensus agreement on the presence of a particular diagnosis based on interviews that elicit concrete information about symptoms and their duration).

There is no reason clinicians working "in the trenches" cannot adopt as rigorous an approach to diagnostic assessment, regardless of the use of formal semi-structured clinical interviews.

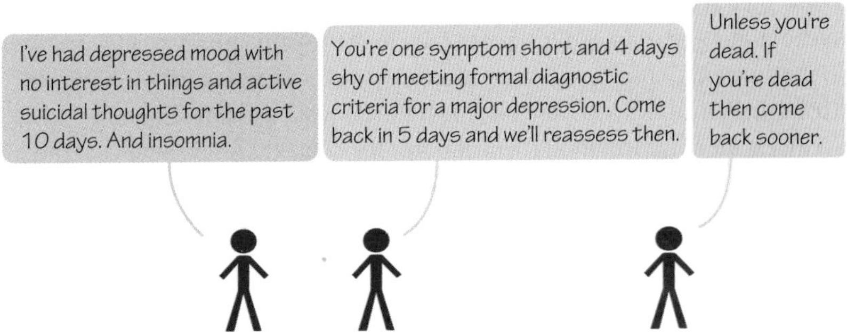

Diagnostic interviews are keyed to the concept of reviewing specific symptom criteria and durations, as well as ruling out other causes that might better account for a clinical presentation. Though detailed and time-consuming, clinical interviewers who undergo formal training to conduct such diagnostic interviews markedly increase the **reliability** with which they can identify specific psychiatric disorders and differentiate them from look-alike mimics. An end result is the determination that a patient either does or does not fulfill the operationally defined criteria for a particular diagnosis. Critics of this approach argue that diagnostic "criteria" are established by committee consensus rather than the laws of nature, and often involve arbitrariness (e.g., defining hypomania by syndromal persistence for at least 4 days, or major depression by at least 2 weeks).

Tip

Reliability means that two or more observers of the same content reach the same conclusion to explain what they see. Diagnostic reliability has nothing to do with validity, a much harder construct, which asks if the observer's conclusions are true and accurate.

Not-so-fun fact

In the DSM-5 field trials, 9 of 23 diagnoses had "questionable" or "unacceptable" reliability of their criteria based on test-retest assessment, including major depressive disorder and generalized anxiety disorder (Regier et al., 2013).

Diagnostic categorization also can change over time in ways that may reflect less science and more the sentiments and vagaries of prevailing opinion (e.g., the construct of somatic symptom disorder replaces the concept of "imagined" or inaccurately perceived health problems in hypochondriasis with the concept of "distress" about health problems, regardless of their objective reality; the emphasis has shifted from misperception or impaired reality testing to a focus mainly on how patients react to or feel about their symptoms).

Nosological systems such as the DSM-5 tend not to be particularly lavish in how they account for the context in which symptoms may arise. Frantic psychomotor agitation could superficially look the same in a patient with psychotic mania as someone trapped in an elevator in a burning building. Attributing an adolescent's poor school efforts "just" to depression may sacrifice a lot of information if one ignores the context of, say, Julie's parents' acrimonious divorce process, Isabel's sexual abuse by a boyfriend, or David's experience of bullying for identifying as LGBTQ+. Contexts influence treatment decisions, both pharmacologically and psychosocially, as elaborated further in Box 1.2.

Box 1.2

How context matters in establishing a diagnostic formulation or treatment recommendation

The particular context in which psychiatric symptoms arise is fundamental to establishing diagnoses. For example, the diagnosis of posttraumatic stress disorder (PTSD) requires an antecedent trauma that poses some threat to one's fundamental safety and well-being, although obviously not all traumas result in PTSD. What exactly was the impact of the trauma? Or: suicidal thinking that arises in the context of intoxication is fundamentally different from sober suicidality in the context of a major depression. Or: relapse of a psychiatric disorder in the context of treatment nonadherence is different from relapse that occurs *despite* ongoing treatment that had, until then, been perceived as effective.

What we might call "Newtonian psychopharmacology" means that an object in motion stays in motion unless an opposing force acts on it. If a clinical condition has been quietly in remission and symptoms re-emerge – or a system otherwise in stable equilibrium falls out of equilibrium – one ideally searches for that opposing force. It can be helpful to pose questions such as the following:

- When exactly did things change? What events or circumstances preceded the change in equilibrium?
- Did a change in medications (such as nonadherence) or psychotherapy precede a clinical change?
- Did a change in work, finances, or social supports coincide with the emergence of psychiatric symptoms? Life stresses can be like pollen's relationship to hay fever – not as the cause of disease, but as its catalyst in someone with a biological predisposition (see also Chapter 5, Box 5.1 for more on the diathesis-stress model in vulnerable individuals)

There are both advantages and disadvantages in adopting a "criteria-based approach" to diagnosis. The most obvious disadvantage involves the notion that operational criteria may be reliable (and even then, not always) but not valid. This latter point makes it rather disingenuous to speak of diagnostic "accuracy," if in fact diagnoses by operational criteria are mainly heuristic constructs that provide a way of organizing narrative information but involve elements of arbitrariness that undermine accuracy. A compelling example might be the categorization of excessive worry as a diagnostic entity. Known as "overanxious disorder" in DSM-III-R (American Psychiatric Association, 1987), the construct was revised in DSM-IV (American Psychiatric Association, 1994) to generalized anxiety disorder (GAD) but criticisms have surrounded both its reliability and validity based on several of its operational criteria. Some authors suggest that determining "excessiveness" of anxiety and worry (an "A" criterion) is subjective and may vary depending on the evaluator; the imposed duration criteria of at least 6 months also has been associated with poorer inter-rater reliability than if a shorter duration (such as 1 month) were acknowledged; and that many of the associated symptoms listed as "C" criteria for GAD are highly nonspecific (e.g., fatigue, poor concentration, insomnia) and unduly overlap with other disorders (such as major depression) (Andrews et al., 2010).

An obvious advantage of using operationally based diagnostic criteria for clinical decision-making is that doing so minimizes subjectivity or ambiguity about how to characterize the phenomenon being treated; the definition is agreed upon, regardless of whether it is accurate. However, without an appreciation for context, this approach could lend itself to overly concrete thinking among practitioners. Imagine if one concluded that because stimulants treat inattention in attention deficit–hyperactivity disorder (ADHD), they might equally improve attention in people with delirium or dementia; or, if tryptans improve migraine headaches, they should expectably improve all other forms of headache; or, if nitrates help chest pain from angina, why not assume they should also alleviate chest pain from a peptic ulcer or rib fracture? Diagnosticians cannot undertake clinical reasoning without ruling out look-alike conditions that might superficially imitate other clinical entities (phenocopies; see Box 1.3) lest we resign ourselves to clinical decision-making as being no more than a wild-West lawless enterprise.

The nature of enrolling patients in a clinical trial hinges on affirming the specificity of diagnosis – for example:

- A patient with suspected major depressive disorder must manifest at least five of nine symptoms for at least 2 weeks, uncontaminated by other factors that might better account for the presenting features (such as, active substance use or clinically meaningful hypothyroidism); or

Box 1.3

What are psychiatric phenocopies?

To the extent that we construe at least some elements of many if not most psychiatric conditions as having some contribution from genetic factors, we refer to the observable manifestations of genetic expression as phenotypes. (Less overt manifestations of genetic forces are sometimes called **endophenotypes**, or "hidden" phenotypes – that is, phenomena that are influenced by genetic factors but are not outwardly visible, or visible only when subjected to tests that elicit a certain behavior or stimulus response, such as poor working memory or an innately diminished capacity to efficiently metabolize certain medications.) The term **phenocopy** is used to describe a genetically influenced observable entity that could resemble a different genetically determined entity. In a phenocopy, the clinical signs and symptoms can outwardly or superficially resemble another clinical entity that is believed to have a different underlying pathology, course, and possible treatment trajectory.

- A patient whose "mood swings" are called "cyclothymia" has never been fully manic, nor had a sufficient number or duration of hypomanic or depressive symptoms to constitute a full syndrome of either polarity; or
- "Panic disorder" connotes the occurrence of specific autonomically driven events with physical (not just psychic) manifestations; or
- PTSD is not a catch-all phenomenon that encapsulates any and all forms of highly stressful events – such as difficult relationship break-ups, job losses, or reversals of financial fortune; in fact, the treatments geared to PTSD focus on its recognized clusters, such as avoidance, autonomic hyperarousal (e.g., exaggerated startle response) or involuntary intrusive thoughts and memories causing physiological distress in response to associated cues; or
- A patient who periodically smokes cannabis would not formally be identified as having cannabis use disorder unless they use for increasingly longer periods in larger amounts, their use adversely affects their work and social functioning, physical or psychological problems ensue from use, and other formal diagnostic criteria are met that differentiate "use" from a "use disorder"

Real-world patients do not always fully meet formal diagnostic definitions of a categorical disorder, and real-world clinicians often do not painstakingly appraise every item within a diagnostic checklist. Nevertheless, for better or worse, there is objective merit behind the phrase "the diagnostic criteria are (or are not) met." Why? In large part, it allows apples-to-apples comparisons between a real-world patient's presentation relative to the patient descriptions found in clinical trials or textbooks. Disparities mean extrapolation, which in turn means that "real-world" outcomes may differ substantially from "prototypical" patients who embody the characteristics of a textbook presentation.

D ARE DSM CRITERIA WRITTEN MAINLY FOR CLINICIANS OR RESEARCHERS?

The operational criteria captured in nosologies such as the DSM or the International Classification of Diseases (ICD) are collections of symptoms and duration criteria arrived at by consensus agreement among experts, rather than "absolute truths" found in nature. They are subject to change and can sometime even become eliminated altogether (as in the case of Asperger syndrome) or "voted" into existence by committee opinion (as in the case of disruptive mood dysregulation disorder or major depressive disorder with mixed features). "Cardinal" symptoms are also subject to greater or lesser importance as consensus opinions about psychiatric diagnoses change over time. For example, neologisms, bizarre delusions, and so-called first-rank symptoms of psychosis (e.g., believing one's thoughts or actions are controlled by outside forces) were once strongly associated with schizophrenia, but eventually were felt to lack diagnostic specificity and consequently "demoted" to the status of holding less pathognomonic importance based on clinical consensus of opinion.

As noted in Section C above, investigators think about psychiatric diagnoses differently than practitioners; like bookkeepers, they focus on whether or not the requisite number and duration of symptoms have been met, and the phrase "the criteria are not met" becomes a ubiquitous refrain when deciding that a patient is ineligible to qualify as a research subject in a clinical trial. Twists occur along the way with regard to problems like "double counting" symptoms that could be attributed to more than one condition. A well-known example is the DSM-5 "mixed features" course specifier, which was conceptually meant to embrace the notion that mania and depressive symptoms could occur on a continuum across all mood disorders. Four particular symptoms – distractibility, irritability, insomnia, and psychomotor agitation ("DIIP") could occur in the context of either a mania or depression and, consequently, crafters of the DSM-5 suggested that none of these symptoms could be used to constitute a "tie-breaker" when deciding on the presence of an opposite affective pole. Critics of this stipulation have argued that DIIP symptoms can be integral to the construct of mixed states, and to exclude them (as polarity-deciding factors) would be akin to excluding fever as a criterion when differentiating an infection from an autoimmune process. Both perspectives are correct in their own way, and underscore the dilemma for the practitioner (who may be altogether less fastidious in even registering DIIP symptoms as casting a decisive diagnostic vote).

E HIERARCHICAL DIAGNOSTIC TREATMENT APPROACHES: HOW TO TRIAGE

It should come as no surprise to in-the-trenches practitioners that most patients with significant psychiatric symptoms often have more than one diagnosable psychiatric condition. Part of the assessment challenge is parsing symptoms that could overlap between two or more disorders in trying to understand "overarching" diagnostic constructs from the collision of multiple separate ailments. When is inattention or distractibility an indication of comorbid ADHD rather than an intrinsic component of depression, anxiety, or psychosis? When are problems with impulse control or emotional self-regulation artifacts of a broader condition such as bipolar disorder rather than manifestations of a comorbidity such as PTSD or a significant personality disorder? And perhaps most important of all, when and how does one determine which is the "core" or predominant psychiatric condition and which are – for want of a better term – subsidiary coexisting conditions?

There is often an implicit assumption that if a predominant or overarching condition is recognized, perhaps its successful treatment will lead to some attenuation of the comorbid or subsidiary conditions. This is an interesting but largely empirically untested hypothesis. Some comorbid conditions may spring from a common underlying process but, once initiated, follow their own trajectories and require their own independent treatment. Outside of psychiatry, diabetes may be the most illustrative example. Diabetic patients who develop neuropathy, retinopathy, nephropathy, poor wound healing, and worsening of cardiovascular disease can ultimately attribute blame to how their body manages glucose – and yet, once the wheels have been set in motion for these end-organ consequences of impaired glucose metabolism, fixing the initial source of the problem will not necessarily repair the collateral downstream damage.

In psychiatry, perhaps substance use disorders represent a comparable dilemma when they are viewed as incidental to some larger, overarching clinical problem. When substance use disorders involve problems with mood or anxiety, patients or their families (and sometimes also their clinicians) sometimes may hypothesize that comorbid substance use might evaporate if only a more effective therapy were in place for the more fundamental problem being "self-medicated." There may very well be instances in which optimal control of mood or anxiety (or other) disorders can help make inroads in active substance use disorders, but a reductive approach such as this discounts the notion that addictions often constitute ailments that exist unto themselves (i.e., disorders of the reward pathway), which typically require their own treatment. Moreover, unmanaged substance use disorders may in turn aggravate and perpetuate a comorbid psychiatric condition such as depression or anxiety. Which condition is subsidiary to which? Or should the preferred rule of thumb be to assume that multidiagnostic clinical presentations are just that, and require separate but coordinated treatments?

Examples of common comorbidities associated with major psychiatric disorders are summarized in Table 1.1. As alluded to above, it is sometimes difficult (and subjective) to classify the "primary" from the "comorbid" condition for many of the scenarios listed below, and it never hurts at least to consider the possibility that many complex/multidiagnostic presentations are two-way streets with traffic that interacts bidirectionally.

Table 1.1 Common comorbidities across major psychiatric disorders

Disorder	Comorbidity
Adult ADHD	Comorbid bipolar disorder in 5%–47% (Wingo and Ghaemi, 2007) Comorbid dysthymia or major depression in 19–53% (NCD Replication; Kessler et al., 2006; Torgersen et al., 2006)
Anxiety disorders	60% of individuals with one anxiety disorder have at least one other anxiety disorder, while 27% have more than three (NCS Replication; Goldstein-Piekarski et al., 2016); major depressive disorder co-occurs with at least one anxiety disorder in about 20% of cases (Goldstein-Piekarski et al., 2016)
Bipolar disorder	Adult ADHD ranges from 10% (NIMH STEP-BD; Nierenberg et al., 2005) to 21% (NCS Replication; Kessler et al., 2006); alcohol use disorder 40% (Hunt et al., 2016) to 60% (Merikangas et al., 2007); other substance use disorders (most notably cannabis use or illicit substance use evident in about 20% of clinical settings (Hunt et al., 2016)); anxiety disorders (about 45%; Pavlova et al., 2015); OCD (about 17%; Amerio et al., 2015)
Eating disorders	Body dysmorphic disorder in about 39% of anorexia nervosa patients (Grant et al., 2002)
Major depressive disorder	2.7-fold increased likelihood of ADHD (NCS Replication; Kessler et al., 2006) About one-third of major depressive disorder patients have comorbid substance use disorders (Davis et al., 2008)
PTSD	About 60% of individuals with PTSD also have major depressive disorder (Goldstein-Piekarski et al., 2016)
Schizophrenia	About one-quarter of schizophrenia patients have comorbid alcohol use disorder, about one-third of the time arising before the onset of schizophrenia (Archibald, 2019); depression prevalence of 25–81% (Abdullah et al., 2020)
Social anxiety disorder	Increased rates of other anxiety disorders and mood disorders (Chartier et al., 2003)

Abbreviations: ADHD, attention deficit-hyperactivity disorder; NCS, National Comorbidity Survey; NIMH STEP-BD, National Institute of Mental Health Systematic Treatment Enhancement Program for Bipolar Disorder; OCD, obsessive-compulsive disorder; PTSD, posttraumatic stress disorder.

F SIGNS AND SYMPTOMS

Signs are objective, outward manifestations of an underlying problem, while symptoms are subjective complaints. In general medicine, a stomach ache is a symptom and abdominal tenderness or grimacing is its corresponding sign. In psychiatry, we expect subjective complaints of sadness or feeling blue to correspond with outward signs of weepiness, a low voice, psychomotor slowing, and exasperation. Patients who identify their mood as depressed would expectably appear unanimated, not so loquacious, and at least somewhat impoverished in their generation of ideas and details, with diminished spontaneity in the course of an interview. In mania, where excess energy and psychomotor activation are fundamental elements, we expect patients to talk fast and be hard to interrupt, use animated gestures, sleep fewer hours, and perhaps make interpersonally provocative or boundary-bending comments to the people with whom they interact; psychomotor retardation with impoverished speech does not reconcile with subjective complaints of euphoria.

> **Tip**
> Always look for concordance versus discordance between signs and symptoms.

Because patients can misidentify their symptoms it is important to clarify the intended meaning of terms they use. Someone who is worried about their cognitive function and reports problems with memory or concentration may be depressed or anxious. Someone who says they feel anxious may mean they have a vague sense of apprehension or anticipation of an imagined catastrophe, or they could mean they are worried their food is being poisoned and someone is following them with malicious intent. Intensity of belief-conviction and the patient's own willingness to consider more than one explanation for their symptoms provide important context for understanding the nature of an underlying problem.

G DEPRESSION AS A DISORDER OF INFORMATION PROCESSING

Fundamentally, clinical depression has less to do with life adversities per se than with how the brain processes emotional information. Perhaps nowhere is that more evident than in the case of an impaired hedonic tone. Think of the capacity to detect and experience pleasure as tantamount to the 13th cranial nerve. It can be tested. The diminished ability to perceive pleasure (anhedonia) when an inherently pleasurable sensation or experience occurs reflects a sensory process, on par with intact olfaction or hearing. Significant forms of depression, where medications can be especially useful, tend to involve impaired hedonic capacity. We can assess whether the reward pathway is intact in an analogous way to testing if the olfactory nerve is intact when we ask someone to smell coffee beans or soap.

Often this is accomplished more by history-gathering than by performance-based in-office testing. Are inherently pleasurable things still as pleasurable as they have ever been? The distinction between the *ability to feel pleasure* versus the extent to which *life itself is inherently enjoyable* is fundamental, inasmuch as clinicians want to differentiate complaints about unfavorable existential circumstances from an impaired capacity to feel positive emotions.

What does this have to do with clinical reasoning and decision-making? In the case of identifying clinical depression, and contemplating the role of pharmacotherapies versus psychotherapies versus, say, prescribing exercise, we are interested in determining if the brain circuits believed relevant to processing pleasurable experiences – the ventral striatum, aka the reward pathway – are intact. This is a critical point when assessing depression as a brain disorder, no different from identifying anosmia or a sinus infection. An impaired capacity to process sensory information lies at the heart of the dysfunctional brain circuitry of depression, and treatment decisions may very much may be targeted to distinct symptom domains such as anhedonia, attentional impairment, or aberrant anxiety processing. Symptom clusters as they may inform differential therapeutics are discussed further in Chapter 9, Section G.

H INTERFACE SYMPTOMS: WHEN DELUSIONS MEET OBSESSIONS

"Overvalued ideas" are isolated, strongly held concepts that take on greater salience for an individual than might seem called for in a given situation. The term may reflect a level of intensity that falls along a continuum influenced by factors such as belief-conviction, awareness of plausibility, insight, idiosyncratic thinking, and cognitive flexibility (where one can consider and vet alternative conclusions behind a given belief). Overvalued ideas move closer to delusions when their content is false, conviction is fixed, and there is generally little to no awareness or recognition about either the falsehood or fixity of thinking. (Contrast this process with either *lying* (where a false proposition is intentionally brought forth not because it accurately reflects someone's interpretation of reality but more for the sake of manipulating someone else's interpretation of reality) or *denial* (in which someone refuses to acknowledge an objective reality because of its undesirable consequences, rather than an inability to perceive objective reality due to psychosis).) Obsessions are persistent intrusive thoughts, ideas, impulses, or images that cause distress. They differ fundamentally from delusions because they tend to make no sense to the individual who experiences them, and in fact may very well conflict directly with their sense of objective reality (in other words,

> **Tip**
> Obsessional thinking is often prefaced by the words "I know this makes no sense, but …"

obsessions involve intact reality testing). Box 1.4 offers further discussion on the concept of schizo-obsessive disorder as a fusion of persistent psychosis with obsessive–compulsive features.

Box 1.4

Is there such a thing as schizo-obsessive disorder?

The term "schizo-obsessive" unofficially entered the psychiatric lexicon many years ago as a conceptual hybrid entity to reflect instances in which obsessions and delusions were hard to disambiguate. Some authors also have used the term to reflect the amalgam of schizophrenia and obsessive-compulsive disorder (OCD) as a singular dual-diagnosis entity. Comorbidity studies suggest that up to one-quarter of schizophrenia patients manifest obsessive-compulsive symptoms, while about 12% would meet diagnostic criteria for both schizophrenia and OCD (Scotti-Muzzi and Saide, 2017). Neurocognitive studies have pointed out that schizophrenia patients tend to manifest marked cognitive impairment in multiple domains (e.g., attention, executive function, working memory, visuospatial functioning) while OCD patients tend to manifest more circumscribed deficits in impulse control and the ability to maintain cognitive set (Scott-Muzzi and Saide, 2017). Little is known about the relative merits (or shortcomings) of pharmacotherapies that focus mainly on the use of dopamine-blocking antipsychotic medications or a combination of these medications when elements of both disorders are present. Though the construct never garnered validity as either a bona fide free-standing entity or a subtype of schizophrenia, it provides at the very least a useful heuristic for thinking about the interface of obsessions and delusions.

THE LONGITUDINAL STABILITY OF PSYCHIATRIC DIAGNOSES

Are psychiatric diagnoses fluid? Obviously, as additional information or new symptoms can become apparent over the long-term course of managing a chronic or recurrent condition, clinicians would be remiss not to periodically reassess their diagnostic formulations. It is never a bad idea for practitioners to wear a clinical investigator hat and attach their own confidence rating to the diagnoses they make (say, "low," "medium," or "high"). Chances are, diagnoses will be less prone to modification the higher one's initial confidence rating is. If we look to the empirical literature on diagnostic stability, we find the results shown in Table 1.2.

Table 1.2 Do psychiatric diagnoses change over time?

Diagnosis	Diagnostic changes
ADHD	Longitudinal follow-up studies show that about 50–60% of children with ADHD will show partial or full persistence of ADHD symptoms into adulthood (Van Meter et al., 2023)
Bipolar disorder	A case registry of 14,577 patients initially diagnosed with bipolar disorder in Madrid between 1980 and 2009 found substantial variability in diagnoses over the course of 10 successive patient visits (only 18% maintained diagnostic stability across the entirety of their follow-up) (Cegla-Schvartzman et al., 2021)
Major depressive disorder	Prospective follow-up studies show that past the age of about 40 years, the probability of diagnostic polarity conversion from unipolar to bipolar disorder is only about 5% (Coryell et al., 1995). On the other hand, up to 20% of major depressive disorder patients with subthreshold mixed features may go on to develop a full mania or hypomania over a mean 17.5-year follow-up (Fiedorowicz et al., 2011)
Personality disorders	Meta-analyses show that a little more than half of personality disorder diagnoses maintain stability across longitudinal follow-ups; antisocial, schizoid, and obsessive-compulsive personality disorder features retained highest stability over time, while others tended to show reductions in criteria over time (d'Huart et al., 2023)
Schizophrenia	At a 10-year follow-up of first-episode psychosis patients, 6.3% of initially identified schizophrenia patients changed diagnoses; of those diagnosed with schizophrenia at follow-up, 23.3% originally were given a different diagnosis (Suárez-Pinilla et al., 2021)

Let us turn next to the interpersonal context in which psychiatric symptoms can present, and the ways in which levels of emotional security or insecurity around important relationships can color the experience of life adversity as well as the experience of symptoms caused by faulty information processing. Here, the concept of attachment theory becomes relevant for diagnostic assessment and subsequent clinical reasoning.

J UNDERSTANDING ATTACHMENT STYLES AS A CLUE TO DIAGNOSTIC FORMULATIONS

British psychiatrist John Bowlby was perhaps the first innovator in the field to draw attention to the ways in which, during development, people form emotional bonds or attachments to identified caregivers with varying degrees of security or insecurity. In adulthood, attachment styles (summarized in

Table 1.3) can influence how people form relationships and interact with others, procure emotional supports, and cope with adversities or negative emotions. Interpersonally, attachment styles can be somewhat like A/B/O blood types – relationship incompatibilities may arise when attachment styles clash. Attachment styles can dramatically influence how individuals present with an interpersonal crisis, or color the presentation of a psychiatric condition such as depression or anxiety as it impacts psychosocial functioning. The attachment style of significant others may also influence collateral information provided when a loved one incurs a psychiatric disorder. For example, avoidant/dismissive family members may minimize the magnitude or significance of emotional distress associated with a loved one's depression; or anxious/preoccupied significant others may overamplify their own sense of distress in response to a loved one's psychiatric disorder when the disorder threatens to make the loved one less emotionally available to the significant other.

Table 1.3 Attachment styles

Attachment style	Description
Secure	Individuals project a sense of warmth and confidence in relationships; they can effectively self-sooth, manage feelings of distress, and self-regulate their emotions; they project healthy self-esteem; they can communicate their needs and both give and receive emotional support
Anxious/preoccupied/ambivalent	Individuals are often preoccupied with expectations of rejection or abandonment; they can be clingy and insecure in relationships and seek constant reassurance, which in turn may drive low self-worth/self-confidence and a basic sense of insecurity over whether their needs will go unmet
Dismissive/avoidant	Individuals project a sense of emotional self-sufficiency, independence, and high self-esteem; they tend not to seek reassurance or express feelings to others; they poorly tolerate emotional or physical intimacy; they may be highly sociable yet tend to avoid relationships that involve emotional closeness or depth
Disorganized/fearful-avoidant	Individuals tend to be mistrustful of others and fearful of responses they expect from people they otherwise emotionally rely on; they tend to both want and fear intimacy, and project a sense of incoherence or confusion in their relationship expectations because they view others as unpredictable

How exactly does an understanding of attachment styles help us make sense of the ways in which a psychiatric problem presents, in order to both better understand the nature of the problem and devise an appropriate treatment? To the extent that both life adversities and psychiatric disorders in and of themselves can evoke distress, the interpersonal ramifications and mode of presentation provide context and colorization to almost any underlying problem. Let us illustrate this with the case of Carlos in Clinical Vignette 1.1.

Clinical Vignette 1.1

Carlos was a 23-year-old single delivery driver with no previous psychiatric history, who had the terrible misfortune of losing in the same week his job of 6 months and his girlfriend of 4 months. He quickly had become deeply invested in the relationship and was devastated by her lack of reciprocity and decision to end it. Waiting outside his ex-girlfriend's apartment building, he made a violent and serious suicide attempt by jumping off the roof of an adjacent building within visibility of her window, timing the event so that she would likely be at home when it occurred. He survived with multiple injuries. When evaluated by the psychiatry consultation-liaison (C–L) team he said that he had never before spoken with a psychiatrist or other mental health professional, and had never in his life experienced symptoms of a major mood disorder, psychotic disorder, or substance use disorder. He related that he felt he could no longer cope with the adversities he was facing and viewed suicide as his only solution. When asked if he still wanted to kill himself, he only said that he could not picture life without his girlfriend. When asked how angry he was at his ex-girlfriend, and whether his attempt to kill himself in front of her might have been misdirected rage meant for her rather than himself, he denied feeling angry. The C–L team placed Carlos on a 1:1 watch yet struggled to find a pharmacologically responsive DSM-5 diagnosis whose criteria Carlos fulfilled other than an adjustment disorder with mixed disturbance of emotions and conduct. No pharmacology was recommended although Carlos was viewed as having a risk for impulsive aggression when feeling interpersonally overwhelmed. The team anticipated his stresses would only worsen as he faced a protracted physical recovery. A dialectal behavior therapy (DBT) intensive outpatient program was ultimately recommended to improve Carlos' range of coping skills and distress tolerance. The hospital administrator was troubled by the team's decision not to recommend any psychopharmacology, asking, "How could there be nothing to medicate after a serious suicide attempt?"

Let us hope Carlos follows through with the C–L team's recommendation; it is not simply a "dispo plan" but more importantly probably the best opportunity for fleshing out missing details. What more lies beneath the surface of Carlos's narrative than we now know? Probably a lot. He could certainly be clinically depressed and, if that is the case, time will help reveal that. He could have an impulse control disorder, although the lack of known previous events makes it hard to draw a pattern, and we are looking for patterns. Collateral history about Carlos would be nice to have. Is he psychotic, and well-compensated (or guarded) enough not to tip his hand on that for the C–L team to appreciate? His attachment style is far from secure. Is he disorganized or preoccupied? Does loss represent to him an unrecoverable catastrophic event, placing him at risk for more of the same depending on what emotional threats await him tomorrow? And is DBT the right psychotherapy modality just for now, or for the long-term? An important point around clinical decision-making will be the extent to which other clinicians find themselves preoccupied with a desire to see Carlos taking *some* medication, at the expense of trying to better elucidate his risk for self-harm and the nature of his distress.

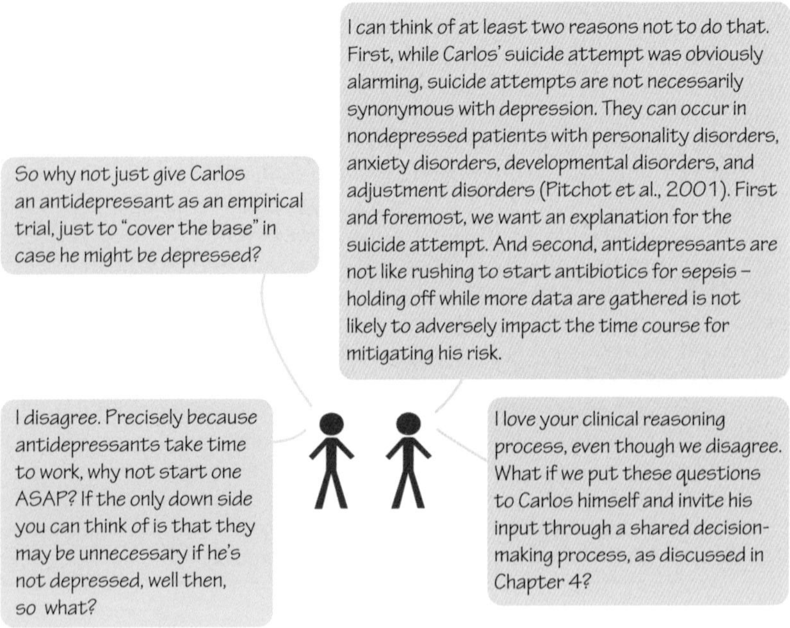

K INFORMATION FLOW

Once we have one or more working diagnostic impressions, we tend to structure the flow of an interview to corroborate (or refute) our developing hypotheses. In suspected depression, we often ask about hopelessness as a precursor to questions about suicide, and we ask about suicidal thoughts before asking about actions because thought precedes action. Questions about a patient's outlook lead to more direct inquiries about negativism and hopelessness, in turn leading to more questions about magnitude of hopelessness and fixed nihilism. In psychosis, we express neutral curiosity about the basis for someone's expressed beliefs – what makes someone so sure about an idea or perception, or is their belief-conviction not so fixed?

Some symptoms within a syndromal constellation also carry more weight than others. If one were assessing depression, suicidal features would have more centrality and gravitas than, say, poor concentration or initial insomnia. Anhedonia, as noted above in Section G, is another cardinal symptom that likely reflects diminished functioning of the ventral striatum and reward pathway.

L THOSE WHO DO NOT LEARN FROM THE PHARMACOLOGICAL PAST ARE DOOMED TO REPEAT IT

A branch of statistics known as Bayesian analytics teaches that subsequent decisions are influenced by prior experiences. Unlike flipping a coin – where the umpteenth toss has the same 50–50 chance for calling "heads" as does the first or second toss – past therapeutic undertakings convey information about the probability of future treatment outcomes. The nature and results of past treatments can inform present and future refinements of a given clinical impression. Table 1.4 summarizes a number of pertinent historical features related to previous treatments that, more often than not, provide useful information about a current working diagnosis and evolving treatment plan.

Table 1.4 Past treatment characteristics that bear on diagnostic formulations and future treatment planning

Historical feature	Why it matters
Has there been more convergence or divergence among past clinicians in their diagnostic impressions (and treatment recommendations for a particular patient)?	Numerous divergent impressions suggest a poorly defined clinical problem and possible haphazard therapeutic undertakings
How stable or peripatetic have patients been in their past treatment engagements?	Lack of stick-to-itiveness or excessive sampling from numerous clinicians bodes poorly for establishing a consistent treatment
How much have previous treatments entailed adequate trials and discontinuations due to true lack of efficacy versus premature cessations due to intolerance or impatience waiting for efficacy	Impatience to judge treatment effects may limit someone's ability to give future treatments enough time to work
Prominent medication side effects in the past have predominated over treatment efficacy	Could the patient be a poor metabolizer for certain catabolic enzymes? Are they predisposed to somatosensory amplification - which could hint at depression, anxiety, autism spectrum disorders, or somatic symptom disorder? What are their attitudes toward medication? Do they fundamentally expect help or harm?
Have many adequate treatment trials failed?	The patient could have a correctly diagnosed treatment-resistant condition; or they may have been treated for the wrong diagnosis; or they may have been poorly adherent to a prescribed regimen; or they may have coexistent medical or psychiatric/substance-related conditions that account for poor treatment responsivity

Tip

Somatosensory amplification is a phenomenon in which some individuals express an inordinate sense of awareness and discomfort in response to normal bodily sensations, and may be exquisitely attuned to subtle perceived physical effects of a treatment that they perceive as noxious.

M THE ART OF INTERPRETING GATHERED CLINICAL INFORMATION

What separates a cub reporter from a seasoned investigative journalist? Consider the inferential and at times forensic qualities that a superb information gatherer must call upon in order to recognize the significance of the very findings they unearth. The essence of clinical decision-making rests on a solid foundation of skills in not simply gathering and ordering relevant information but interpreting it and using the conclusions as a kind of launching pad for knowing pertinent next steps. In medical education, the so-called "RIME" framework has been established to describe the phases of professional growth and development for physicians in training. Formulated originally by Pangaro (1999) for evaluating the development of professional expertise among medical student clerks, the core tenets of the RIME mnemonic focus on transitioning a clinician from a data gatherer to a data interpreter to a problem solver capable of devising strategies to remedy clinical problems, as summarized in Table 1.5.

Let us see how these concepts surrounding clinical reasoning play out in the case of Warren (Clinical Vignette 1.2).

Clinical Vignette 1.2

Warren is a 43-year-old single unemployed man with chronic depression and alcohol use disorder. For the past 2 years he has been taking duloxetine 120 mg/day along with quetiapine 25–50 mg at night, buspirone 120 mg/day and hydroxyzine 25 mg three times daily. Now he has brought himself to the emergency department complaining of vertigo and electrical sensations running through his body. His blood alcohol level is 50 mg/dL (mild intoxication) and he is mildly tremulous. A psychiatric consultation has been requested.

What does the RIME manager or educator notice about Warren? His SNRI (serotonin–norepinephrine reuptake inhibitor) dose has been optimized for more than long enough to judge its success, placing him in the categories of both chronic depression and treatment-resistant depression. The RIME reporter or interpreter may fail to recognize Warren's physical symptoms as probable discontinuation effects from duloxetine, which he likely has either stopped (if his bodily sensations are recent) or taken erratically (if they have been occurring for an extended period of time). They might also innocently wonder about the possibility of serotonin syndrome until the RIME educator advises them to perform a MedLine search linking the terms "buspirone" + "SNRI" + "serotonin

Table 1.5 The RIME framework

Role	Task	Example
Reporter	Gathering factual information with consistent accuracy and reliability	Dr. Smith identifies that Tammy, a 27-year-old woman in the emergency department, complains of suicidal thoughts, has twice previously overdosed, takes no medicines currently, and says she is depressed
Interpreter	Applying medical knowledge and weighing evidence in order to apply knowledge and interpret the clinical meaning and significance of observable phenomena (e.g., generating a differential diagnosis, offering an explanatory hypothesis for symptoms)	Dr. Jones determines that Tammy is distraught about the recent break-up of a brief relationship, which may have precipitated the exacerbation of an underlying depression; notes that Tammy historically stops and starts both pharmacotherapy and psychotherapy and then relapses
Manager	The ability to organize and prioritize evidence in order to proactively problem-solve and devise a cogent and strategic treatment plan	Dr. Watson wonders aloud whether Tammy's decision to stop her prior treatment was a way of abandoning her own self-care, and asks if on some level she may have sabotaged herself because she feels she deserves to suffer
Educator	The ability to articulate known facts, identify gaps in knowledge, translate medical concepts into lay language, and vice-versa	Dr. Conan tells Dr. Watson to skip the psychobabble, regardless of whether or not it may be accurate, because it is a prematurely formulated hypothesis that needs more data. Instead, he suggests explaining to Tammy that she has a known biological vulnerability to the illness of depression, that certain kinds of stressful life events could aggravate that vulnerability, and that resuming treatment could both protect her from the pain and suffering caused by her vulnerability and simultaneously improve her ability to problem-solve and find solutions for the difficulties she is facing

syndrome" or "high-dose buspirone" and "serotonin syndrome" and they discover there are no relevant entries. Hierarchical prioritization demands ruling in or out life-threatening conditions. The RIME reporter/interpreter thinks Warren's tremor cannot reflect alcohol withdrawal given his more-than-respectable blood alcohol level in the emergency department, but the educator wonders if chronic alcohol use places Warren's usual blood alcohol level at much higher than 50 mg/dL, meaning that a dip downward from a higher norm could certainly equate to acute withdrawal.

The RIME reporter orders a toxicology screen to see what other substances Warren may have ingested, while the interpreter readies a benzodiazepine test dose to see if his tremor and autonomic signs improve (with an eye toward – depending on the results – likely admitting Warren for alcohol detoxification and gearing up fluid hydration, supplemental thiamine and folate, and an aftercare dual-diagnosis intensive outpatient program). Meanwhile, the RIME manager/educator wonders why Warren has remained for so long on a medication regimen that clearly has done nothing to improve his condition. Does that reflect disengagement or nihilism on the part of the prescriber? Or has the prescriber encouraged changes to his regimen that Warren may not have followed through on? The outpatient prescriber was clearly impressed enough with Warren's alcohol use and/or risk for gobbling up controlled substances to construct an aggressive regimen of lowish-potency anxiolytic medications that steers clear of sedative-hypnotics. Are we sure Warren has not gotten a hold of benzodiazepines elsewhere?

Unless Warren's prior follow-through has been poor, his prescriber must have been underwhelmed with Warren's depression to have left his optimally dosed duloxetine unchanged for so long. There have been no past hospitalizations or suicide attempts to up the ante of how impressive his depression symptoms come across as standout features. But the history also does not reflect aggressive attention being paid to comorbid alcohol use disorder. Where are the prior detoxes? Why no trail of failed naltrexone or disulfiram or acamprosate or even topiramate trials? Is this really Warren's first rodeo when it comes to addressing his alcohol use, and implicating it as a potential exacerbator, if not even a cause, of his persistent depression?

Detoxing Warren from alcohol is probably the easiest part of this case. The remaining threads are left hanging without so clear a narrative, at least as yet, in order to construct a more cogent and comprehensive treatment plan.

TAKE-HOME POINTS

- Gather comprehensive factual information as a "first pass," looking for cohesive themes that are consistent with testable hypotheses about the nature of a suspected clinical problem set
- Take advantage of all credible sources of information; vet the credibility of a source based on their depth of knowledge and detail, plausibility of facts, and any personal agendas that may bias their observations
- Strive to identify and organize pertinent clinical information beyond the sheer level of reporting observations; formulate hypotheses that offer viable and compelling explanations for the data gathered
- Diagnoses are not necessarily static; they can evolve over time and are subject to revision as additional data become available
- Formulate initial treatment plans only after initial working diagnostic hypotheses have been made; use the results of interventions as feedback to help affirm, refute, and revise diagnostic working hypotheses

References

Abdullah HM, Shahul HZ, Hwang MY, et al. Comorbidity in schizophrenia: Conceptual issues and clinical management. Focus (Am Psychiatr Publ) 2020; 18: 386–390

American Psychiatric Association. Diagnostic and Statistical Manual of Mental Disorders, 3rd edition, revised. Washington, DC: American Psychiatric Association, 1987

American Psychiatric Association. Diagnostic and Statistical Manual of Mental Disorders, 4th edition. Washington, DC: American Psychiatric Association, 1994

American Psychiatric Association. Diagnostic and Statistical Manual of Mental Disorders, 5th edition. Washington, DC: American Psychiatric Association, 2013

Amerio A, Stubbs B, Odone A, et al. The prevalence and predictors of comorbid bipolar disorder and obsessive–compulsive disorder: A systematic review and meta-analysis. J Affect Disord 2015; 186: 99–109

Andrews G, Hobbs MJ, Borkovec TD, et al. Generalized worry disorder: A review of DSM-IV generalized anxiety disorder and options for DSM-V. Depress Anxiety 2010; 27: 134–147

Archibald L. Alcohol use disorder and schizophrenia or schizoaffective disorder. Alcohol Res 2019; 40: arcr.v40.1.06

Cegla-Schvartzman F, Ovejero S, López-Castroma J, et al. Diagnostic stability in bipolar disorder: A follow-up study in 130,000 patient-years. J Clin Psychiatry 2021; 82: 20m13764

Chartier MJ, Walker JR, Stein MB. Considering comorbidity in social anxiety phobia. Soc Psychiatry Psychiatr Epidemiol 2003; 38: 728–734

Coryell W, Endicott J, Maser JD, et al. Long-term stability of polarity distinctions in the affective disorders. Am J Psychiatry 1995; 152: 385–390

Davis L, Uezato A, Newell JM, et al. Major depression and comorbid substance use disorders. Curr Opin Psychiatry 2008; 21: 14–18

d'Huart D, Seker S, Bürgin D, et al. The stability of personality disorders and personality disorder criteria: A systematic review and meta-analysis. Clin Psychol Rev 2023; 102; 102284

Fiedorowicz JG, Endicott J, Leon AC, et al. Subthreshold hypomanic symptoms in progression from unipolar major depression to bipolar disorder. Am J Psychiatry 2011; 168: 40–48

Goldstein-Piekarski AN, Williams LN, Humphreys K. A trans-diagnostic review of anxiety disorder comorbidity and the impact of multiple exclusion criteria on studying clinical outcomes in anxiety disorders. Transl Psychiatry 2016; 6: e47

Grant J, Kim SW, Eckert ED. Body dysmorphic disorder in patients with anorexia nervosa: Prevalence, clinical features, and delusionality of body image. Int J Eat Disord 2002; 32: 291–300

Hunt GE, Malhi GS, Cleary M, et al. Prevalence of comorbid bipolar and substance use disorders in clinical settings, 1990–2015: Systematic review and meta-analysis. J Affect Disord 2016; 206: 331–349

Kessler RC, Adler L, Barkley R, et al. The prevalence and correlates of adult ADHD in the United States: Results from the National Comorbidity Survey Replication. Am J Psychiatry 2006; 163: 716–723

Merikangas KR, Akiskal HS, Angst J, et al. Lifetime and 12-month prevalence of bipolar spectrum disorder in the national comorbidity survey replication. Arch Gen Psychiatry 2007; 64: 543–552

Nierenberg AA, Miyahara S, Spencer T, et al. Clinical and diagnostic implications of lifetime attention-deficit/hyperactivity disorder comorbidity in adults with bipolar disorder: Data from the first 1000 STEP-BD participants. Biol Psychiatry 2005; 57; 1467–1473

Pangaro LN. A new vocabulary and other innovations for improving descriptive in-training evaluations. Academic Medicine 1999; 74: 11

Pavlova B, Perlis RH, Alda M, et al. Lifetime prevalence of anxiety disorders in people with bipolar disorder: A systematic review and meta-analysis. Lancet Psychiatry 2015; 2: 710–717

Pitchot W, Hansenne M, Ansseau M. Role of dopamine in non-depressed patients with a history of suicide attempts. Eur Psychiatry 2001; 16: 424–427

Regier DA, Narrow WE, Clarke DE, et al. DSM-5 field trials in the United States and Canada. Part II: Test-retest reliability of selected categorical diagnoses. Am J Psychiatry 2013; 170: 59–70

Scotti-Muzzi E, Saide OL. Schizo-obsessive spectrum disorders: An update. CNS Spectrums 2017; 22: 258–272

Suárez-Pinilla P, Suárez-Pinilla M, Setién-Suero E, et al. Stability of schizophrenia diagnosis in a 10-year longitudinal study on first episode of non-affective psychosis: Conclusions from the PAFIP cohort. Acta Psychiatr Scand 2021; 144: 342–357

Torgersen T, Gjervan B, Rasmussen K. ADHD in adults: A study of clinical characteristics, impairment and comorbidity. Nordic J Psychiatry 2006; 60: 48–43

Van Meter AR, Sibley MH, Vandana P, et al. The stability and persistence of symptoms in childhood-onset ADHD. Eur Child Adolesc Psychiatry 2023; https://doi.org/10.1007/s00787-023-02235-3

Wingo AP, Ghaemi SN. A systematic review of rates and diagnostic validity of comorbid adult attention-deficit/hyperactivity disorder and bipolar disorder. J Clin Psychiatry 2007; 68: 1776–1784

2 The Approach to Diagnostic Ambiguity

LEARNING OBJECTIVES

- [ ] Recognize the role of symptoms, longitudinal course, family history, epidemiological context, treatment response, and laboratory assessments that can help to corroborate the validity of a psychiatric diagnosis
- [ ] Recognize the nonoverlapping symptoms among psychiatric disorders that share phenomenological features
- [ ] Appreciate both the utility and limitations of pharmacological assays to corroborate clinical diagnostic impressions
- [ ] Formulate working diagnostic hypotheses that are subject to revision over time as additional information becomes available through longitudinal course and treatment outcome

A WHAT TO DO IF YOU DON'T KNOW WHAT YOU'RE TREATING

Clarity about the intended targets of treatment is, by necessity, a prerequisite for any psychiatric or other medical intervention. One cannot make sensible treatment decisions unless one knows with some degree of confidence what exactly constitutes the object of treatment. Yet, by and large, psychiatric diagnoses are made on purely clinical grounds – meaning, they derive from collections of signs and symptoms that cohere in an organized fashion, seldom with definitive corroboration by an external biomarker. (Some exceptions to this might include positive blood or urine toxicology screens to affirm the diagnosis of alcohol or other substance intoxications; low cerebrospinal fluid levels of orexin to diagnose narcolepsy; or neuroimaging or other laboratory tests that affirm an underlying nonpsychiatric medical condition (such as a brain malignancy, or metabolic derangement) that might explain an acute mental status change.) Herein lies a dilemma: while evidence-based treatment means identifying a plausible working diagnosis, categorical diagnoses cannot always be made with the degree of exactitude one might otherwise hope for. In clinical trials, consensus-based diagnostic teams often review all available information from semi-structured interviews and past records to arrive at "low," "medium," and "high" probability levels for a suspected diagnosis, recognizing that cases which stray too far from "high" diagnostic probability invite extrapolation and variability from the treatment effects seen in more clear-cut presentations of a suspected disorder.

> **Tip**
>
> It is generally more useful to acknowledge diagnostic ambiguity when the clinical elements of a given patient's presentation seem not to add up to a recognizable clinical profile, rather than to "force fit" a diagnosis (or consequent treatment) when key features may not be evident.

The idea of diagnostic "accuracy" may be a more relative than absolute construct, insofar as the operational criteria for some psychiatric disorders may change over time, and are often based more on committee consensus than empirical discovery; some diagnoses become "voted" into favor (e.g., disruptive mood dysregulation disorder) or altogether out of existence (e.g., Asperger syndrome) based on prevailing sentiments among experts at any given time. Fuzzy treatment targets can beget murky therapies, and the process of differential decision-making across viable strategies (and their evidence base) becomes a slippery slope. Yet, without coherent operational criteria for defining a clinical entity, it may be next to impossible to apply any kind of objective decision-making calculus to differential therapeutics.

Pattern recognition and the related notion of **template matching**, as discussed in Chapter 7, Section B, offers one approach for clinicians to identify a coherent clinical entity (say, major depression), and its possible subtypes (say, melancholic versus atypical). The basic concept here means trying to identify a constellation of recognizable signs and symptoms that fits within an expected epidemiological framework (see Table 2.1 in Section D) and can help clinicians formulate cogent diagnostic impressions and consequent therapeutic targets; that process, in turn, should then align with evidence-based treatment options. Certain clinical elements are expected to congeal for particular diagnostic entities, and their presence or absence may strengthen or weaken the confidence with which one establishes a working diagnosis, as well as a plan of viable therapeutic options. For instance:

- One would expect a manic patient to manifest signs of high energy and psychomotor acceleration (in speech, thought, and movement)
- One would expect someone with schizophrenia to demonstrate concrete and impoverished thinking as well as poor affective relatedness
- Suspected autism usually involves preoccupations with restricted interests and poor reciprocal social skills
- Personality disorders involve persistent (non-episodic) traits that can be provoked at any given point in time in response to the right interpersonal context or stressor; as lifelong phenomena, they are likely to become manifest sooner than later

Certain psychiatric symptoms can be highly nonspecific and, in themselves, lead toward no particular diagnostic impression unless contextualized by associated symptoms. Examples include inattention; mood instability; anhedonia; poor impulse control; aggression; idiosyncratic thinking; and even psychosis.

B SYMPTOMATIC OVERLAP

Symptoms that overlap across multiple diagnoses are nonpathognomonic. In fact, modern nosological systems such as the DSM-5 (American Psychiatric Association, 2013) prohibit the "counting" of an identified symptom as being a component of one disorder if it can be better accounted for by another. For example, in the medically ill, it can be problematic to attribute vegetative signs such as fatigue or loss of appetite to depression versus a chronic medical condition. Socially avoidant behavior could occur for different reasons in someone with schizophrenia or social anxiety disorder. Similarities and differences between depression and negative symptoms in schizophrenia may seem to involve nuanced distinctions but their phenomenological discrimination can be identified (Krynicki et al., 2018). Several examples of conditions with overlapping symptoms, for which the nonoverlapping features may be fruitfully differentiated, are illustrated in Figures 2.1–2.4.

Figure 2.1 Overlapping versus nonoverlapping features in bipolar disorder and attention deficit-hyperactivity disorder (ADHD)

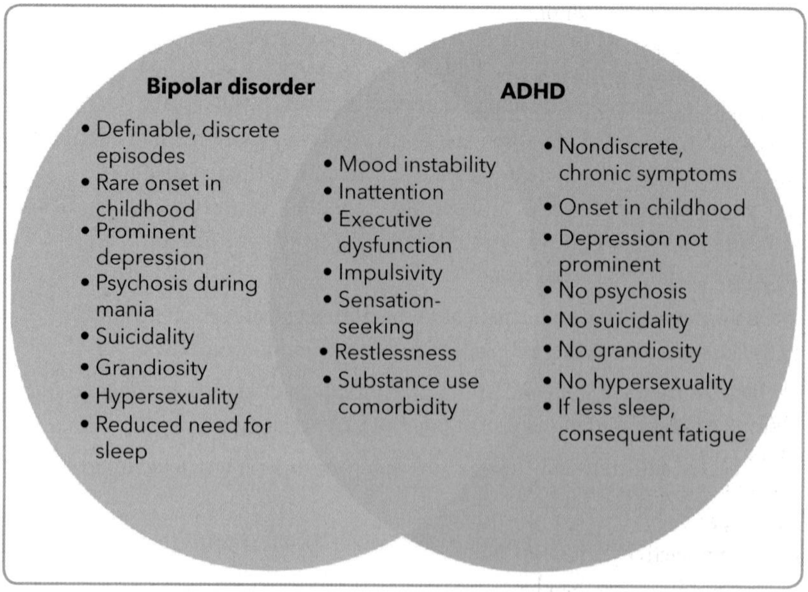

Figure 2.2 Overlapping versus nonoverlapping features in bipolar disorder and borderline personality disorder

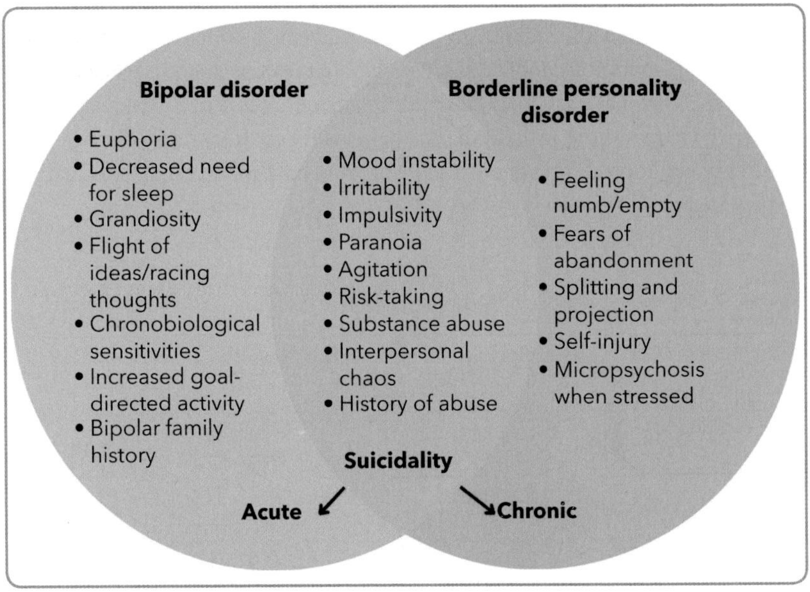

Constructs such as "mood instability" have been shown to have little diagnostic value for discriminating bipolar disorder from other conditions that may involve high emotional variability (Goldberg et al., 2012) – not just borderline personality disorder as noted in Figure 2.2, but also substance use disorders, posttraumatic stress disorder (PTSD), developmental disabilities, and cognitive impairment disorders (e.g., dementia), among others. Some authors have rather controversially proposed that common underlying mechanisms might account for swift mood changes and problems with impulse control in people with bipolar disorder or borderline personality disorder (and the use of medications studied in bipolar disorder as plausible treatments for symptoms of borderline personality disorder) (MacKinnon and Pies, 2006). We would instead encourage more of a focus on their *nonoverlapping features* to better guide their phenomenological discrimination – as illustrated in Figure 2.2. Notably, emotional dysregulation in borderline personality disorder tends to be triggered by interpersonal events whose impact lasts on the order of minutes to hours, whereas mood changes in people with bipolar disorder less clearly arise in response to such provocations, last more on the order of days to weeks or months, and are by definition accompanied by changes in the sleep–wake cycle and energy–activity levels. *Abrupt* rather than *gradual* changes in mood also are evident in a little less than half of individuals with bipolar disorder (and may be a phenomenon also evident in their first-degree relatives) (MacKinnon et al., 2003), whereas sudden and dramatic mood shifts are nearly universally observed when describing patterns of affective instability in borderline personality disorder.

The nature of mood instability in itself also appears qualitatively different between both conditions: individuals with bipolar disorder tend to experience mood states that may vary from euthymic to anxious, depressed, irritable, or euphoric, whereas those with borderline personality disorder rarely display features of euphoria and tend much more often to have mood excursions that involve anger and rage (Henry et al., 2001).

Figure 2.3 Overlapping versus nonoverlapping features in depression and anxiety disorders

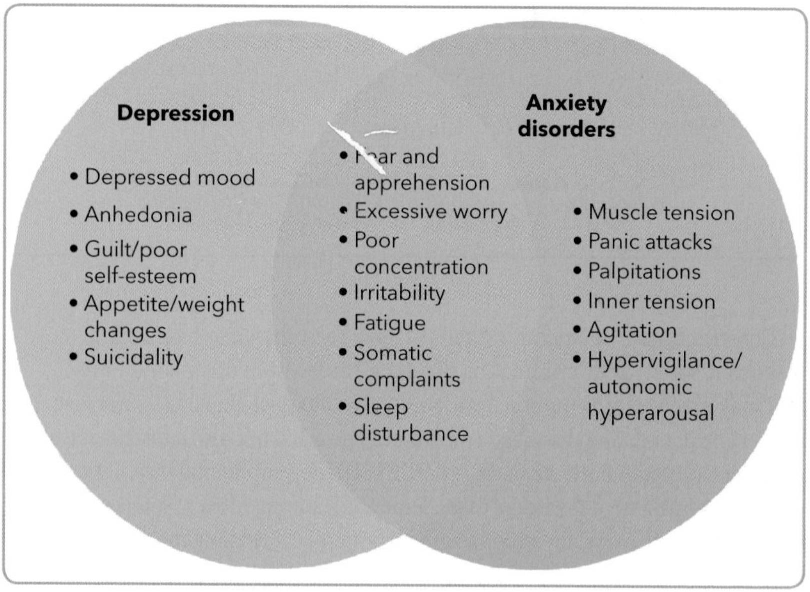

Efforts to define "mixed anxiety and depression" as a unique clinical entity failed to achieve inter-rater reliability in field trials for the DSM-IV (American Psychiatric Association, 1994), in large part because nonspecific patterns of anxious and depressive symptoms were highly prevalent across the primary care and mental health outpatient centers being studied (Zinbarg et al., 1994). Nevertheless, conglomerations of prominent anxiety and depression unambiguously exist – by whatever name one prefers – and generally pose a more daunting therapeutic task than when either set of features presents without the other.

Figure 2.4 Overlapping versus nonoverlapping features in depression and schizophrenic negative symptoms

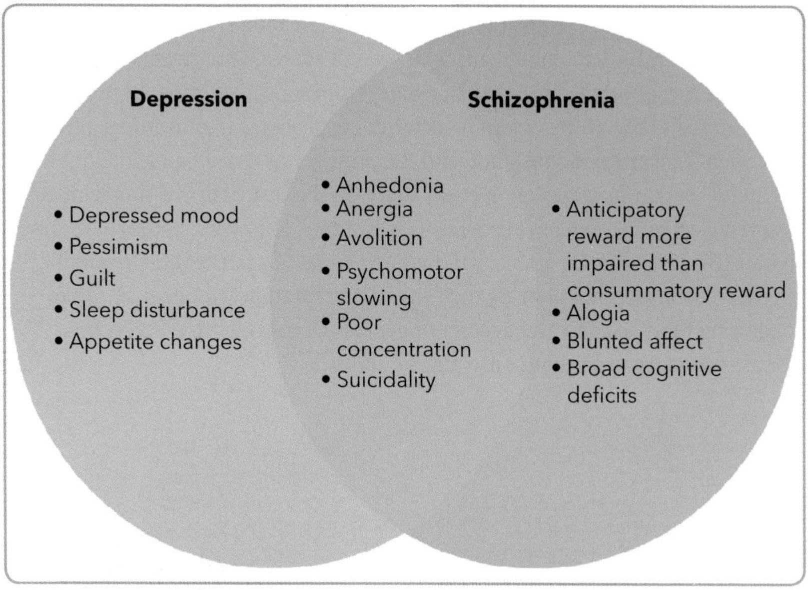

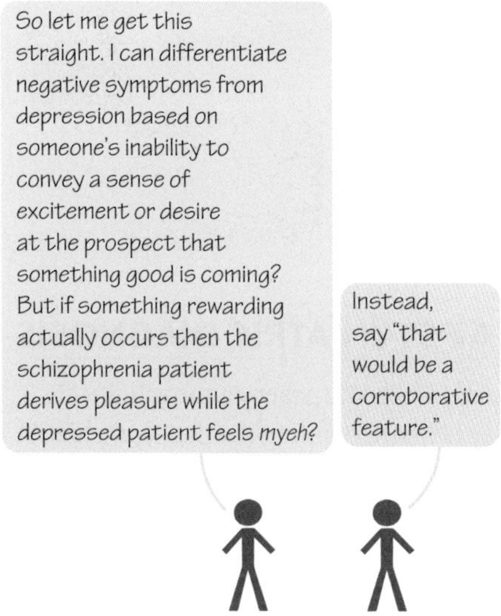

Tip

Anticipatory reward refers to the value associated with expecting a pleasurable experience (believed to be driven by striatal dopaminergic circuitry), while consummatory reward describes the delivery or actual receipt of a pleasurable stimulus (believed to be linked with orbitofrontal and ventromedial prefrontal cortical structures) (Galtress et al., 2012).

C SUBSTANCE USE AS A DIAGNOSTIC CONFOUNDER

A further challenge when diagnosing primary psychiatric conditions in general involves the chronology of seemingly comorbid conditions, particularly substance use disorders. Significant (even intermittent) alcohol or substance use disorders cause mood dysregulation, irritability, problems with impulse control, and a host of psychosocial consequences, as well as impaired cognition and judgment. At the same time, substance use disorders can be common comorbidities across a range of psychiatric disorders. In patients who present acutely with psychosis and active substance use, efforts to tease apart primary from substance-induced psychosis have pointed to the utility of family histories of substance use disorders, physical dependence on any one substance, and the presence of visual hallucinations as useful for discrimination (Caton et al., 2005). In the case of depression with co-occurring active alcohol or substance use disorders, follow-up studies have shown that nearly 90% of such patients will manifest signs of persistent depression over the 1-year period following their initial presentation (Nunes et al., 2006) – suggesting that the clinical trajectory of depressive episodes that are "primary" versus secondary to substance use may be similar.

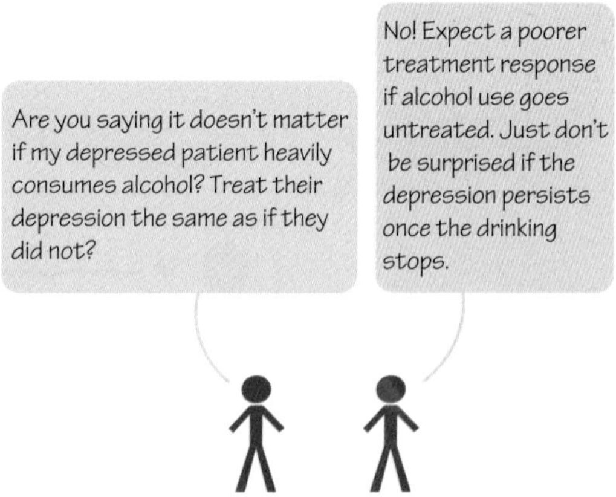

D CORROBORATORS OF A PSYCHIATRIC DIAGNOSIS

Figure 2.5 expands on the ideas presented in a classic paper on the validity of psychiatric diagnoses by Robins and Guze (1970), pointing out that a psychiatric diagnosis depends not only on current and past symptoms but also a predictable trajectory over time, an expectable time frame over the lifespan for symptoms to arise, and corroboration by supportive features such as family history, treatment response, and laboratory testing if it exists. Let us elaborate on each of these features as useful tools for clinical reasoning when formulating diagnostic impressions and targets of therapeutic intervention.

D.1 Expected Epidemiology

Fortunately for the diagnostician, certain psychiatric conditions arise at more-or-less expectable time points in the lifespan. Table 2.1 provides information about

Figure 2.5 Corroborators of a psychiatric diagnosis

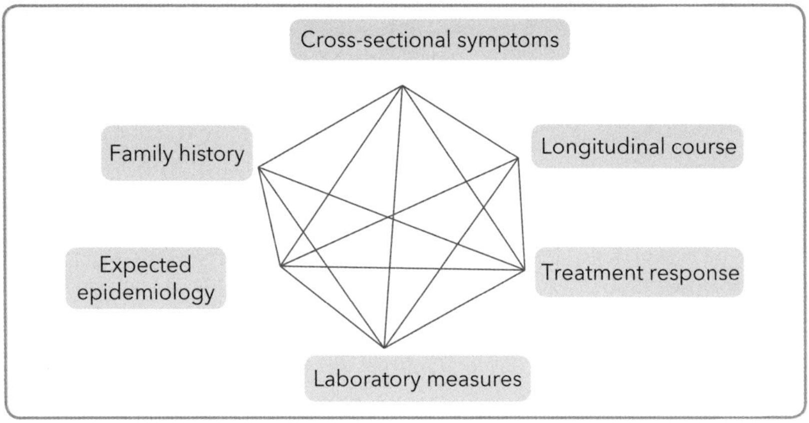

the modal age at onset for a number of major psychiatric disorders (findings are based on reported meta-analyses or large-scale epidemiological studies, as cited), which can help clinicians as they reason through likely differential diagnostic considerations. Notably, most major psychiatric disorders usually begin in late adolescence and young adulthood.

We would add one caveat to Table 2.1, with respect to PTSD. The idea of "age at onset" for PTSD is rather disingenuous insofar as symptoms arise *at any age* in proximity to a discrete life-threatening trauma that occurs at any point in the life cycle. Typically, symptoms become manifest within 1 year of trauma exposure (delayed onset is rare). However, it is tempting to speculate about risk windows for people who are genetically predisposed to develop PTSD (or who may have genetic protection through resilience factors). If a given level of traumatic stress in a given individual has not led to PTSD by a certain age, can they be considered protected from the risk for developing PTSD in the setting of future traumatic stresses? And if that were true – as we speculate here – how much does the magnitude of traumatic stress (chronic? catastrophic?) exert influence in older versus younger patients based on both their genetic risk and cumulative past exposure to previous traumatic stress? Trauma exposure before the end of adolescence also carries an elevated risk for other forms of psychopathology in addition to (and independent of) PTSD, including major depression, conduct disorders, self-harming behaviors, and substance use disorders (Lewis et al., 2019). The majority of trauma-exposed individuals do not develop PTSD (Weisaeth, 1998), and the interplay between possible age-based risk windows and genetic or other factors that confer risk versus protection from PTSD after traumatic stress remain poorly understood.

Table 2.1 Modal age at onset for major psychiatric or substance use disorders

Condition	Modal age at onset
Social anxiety disorder	10.6 years (95% CI = 6.4–14.9 years) (de Lijster et al., 2017)
Simple phobias	11 years (Solmi et al., 2022)
ADHD	In the National Comorbidity Survey Replication study, only 50% of adults recalled ADHD symptoms before age 7 whereas 95% recalled symptoms before age 12 as did 99% before age 16 (Kessler et al., 2005)
Cannabis use disorder	15–18 years (Behrendt et al., 2012)
Anorexia nervosa	17 years (Solmi et al., 2022)
Bulimia nervosa	18 years (Solmi et al., 2022)
Alcohol use disorder	Peaks at age 18–19, then declines rapidly after age 25 (Reich et al., 1998; Li et al., 2004)
OCD	19.5 years (men earlier than women; new cases are rare after age 30) (Ruscio et al., 2010; Solmi et al., 2022)
Schizophrenia	Peak incidence = ages 20–24 in men, 25–35 in women (Welham et al., 2004; Ochoa et al., 2012)
Major depressive disorder	20s to early 30s (Kessler et al., 2005)
PTSD	26.6 years (95% CI = 22.1–31.6 years) (de Lijster et al., 2017)
Panic disorder	30.3 years (95% CI = 26.1–34.6 years) (de Lijster et al., 2017)
Bipolar disorder	Median age 33 (Solmi et al., 2022); a meta-analysis of 22,981 subjects across 21 studies found that 45% of patients had a mean age at onset of 17.3 $\pm$ 1.9 years (Bolton et al., 2021)
Generalized anxiety disorder	34.9 years (95% CI = 30.9–39.0 years) (de Lijster et al., 2017)

Abbreviations: ADHD, attention deficit-hyperactivity disorder; CI, confidence interval; OCD, obsessive-compulsive disorder; PTSD, posttraumatic stress disorder.

Exceptions to the rule obviously occur, and the quality of information obtained in a patient's history may not fully reveal a true age at onset. For example, individuals with bipolar disorder who initially present later in life may very well have experienced previous hypomanias or even manias that either went undetected, were misidentified, or were disavowed as being clinically important. Some patients may have experienced a chronic psychiatric condition that was never brought to clinical attention because of denial, concerns about stigma, or a family system that tolerated, managed, or otherwise compensated for the presence of symptoms; if the equilibrium state of the family system changes,

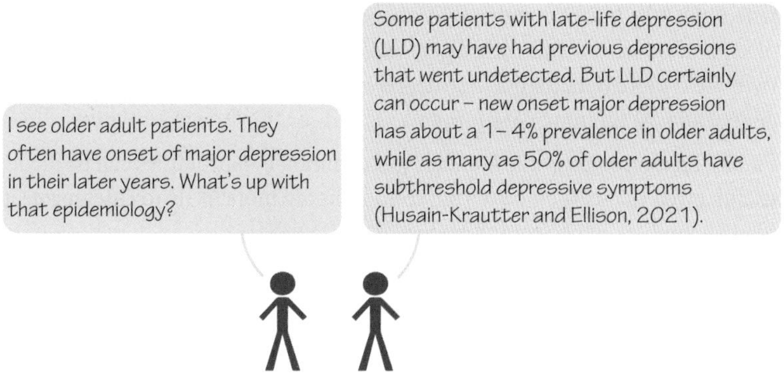

clinical casehood becomes detected long after the onset of a chronic psychiatric condition has become ensconced and a set of "compensatory" norms and expectations about daily functioning has become established.

D.2 Family History

As much as genetic factors are known contributors to psychiatric disorders, it is difficult to quantify that risk or appreciate its impact alongside other clinical features for several reasons. Psychiatric disorders do not follow the rules of so-called Mendelian genetics. That means that unlike diseases such as cystic fibrosis or muscular dystrophy, where a single gene variant is the known cause of a disorder, the features that comprise psychiatric conditions are regarded as complex traits, where multiple genes confer small effects that contribute to an overall clinical outcome. Consider the following:

- Transmissible traits may not necessarily involve complete syndromes but, rather, distinct traits such as inattention, impulsivity, sleep–wake cycle disturbances, or creativity
- Quality of information that is often obtained second-hand from a patient about the psychiatric symptoms of a relative may not be accurate. In order to properly and rigorously assess the presence or absence of psychopathology in family members, clinical trials utilize formal psychiatric tools such as the Diagnostic Interview for Genetic Studies (Nurnberger et al., 1994), a "gold standard" but rather complex measure that can take many hours to administer, and only after assessors have received formal training in its implementation (further discussed in Chapter 3, Section C)

Tip

A polygenic risk score (PGS) is a cumulative or aggregate rating from genome-wide assessments of minor allele frequencies for genes associated with a particular complex trait. PGSs are continuous numbers that reflect an area under the curve falling between 0 and 1; larger numbers suggest higher predictive value.

- One must take into account a dilutional effect of genetic factors across degrees of separation across and within generations; observations in a monozygotic twin yield more data than a first-degree relative, which in turn holds more genetically useful information than a second- or third-degree relative
- Finally, an awareness of the familiality of common comorbidities can be useful, given that certain comorbid conditions are more likely to cosegregate in family members of probands who have a particular psychiatric condition, as shown in the examples provided in Table 2.2. (And likewise, some conditions show little patterning of familial cosegregation; for example, probands with panic disorder or social anxiety disorder tend to have relatives with those disorders but not mood disorders, alcohol use disorder, or other anxiety disorders (Low et al., 2008))

Tip

Cosegregation means that two or more linked genes originate from the same parental chromosome and thus may account for inheritance of linked traits.

Table 2.2 Examples of heritable comorbid psychiatric conditions across major psychiatric disorders

Primary disorder	Common associated familial disorders
Alcohol use disorder	Strong familial association with anxiety disorders (Merikangas et al., 1998)
ADHD	Strong familial association with both major depressive disorder and bipolar disorder (Biederman et al., 1991; Faraone and Biederman, 1997; Chen et al., 2019) as well as autism spectrum disorders (Chen et al., 2019)
Bipolar disorder	Increased risk in first-degree relatives for recurrent depression (Fisfalen et al., 2005), panic disorder (MacKinnon et al., 2002), state and trait anxiety (Contreras et al., 2010), suicide attempts (Fisfalen et al., 2005; Ballard et al., 2019), cannabis use disorder (Quick et al., 2022), alcohol use disorder (Fisfalen et al., 2005), and any substance use disorder (Wilens et al., 2007 - although some studies find no increased risk (e.g., Sbrana et al., 2007)). Unaffected relatives of bipolar probands demonstrate cognitive problems (verbal ability, executive functioning, psychomotor processing speed) (Antila et al., 2007) without necessarily meeting criteria for ADHD
Major depressive disorder	In relatives of probands with early onset depression: increased risk for alcohol (Puig-Antich et al., 1989) and substance use disorders or antisocial behavior (Goldstein et al., 1994) as well as suicide attempts (Mann et al., 2005)
OCD	Relatives show increased rates of schizophrenia, major depression, bipolar disorder, autism spectrum disorders, and ADHD (Huang et al., 2021)

Table 2.2 (cont.)

Primary disorder	Common associated familial disorders
Panic disorder	Offspring of parents with panic disorder have increased risk for multiple anxiety disorders, panic disorder, agoraphobia, social anxiety disorder, and OCD (Hirschfeld-Becker et al., 2012)
Schizophrenia	Offspring of parents with schizophrenia demonstrate higher rates of ADHD (Sanchez-Gistau et al., 2015; Cheng et al., 2018) as well as major depression and bipolar disorder (Cheng et al., 2018)
Social anxiety disorder	Increased risk for suicide attempts in first-degree relatives (Ballard et al., 2019)

Abbreviations: ADHD, attention deficit-hyperactivity disorder; OCD, obsessive-compulsive disorder.

D.3 Laboratory Measures

When Robins and Guze (1970) initially included "laboratory measures" as a component of diagnostic validation, they acknowledged that "consistent and reliable laboratory findings have not yet been demonstrated in the more common psychiatric disorders." While in some respects the search for biomarkers or other laboratory-based corroborators of most psychiatric diagnoses remains just as elusive half a century later, there are a number of instances in which laboratory data can be helpful to rule out (if not rule in) components of a psychiatric differential diagnosis. Examples are depicted in Table 2.3.

Table 2.3 Pertinent laboratory measures for diagnostic purposes in psychiatry

Test	Purpose
Thyroid function tests	Can rule out mood disorders secondary to hypo- or hyperthyroidism
Neuroimaging	Useful when a clinical presentation raises concerns about a possible underlying neurological explanation (e.g., mass lesion, infarction, age-inappropriate atrophy) for new-onset psychiatric symptoms
EEG	Useful mainly in the evaluation of major cognitive disorders, suspicions of epilepsy, or sudden changes in mental status such as a suspected delirium
Pharmacogenetic testing	Can help to identify patients who may poorly convert some drugs to their active metabolites or accrue excessive side effects because of inefficient breakdown of parent drugs, or patients who may metabolize drugs too rapidly and consequently derive little or no benefit; not necessarily so pertinent to psychiatric diagnostics
Toxicology screens	Fundamental when a history of substance use or other environmental exposure (e.g., heavy metals) is suspected in accounting for a change in mental status

Vitamin deficiencies are uncommon causes for common psychiatric disorders. Some authors have expressed concerns in the literature that because deficiencies of vitamin B_{12} or folic acid (Coppen and Bolander-Gouaille, 2005) and vitamin D (Anglin et al., 2013) can be associated with clinical depression, they may be under-recognized and correctable causes for it. However, before routinely looking for vitamin deficiencies in patients without known risk factors (e.g., strict vegans, heavy alcohol consumers, or people chronically taking proton pump inhibitors), clinicians should recognize that vitamin deficiencies usually present with physical as well as potential psychiatric signs. Clinically meaningful vitamin B_{12} deficiency usually presents with megaloblastic anemia and/or paresthesias or areflexia. Clinically meaningful vitamin D deficiency usually presents with muscle weakness, bone pain, and fatigue. The direction of causality is also often unclear between some vitamin deficiencies and depression – that is, do low vitamin D levels lead to depression, or does depression lead to poor dietary intake and less exposure to outdoor sunlight, with consequent reductions in vitamin D levels?

D.4 Treatment Response

How much is treatment response a reliable or valid informant about the nature of an underlying psychiatric condition? This is a difficult question, given the uncoupling that exists between the largely unknown etiologies and pathophysiological mechanisms behind most psychiatric conditions and treatments that are largely meant to give symptomatic relief. Many psychotropic medications can exert multiple pharmacodynamic effects, further preventing causal inferences about an underlying pathology based simply on drug response (e.g., if feelings of distress improve with a drug that happens to possess antipsychotic properties, that does not mean the distress was caused by psychosis). On the other hand, response to certain drugs can sometimes be viewed as consistent with a diagnostic impression, or can be used as an assay to help rule out suspected underlying processes. Examples appear farther ahead in Clinical Vignettes 2.3 and 2.4.

D.5 Longitudinal Course

There is nothing wrong with formulating a working diagnosis from cross-sectional symptom information, but the evolution of symptoms and course over time are well-recognized corroborators of a diagnosis. Certain ailments have predictable time courses. Mood episodes in bipolar disorder, for example, on average last about 13 weeks (Solomon et al., 2010). This does not mean that a mania or depression cannot have a much shorter or longer duration, but it does raise suspicion if a purported manic episode leads to hospitalization on a Friday night and all symptoms seem completely resolved by Monday morning. Developmental windows also bear on the corroboration of many diagnoses. Attention deficit–hyperactivity disorder (ADHD) is considered a childhood/

preadolescent disorder that can persist into adulthood in half or fewer of cases; it is not thought to arise de novo in adults. Psychosis is possible, but quite rare, in children, as is bipolar disorder. Prodromal features can reflect nonspecific rudiments of a psychiatric disorder in the making, which has not yet fully blossomed.

Mood symptoms in an adolescent may not present with sufficient clarity to rule in or out distinctions about polarity, psychosis, comorbidity, or personality – but the course over time may help crystallize an initial impression, which in turn can help to inform best treatment decisions. That example is illustrated with Jack in Clinical Vignette 2.1.

Clinical Vignette 2.1

Jack was a previously-untreated 15-year-old boy with a 6-month history of depression manifested by irritability, depressed mood, oversleeping, low motivation, and social isolation. There was no substance misuse and no conduct or other behavioral problems. His mother was reportedly diagnosed with bipolar II disorder and treated with topiramate 200 mg/day. The consulting psychiatrist advised a selective serotonin reuptake inhibitor (SSRI) trial as an initial step but Jack's mother was worried about a risk for inducing mania or worsening suicidal thinking, and preferred that a mood stabilizer be tried first. How should one think about next steps?

There are a few elements of Jack's case that are not so straightforward, making it harder for the clinician to sort through what course of action makes the most sense. (And for the sake of simplicity, let us not yet read ahead to Chapter 4 on the topic of shared decision-making, which introduces a thornier proposition if the clinician does not have a clear sense in his or her own mind about their own formulation and treatment plan.) First, it is certainly possible that Jack may some day develop bipolar disorder. *If* indeed Jack's mother was correctly diagnosed (and why exactly does her pharmacology for purported bipolar disorder consist solely of a drug that has only negative randomized trial data for that condition?), that datapoint alone would confer anywhere from a 15% to a 25% risk, depending on the source one reads, as compared to the 1–2% risk in the general population. Although early-onset depression adds another potential risk factor for eventually developing mania or hypomania, Jack is currently on the young side for developing a first lifetime mania. Recall also from Table 2.2 that Jack's family history places him at risk for a range of psychiatric problems besides possible future bipolar disorder, including unipolar depression, anxiety disorders, cognitive disorders, and substance use disorders – should he be treated prophylactically for all of those? Herein lies a big uncertainty: if and until Jack ever develops a mania or hypomania, there is no evidence base to support treating his current depression with medicines that have not been studied for youth who are only *at risk* for bipolar disorder. In fact, the sole published randomized trial of lithium for prepubescent (thus-far unipolar) depressed offspring of bipolar parents found no significant difference from placebo over a 6-week treatment period (Geller et al., 1998). Whatever intervention one might choose for Jack, longitudinal follow-up becomes especially important – not just to assure treatment efficacy and avoid worsening of his depression but, moreover, to provide corroborative data regarding possible evolution of his diagnosis over time.

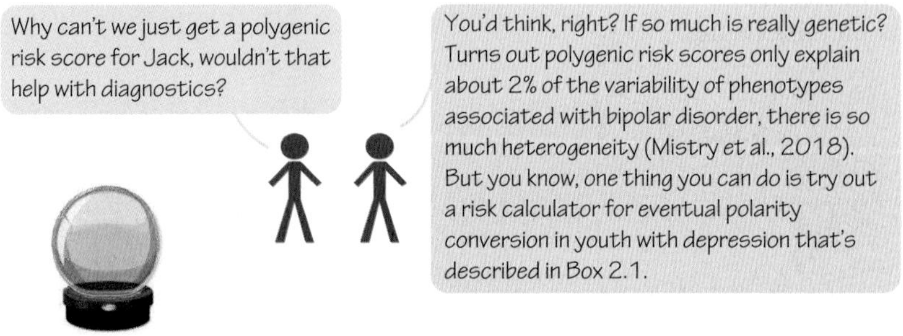

Box 2.1

A risk calculator for polarity conversion in depression?

In the spirit of machine learning and applications of big data - discussed in depth later on in Chapter 6, Section J - one might consider the possible utility of a risk calculator developed at Queen's University for estimating the probability of eventual polarity conversion from major depression to bipolar disorder in at-risk youth (www.queensu.ca/u-flourish/bipolar-calculator/calculator/). Data from an original study cohort (a "training sample") was used to devise likelihoods for estimating risk for future patients based on a number of simple baseline characteristics, including parental age at bipolar onset and treatment response. The model had a 70% chance for predicting which of two 15-year-olds was more likely to have a future manic or hypomanic episode (Keown-Stoneman et al., 2021). Using data from Jack and his mother, we can calculate a 5-year risk of 22% (95% CI = 7% to 41%) and a 10-year risk of 42% (95% CI = 15% to 70%).

In general, when we speak of an "expectable clinical course," we imply a certain likelihood or probability of future events that follow with some degree of predictability from an initial event. While recovery, to varying degrees, can occur for most patients diagnosed with schizophrenia, it is rare for there to occur a complete absence of positive and negative symptoms over the long term. Similarly, in mood disorders, even with the best of treatments it is rare to encounter patients who report having had only a single lifetime affective episode in the distant past with no recurrences. (A 25-year longitudinal follow-up in a well-characterized Swiss cohort identified a recurrence risk of 0.40 annual episodes among bipolar patients and 0.20 annual episodes in (unipolar) major depressive disorder patients (Angst et al., 2003).) With this in mind, consider the case of Tanya in Clinical Vignette 2.2.

Clinical Vignette 2.2

Tanya was a 73-year-old divorced woman, who initially presented with a hospitalized manic episode in her 30s when she abruptly stopped sleeping and began purchasing endless quantities of skin care products as part of an impulsive whim to start a resale business. There was no substance use disorder or identifiable nonpsychiatric/medical explanation for her new-onset noninsidious symptoms. Begun on lithium, which reportedly was beneficial for her mother's diagnosis of bipolar disorder, she remained well for a few years until deciding to stop. When she then became depressed, she was prescribed paroxetine 30 mg/day along with low-dose lorazepam, which she then remained on for 25 years with reportedly no affective recurrences.

By all expectations, Tanya should have had at least one or more additional manic episodes over the course of 25 years, especially in the absence of a mood-stabilizing drug, and in the presence of an unopposed SSRI. Does her longitudinal course call into question the veracity of her original diagnosis? Is hers simply an atypical presentation? And, if she has indeed been euthymic for over two decades mainly on just paroxetine, would the traditional rules of pharmacological hygiene argue for encouraging her to discontinue the paroxetine? It would be hard to claim that unopposed paroxetine in a bipolar I disorder patient is posing a threat to Tanya's sustained euthymia, based on her personal history. There are a handful of curious reports that abrupt cessation of antidepressant medications in euthymic patients with bipolar disorder could paradoxically trigger mania because of disruption to a stable equilibrium state (Goldstein et al., 1999). Should we turn Tanya into a science-fair project and encourage her to stop taking paroxetine because it may be unnecessary, or as an evocative test to try to see if she becomes manic and add to the above paradoxical case literature? Or do we leave everything alone because there is no compelling reason to change anything other than for the sake of diagnostic curiosity?

E STRENGTHS AND LIMITATIONS OF DIAGNOSTIC SCREENS

Screening for disorders within all of medicine is a strategy to identify potential cases. From a public health standpoint, screening is meant to be a more over- than underinclusive endeavor because the primary objective is to not miss true cases. However, by intentionally casting a wide net for such purposes, screening is not necessarily so useful a method to discriminate true cases from false cases that may bear a faint resemblance, or for teasing apart complex presentations in which comorbidities or atypical features may require a much more fine-grained analysis in order to render a more formal diagnostic impression. Screens are thus not proxies for diagnoses, but they are useful starting points. Just as a positive pap smear does not equate to the diagnosis of cervical cancer, or a positive antinuclear antibody test alone does not designate lupus, an above-threshold score on a psychiatric diagnostic screen indicates the need for further evaluation and comparative diagnostic assessment.

Chapter 6, focused on measurement-based care, provides a more detailed discussion about specific diagnostic screening tools in psychiatry. In particular, Table 6.7 in Chapter 6 summarizes a number of commonly used measures, alongside their relative strengths and limitations.

F WORKING WITH DIAGNOSTIC AMBIGUITY: THE ROLE FOR HYPOTHESIS-TESTING AND PHARMACOTHERAPY AS A DIAGNOSTIC ASSAY

When evaluating and treating patients whose symptom profiles do not fit neatly into a predefined diagnostic category, an empirical approach with a working diagnosis often makes sense. Sometimes it may also make even more sense to sidestep the issue or relevance of finding a shorthand name that captures the essential elements of a clinical problem, and instead just describe and treat the salient signs, symptoms, or behavioral manifestations, with an eye toward using a longitudinal course as an eventual corroborator of an initial working diagnosis or hypothesis. Like managing a fever of unknown origin, one might empirically treat for a suspected condition – say, to help parse the distinction between anxiety and hypomania, or undertake a stimulant trial for complaints of inattention that have no obvious alternative explanation when a diagnosis of adult ADHD is suspected but not confirmed from a childhood history. These instances are illustrated, respectively, in Clinical Vignettes 2.3 and 2.4.

Clinical Vignette 2.3

Sandy was a 38-year-old woman who had long struggled with feelings of inner tension, anxiety, "raciness," and insomnia, with what one psychiatrist called a "soft spectrum" bipolar diagnosis. She had a sibling with bipolar disorder and second-degree relatives with various forms of anxiety and depression. She had been maintained on lithium carbonate 300 mg/day, and in the past also took low-dose sertraline (75 mg/day) but stopped due to sexual side effects. In recent months she reported waking up at 3 A.M. with anxious ruminations and apprehension about obligations for the next day. A variety of sleep medications ("z"-drugs, ramelteon, and dual orexin receptor antagonists) had not yielded substantial improvement. Low-dose lorazepam at bedtime had helped her to maintain sleep continuity but left her feeling drowsy the next day. Similar experience came from taking quetiapine 25–50 mg at bedtime. She was not especially fatigued from disrupted sleep but denied feeling "over energized." She identified her current mood as "worried" more than "elevated," "irritable" or "depressed."

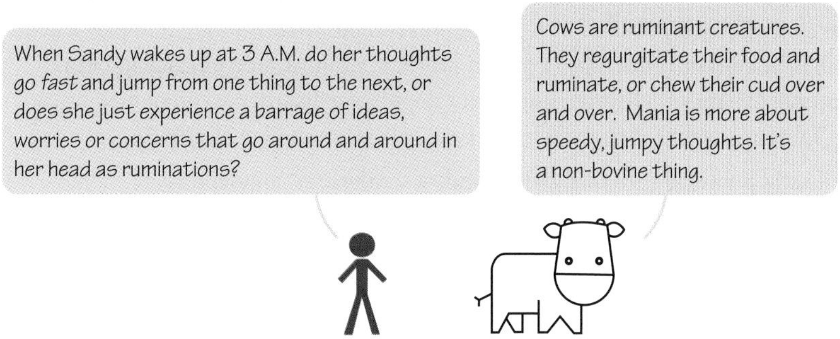

The differential diagnostic question for Sandy involves whether her signs of psychomotor activation reflect predominantly an anxiety disorder (with prominent autonomic hyperarousal) or a mood disorder (versus their combination). Which conceptual model best explains her inner tension, restlessness, and sleep disruption? We can devise an experiment to help clarify this question. Let us begin with the hypothesis that hypomania is keeping her awake and agitated. We can test that hypothesis by raising her lithium dose to a more standard therapeutic level. After no more than a 3–4-week period, we would expect either to see or not see some improvement in her symptoms. Let us define what clinical trialists call the primary outcome measure of this experiment (meaning, the main thing we are looking at from which to judge efficacy), and we will pick two ("co-primary outcomes"): (a) *time of waking* and (b) *sense of inner tension and agitation*. If essentially tripling Sandy's lithium dose, progressively, from 300 to 600 to 900 mg/day fails to impact either primary outcome measure even to a modest degree, that does not necessarily disprove that hypomania was the cause, but it would certainly lend less support to that hypothesis. On the other hand, if the increased lithium dose *did* noticeably impact either outcome measure, that would be consistent with, and corroborative of, the hypothesis that hypomania is the culprit.

Suppose our test of the "hypomania" hypothesis was unsupported by our lithium dose experiment. Then what? Our alternative hypothesis is that anxiety is more the driver of her symptoms. If lithium – which has really no known anxiolytic properties – did nothing to alter the primary outcome measures, then our alternative plan would be to deploy a medication that was more specifically anxiolytic. That could be a higher dose benzodiazepine, but that carries two limitations: (a) benzodiazepines can simply be soporific without necessarily informing about separate anxiolytic effects; and (b) Sandy found low-dose lorazepam hard to tolerate in terms of sedation, making a higher-dose experiment not so practical. It can be awfully hard, in general, to identify an effective anxiolytic that has no adverse effects on alertness. We could pick something else that is a known anxiolytic that is less soporific for this experiment. What are viable options? They might include (a) gabapentin, (b) pregabalin, or (c) an anxiolytic serotonergic drug other than sertraline – say, vilazodone, which has potent binding at the 5-HT_{1A} serotonin receptor that is thought to play a key role in anxiolysis (Toth, 2003), and in fact has demonstrated efficacy in both generalized anxiety disorder and major depressive disorder accompanied by prominent baseline anxiety (Thase et al., 2014; Gommoll et al., 2015).

Lastly, how likely is it that giving Sandy a serotonergic antidepressant might worsen her condition if she has bipolar disorder? Contrary to popular perception, the likelihood that traditional monoaminergic antidepressants can induce manic or hypomanic symptoms pertains to a rather small minority of bipolar disorder patients – about 12% according to prospective randomized trials (Fornaro et al., 2018). That risk also seems especially salient in people with bipolar I rather than bipolar II disorder, those with recent mania or hypomania, those with current mixed features, and those with a history of antidepressant-induced mania/hypomania (Goldberg, 2019) – none of which are characteristics that apply to Sandy.

Now consider Lindsay from Clinical Vignette 2.4. While a cognitively organizing response to simulants is not necessarily diagnostic of ADHD, it is consistent with

Clinical Vignette 2.4

Lindsay was a 43-year-old married woman who had intermittently been in and out of psychotherapy and off and on brief trials of SSRIs over may years for complaints of "mood instability, depression, and irritability." Somewhat randomly, she one day told her psychiatrist that she thought she might have adult ADHD because she often felt flustered, inefficient, and inattentive, and she thinks that causes her to become impatient with her children and lose her temper. Her psychiatrist quizzed her about childhood features of inattention or academic problems to which she said only that she often daydreamed. He insisted that ADHD does not arise in adults for whom it was not evident in childhood, and that "inattention" is a very broad phenomenon that can likely be found in almost all psychiatric conditions, including depression and anxiety. Dissatisfied with that response, she sought a second opinion from another psychiatrist, Dr. Compromesso. Dr. Compromesso proposed that it would take no more than a few days to test her hypothesis by prescribing a small quantity of amphetamine salts and tracking the result. He suggested that if Lindsay did *not* notice a rather abrupt calming and organizing effect, that would lessen support for Lindsay's hypothesis about adult ADHD and prompt the need to explore alternative hypotheses for her inattention and mood instability.

and supportive of the diagnosis – particularly if the recipient is less aware of a nonspecific "energizing" effect. Rather than commit to a diagnostic formulation, Dr. Compromesso's suggestion to use a pharmacological assay as a probe for differential diagnostics offers a time-limited and empirical approach for clarifying the nature of Lindsay's problem. Suppose that Lindsay reports back that she was pleased by a mood-elevating effect and general sense of well-being with the 5-day prescription she received for 10 mg of mixed amphetamine salts and wanted to try a higher dose. Dr. Compromesso might then observe that if she mainly experienced a mood-enhancing effect, it may be worth moving to the next part of the experiment, in which a more dedicated assay for depression could help tease apart the nonspecific cognitive complaints of depression from freestanding ADHD. Her Patient Health Questionnaire-9 score was 9, suggesting at most a mild degree of depressive symptom severity. The longevity of her complaints involving depressed mood, poor concentration, and irritability corresponded most closely to a diagnosis of dysthymic disorder. Dr. Compromesso next suggested a 4-week trial of vortioxetine, given the database showing its efficacy for slowed attentional processing associated with depression (McIntyre et al., 2014), its potential superiority to other catecholaminergic antidepressant medications for targeting psychomotor processing speed in depression (Rosenblat et al., 2015), and a (usefully) *negative* database for vortioxetine in adult ADHD in the absence of major depression (Biederman et al., 2019). In other words, vortioxetine could provide an assay for attentional symptoms related to depression without targeting ADHD per se.

Speaking of adult-onset ADHD, the diagnosis in itself remains controversial if and when evidence of childhood symptoms cannot be established; read more about this in Box 2.2.

Box 2.2

Is adult-onset ADHD a real thing?

Traditionally and "officially" regarded as a childhood disorder that may persist into adulthood for a sizable minority of patients, adult ADHD has, in recent years, been a subject of debate with regard to the possibility of de novo onset in adulthood. A handful of longitudinal cohort studies have proposed that adult-onset ADHD is a distinct clinical entity in which functionally disabling problems with attentional processing and distractibility were absent in childhood and present in adulthood and are not better accounted for by another psychiatric explanation (e.g., Agnew-Blais et al., 2016; Caye et al., 2016). Critics of such reports raise concerns about possible recall bias and question the value of patient self-report versus informant report regarding childhood symptoms – arguing that subthreshold signs of childhood ADHD may have been present but poorly recollected. The pragmatic concern for practitioners involves how to evaluate adult patients who self-diagnose adult ADHD, may have poor recall of childhood cognitive processing, and may not necessarily ascribe adult attentional problems to other plausible explanations besides ADHD.

How about the reverse situation from adding a medication as a potential diagnostic assay: does *eliminating* a drug support the hypothesis that a diagnosis was present if clinical deterioration ensues? This approach can be problematic because there is no way to know with confidence the time course for expectable deterioration – if that even happens – once a relevant medication is withdrawn. (Exceptions to that rule might be stimulants or benzodiazepines, whose pharmacodynamic effects make themselves known fairly quickly and buildup over time is generally not necessary to judge efficacy.) For most psychotropic medications that do require several weeks or longer to judge an effect, the time frame for observing potential relapse after treatment cessation may also vary depending on drug dosage, adherence, baseline severity, chronicity, and the length of initial exposure.

G INPATIENT ADMISSION FOR DIAGNOSTIC ASSESSMENT AND "ACUTE STABILIZATION"

In Chapter 10 we discuss at some length the matchup between treatment setting (or intensity and level of care) with the degree of symptoms and severity in a given patient's presentation. Here, let us consider more briefly the idea of implementing a higher level of care (say, psychiatric hospitalization) as a proposed means by which to gain greater clarity about diagnostic ambiguity, or, as sometimes occurs, the idea that a hospital stay can deliver a kind of stabilization to a clinical problem that is often complex, longstanding, and not so easily rectified on a short-term basis. Consider Clinical Vignette 2.5.

Clinical Vignette 2.5

Chloë was a 40-year-old woman with longstanding complex psychopathology that involved chronic mood instability, periods of paranoid thinking, social isolation and withdrawal, and poor work functioning despite completing an advanced degree. Trials of numerous pharmacotherapies for depression, anxiety, agitation, psychosis, inattention, and mood instability were undertaken over several years with little more than brief spurts of fleeting improvement. Her psychiatrist, Dr. Accomodante, had in mind a working diagnosis of chronic PTSD related to a lengthy period of sexual abuse during adolescence. A new therapist trained in eye-movement desensitization and reprocessing expressed alarm about Chloë's persistently poor functioning and level of psychopathology. She called Dr. Accomodante to voice concerns that Chloë was "severely ill" and needed to be in the hospital for a "thorough workup and stabilization of her condition."

Perhaps the most concerning aspect of Chloë's treatment is not the question of whether her chronic symptoms have become more acute, whether she needs more evaluation than she has already undergone, or whether a hospital is the right environment to render "stabilization," but rather, the glaring mismatch between the two members of her treatment team in their appraisal of her condition and the perceived appropriate or necessary level of care. Dr. Accomodante knows Chloë well and suggested a trauma-oriented behavioral therapy as a strategy to address her mood dysregulation and complex associated features. While her symptoms and functional deficits may be dramatic, they may very well also be "stably unstable." In the absence of a particular unique therapeutic approach or occult diagnostic element, hospitalization may not be the kind of intervention that would be of much help to improve Chloë's problems.

H WHEN ORDERING PSYCHOLOGICAL TESTING MAY BE HELPFUL

Like any ordered test, psychological testing can be utilized to answer specific questions that may, in certain instances, help to shed light on diagnostic issues or treatment recommendations. Neuropsychological testing, specifically, can help to clarify the nature and extent of cognitive complaints, particularly if the clinical impression is that subjective complaints may not simply reflect undertreated psychopathology such as depression or anxiety. An initial "bedside" objective assessment might utilize a simple instrument such as the Montreal Cognitive Assessment (commonly known as the MoCA; Nasreddine et al., 2005); scores below 26 out of 30 likely warrant more detailed and formal evaluation.

Projective testing and measures of personality structure can be helpful adjuncts toward diagnostic assessment, addressing attitudes, perceptions, inner emotions, and styles of interpersonal relatedness that can provide additional data beyond direct clinical interviews.

I LINGERING SYMPTOMS

Situations arise in which the syndromal features of a disorder, such as major depression, resolve except for one or more low-grade residual symptoms, such as insomnia or fatigue. From the standpoint of diagnostic assessment, practitioners must differentiate true residual symptoms from iatrogenic features confusable with primary symptoms. It therefore becomes especially important to carefully assess the chronology of "symptom" onset relative to medication introductions or dosage changes. Cognitive complaints can be especially challenging to assess insofar as they are often multideterminate and may reflect core elements of depression or anxiety versus both psychotropic and nonpsychotropic medication effects (are any medications with anticholinergic, antihistaminergic, or sedative–hypnotic action in the clinical picture?) versus alcohol or substance use (is the quantity of reported consumption reliable?) or potential underlying medical/neurological etiologies. A critical component of diagnostic assessment and treatment planning involves teasing apart entrenched from modifiable aspects of psychopathology and core psychiatric symptoms from drug side effects or other spurious factors. Elements such as these will surface time and time again as we further embark on the more formal process of clinical decision-making in the chapters ahead.

TAKE-HOME POINTS

- Psychiatric diagnoses should not be based solely on diagnostic screens or cross-sectional symptoms but involve corroboration from family history, longitudinal course, and treatment response
- Formulate initial working hypotheses that are subject to revision as more data become available thorough longitudinal observation as well as the traversing of developmental milestones among younger patients
- *Reliably* identified diagnoses may not necessarily be *valid*
- Family history data can provide far more useful forms of information than just the categorical presence or absence of a specific psychiatric diagnosis; explore the potential cosegregation of common comorbidities or trait features that might help to refine an initial diagnostic impression
- Treatment response can corroborate, but not stand as proxy for, diagnostic impressions

References

Agnew-Blais JC, Polanczyk GV, Danese A, et al. Evaluation of the persistence, remission, and emergence of attention-deficit/hyperactivity disorder in young adulthood. JAMA Psychiatry 2016; 73: 713–720

American Psychiatric Association. Diagnostic and Statistical Manual of Mental Disorders, 4th edition. Washington, DC: American Psychiatric Association, 1994

American Psychiatric Association. Diagnostic and Statistical Manual of Mental Disorders, 5th edition. Washington, DC: American Psychiatric Association, 2013

Anglin RES, Samaan Z, Walter SD, et al. Vitamin D deficiency and depression in adults: Systematic review and meta-analysis. Br J Psychiatry 2013; 202: 100–107

Angst J, Gamma A, Sellaro R, et al. Recurrence of bipolar disorders and major depression. A life-long perspective. Eur Arch Psychiatry Clin Neurosci 2003; 253: 236–240

Antila M, Tuulio-Henrikkson A, Kieseppä T, et al. Heritability of cognitive functions in families with bipolar disorder. Am J Med Genet B Neuropsychiatr Genet 2007; 144B: 802–808

Ballard ED, Cui L, Vandeleur C, et al. Familial aggregation and coaggregation of suicide attempts and comorbid mental disorders in adults. JAMA Psychiatry 2019; 76: 826–833

Behrendt S, Beesdo-Baum K, Höfler M, et al. The relevance of age at first alcohol and nicotine use for initiation of cannabis use and progression to cannabis use disorders. Drug Alcohol Depend 2012; 123: 48–56

Biederman J, Faraone SV, Keenan K, et al. Evidence of familial association between attention deficit disorder and major affective disorders. Arch Gen Psychiatry 1991; 48: 633–642

Biederman J, Lindsten A, Sluth LB, et al. Vortioxetine for attention deficit hyperactivity disorder in adults: A randomized, double-blind, placebo-controlled, proof-of-concept study. J Psychopharmacol 2019; 33: 511–521

Bolton S, Warner J, Harriss E, et al. Bipolar disorder: Trimodal age-at-onset distribution. Bipolar Disord 2021; 23: 341–356

Caton CLM, Drake RE, Hasin DS, et al. Differences between early-phase primary psychotic disorders with concurrent substance use and substance-induced psychoses. Arch Gen Psychiatry 2005; 62: 137–145

Caye A, Rocha T B-M, Anselmi L, et al. Attention-deficit/hyperactivity disorder trajectories from childhood to young adulthood: Evidence from a birth cohort supporting a late-onset syndrome. JAMA Psychiatry 2016; 73: 705–712

Chen M-H, Pan T-L, Huang K-L, et al. Coaggregation of major psychiatric disorders in first-degree relatives of individuals with attention-deficit/hyperactivity disorder: A nationwide population-based study. J Clin Psychiatry 2019; 80(3): 18m12371

Cheng C-M, Chang W-H, Chen M-H, et al. Co-aggregation of major psychiatric disorders in individuals with first-degree relatives with schizophrenia: A nationwide population-based study. Mol Psychiatry 2018; 23: 1756–1763

Contreras J, Hare E, Pachico A, et al. Is subclinical anxiety an endophenotype for bipolar I patients? A study from a Costa Rican sample. J Affect Disord 2010; 122: 267–272

Coppen A, Bolander-Gouialle C. Treatment of depression: Time to consider folic acid and vitamin B_{12}. J Psychopharmacol 2005; 19: 59–65

de Lijster J, Dierckx B, Utens EMWJ et al. The age of onset of anxiety disorders. Can J Psychiatry 2017; 62: 237–246

Faraone SV, Biederman J. Do attention deficit hyperactivity disorder and major depression share familial risk factors? J Nerv Ment Dis 1997; 185: 533–541

Fisfalen ME, Schulze TG, DePaulo Jr. JR, et al. Familial variation in episode frequency in bipolar affective disorder. Am J Psychiatry 2005; 162: 1266–1272

Fornaro M, Anastasia A, Novello S, et al. Incidence, prevalence and clinical correlates of antidepressant-emergent mania in bipolar depression: A systematic review and meta-analysis. Bipolar Disord 2018; 20: 195–227

Galtress T, Marshall AT, Kirkpatrick K. Motivation and timing: Clues for modeling the reward system. Behav Processes 2012; 90: 142–153

Geller B, Cooper TB, Zimerman B, et al. Lithium for prepubertal depressed children with family history predictors of future bipolarity: A double-blind, placebo-controlled study. J Affect Disord 1998; 51: 165–175

Goldberg JF. Determining patient candidacy for antidepressant use in bipolar disorder. Psychiatr Ann 2019; 49: 386–391

Goldberg JF, Garakani A, Ackerman SH. Clinician-rated versus self-rated screening for bipolar disorder among inpatients with mood symptoms and substance misuse. J Clin Psychiatry 2012; 73: 1525–1530

Goldstein RB, Weissman MM, Adams PB, et al. Psychiatric disorders in relatives of probands with panic disorder and/or major depression. Arch Gen Psychiatry 1994; 51: 383–394

Goldstein TR, Frye MA, Denicoff KD, et al. Antidepressant discontinuation-related mania: Critical prospective observation and theoretical implications in bipolar disorder. J Clin Psychiatry 1999; 60: 563–567

Gommoll C, Durgam S, Mathews M, et al. A double-blind, randomized, placebo-controlled, fixed-dose phase III study of vilazodone in patients with generalized anxiety disorder. Depress Anxiety 2015; 32: 451–459

Henry C, Mitropoulou V, New AS, et al. Affective instability and impulsivity in borderline personality and bipolar II disorders: Similarities and differences. J Psychiatr Res 2001; 35: 307–312

Hirschfeld-Becker DR, Micco JA, Henin A, et al. Psychopathology in adolescent offspring of parents with panic disorder, major depression, or both: A 10-year follow-up. Am J Psychiatry 2012; 169: 1175–1184

Huang M-H, Cheng C-M, Tsai S-J, et al. Familial coaggregation of major psychiatric disorders among first-degree relatives of patients with obsessive–compulsive disorder: A nationwide study. Psychol Med 2021; 51: 680–687

Husain-Krautter S, Ellison JM. Late-life depression: The essentials and the essential distinctions. Focus (Am Psychiatr Publ) 2021; 19: 282–293

Keown-Stoneman CDG, Goodday SM, Preisig M, et al. Development and validation of a risk calculator for major mood disorders among the offspring of bipolar parents using information collected in routine clinical practice. EClincalMedicine 2021; 39: 101083

Kessler RC, Berglund P, Demler O, et al. Lifetime prevalence and age-of-onset distributions of DSM-IV disorders in the National Comorbidity Survey Replication. Arch General Psychiatry 2005; 62: 593–602

Krynicki CR, Upthegrove R, Deakin JFW, et al. The relationship between negative symptoms and depression in schizophrenia: A systematic review. Acta Psychiatr Scand 2018; 137: 380-390

Lewis SJ, Arseneault L, Caspi A, et al. The epidemiology of trauma and post-traumatic stress disorder in a representative cohort of young people in England and Wales. Lancet Psychiatry 2019; 6: 247–256

Li TK, Hewitt BG, Grant BF. Alcohol use disorders and mood disorders: A National Institute on Alcohol Abuse and Alcoholism perspective. Biol Psychiatry 2004; 56: 718–720

Low NCP, Cui L, Merikangas KR. Specificity of familial transmission of anxiety and comorbid disorders. J Psychiatr Res 2008; 42: 596–604

MacKinnon DF, Pies R. Affective instability as rapid cycling: Theoretical and clinical implications for borderline personality and bipolar spectrum disorders. Bipolar Disord 2006; 8: 1-14

MacKinnon DF, Zandi PP, Cooper J, et al. Comorbid bipolar disorder and panic disorder in families with a high prevalence of bipolar disorder. Am J Psychiatry 2002; 159: 30-35

MacKinnon DF, Zandi PP, Gershon E, et al. Rapid switching of mood in families with multiple cases of bipolar disorder. Arch Gen Psychiatry 2003; 60: 921–928

Mann JJ, Bortinger J, Oquendo MA, et al. Family history of suicidal behavior and mood disorders in probands with mood disorders. Am J Psychiatry 2005; 162: 1672–1679

McIntyre RS, Lophaven S, Olsen CK. A randomized, double-blind, placebo-controlled study of vortioxetine on cognitive function in depressed adults. Int J Neuropsychopharmacol 2014; 17: 1557–1567

Merikangas KR, Stevens DE, Fenton B, et al. Co-morbidity and familial aggregation of alcoholism and anxiety disorders. Psychol Med 1998; 28: 773–788

Mistry S, Harrison JR, Smith DJ, et al. The use of polygenic risk scores to identify phenotypes associated with genetic risk of bipolar disorder and depression: A systematic review. J Affect Disord 2018; 234: 148–155

Nasreddine ZS, Phillips NA, Bédirian V, et al. The Montreal Cognitive Assessment, MoCA: A brief screening tool for mild cognitive impairment. J Am Geriatr Soc 2005; 53: 695–699

Nunes EV, Liu X, Samet S, et al. Independent versus substance-induced major depressive disorder in substance-dependent patients: Observational study of course during follow-up. J Clin Psychiatry 2006; 67: 1561–1567

Nurnberger JI Jr., Blehar MC, Kauffman CA, et al. Diagnostic interview for genetic studies. Rationale, unique features, and training. NIMH Genetics Initiative. Arch Gen Psychiatry 1994; 51: 849–859

Ochoa S, Usall J, Cobo J, et al. Gender differences in schizophrenia and first-episode psychosis: A comprehensive literature review. Schiz Res Treat 2012; 916198

Puig-Antich J, Goetz D, Davies M, et al. A controlled family history study of prepubertal major depressive disorder. Arch Gen Psychiatry 1989; 46: 406–418

Quick CR, Conway KP, Swendsen J, et al. Comorbidity and coaggregation of major depressive disorder and bipolar disorder and cannabis use disorder in a controlled family study. Arch Gen Psychiatry 2022; 79: 727–735

Reich T, Edenberg HJ, Goate A, et al. Genome-wide search for genes affecting the risk for alcohol dependence. Am J Med Genet 1998; 81: 207–215

Robins E, Guze SB. Establishment of diagnostic validity in psychiatric illness: Its application to schizophrenia. Am J Psychiatry 1970; 126: 983–987

Rosenblat JD, Kakar RM, McIntyre RS. The cognitive effects of antidepressants in major depressive disorder: A systematic review and meta-analysis of randomized clinical trials. Int J Neuropsychopharmacol 2015; 19: pyv082

Ruscio AM, Stein DJ, Chiu WT, et al. The epidemiology of obsessive–compulsive disorder in the National Comorbidity Survey replication. Mol Psychiatry 2010; 15: 53–63

Sanchez-Gistau V, Romero S, Moreno D, et al. Psychiatric disorders in child and adolescent offspring of patients with schizophrenia and bipolar disorder: A controlled study. Schizophr Res 2015; 168(1-2): 197–203

Sbrana A, Bizzarri JV, Rucci P, et al. Family history of psychiatric disorders and alcohol and substance misuse in patients with bipolar I disorder, substance use disorder, or both. Am J Addict 2007; 16: 227-231

Solmi M, Radua J, Olivola M, et al. Age at onset of mental disorders worldwide: Large-scale meta-analysis of 192 epidemiological studies. Mol Psychiatry 2022; 27: 281–295

Solomon DA, Leon AC, Coryell WH, et al. Longitudinal course of bipolar I disorder: Duration of mood episodes. Arch Gen Psychiatry 2010; 67: 339–347

Thase ME, Chen D, Edwards J, et al. Efficacy of vilazodone on anxiety symptoms in patients with major depressive disorder. Int Clin Psychopharmacol 2014; 29: 351–356

Toth M. 5-HT1A receptor knockout mouse as a genetic model of anxiety. Eur J Pharmacol 2003; 463(1–3): 177–184

Weisaeth L. Vulnerability and protective factors for posttraumatic stress disorder. Psychiatry Clin Neurosci 1998; 52: S39–S44

Welham JL, Thomis RJ, McGrath JJ. Age-at-first-registration for affective psychosis and schizophrenia. Schiz Bull 2004; 30: 849–853

Wilens TE, Biederman J, Adamson J, et al. Association of bipolar and substance use disorders in parents of adolescents with bipolar disorder. Biol Psychiatry 2007; 62: 129–134

Zinbarg RE, Barlow DH, Liebowitz M, et al. The DSM-IV field trial for mixed anxiety–depression. Am J Psychiatry 1994; 151: 1153–1162

3 What the Patient Isn't Telling You: When Seeing is Not Believing

LEARNING OBJECTIVES

- ☐ Adopt a forensic mindset for sifting through clinical information; recognize coherent themes versus logical inconsistencies when deciding if a clinical narrative is compelling and credible or leaves too many unanswered questions
- ☐ Recognize malingering and secondary gain when it exists but maintain a thoughtful and nonjudgmental approach when evaluating the information patients relate
- ☐ Differentiate when patients distort information because of misinformation versus subterfuge
- ☐ Appreciate the often under-recognized contribution of alcohol or substance misuse as contributors to clinical presentations that do not improve with standard therapies
- ☐ Understand how alexithymia, psychosis, and anosognosia can color a patient's self-report
- ☐ Understand the basic tenets of motivational interviewing not only as a therapeutic technique but as a strategy to help clarify patients' own treatment goals

Part of the intellectual intrigue for many people who choose a career in mental health is the challenge of reading between the clinical lines and sussing out information that transcends the obvious. Do patients' words and behaviors align? Are subjective symptoms consistent with overt functioning? Does a clinical narrative conform to a set of circumstances? How does a clinician know when someone is lying, concealing key information, embellishing facts, or otherwise operating with an agenda? Or what if the patient has no vocabulary for accurately communicating their internal experience, and it is left to the clinician to deduce what may actually be happening for them internally? A clinician's ability to recognize the unspoken parameters of psychiatric communication pertains to many if not most forms of mental illness, either by intention or happenstance, since patients themselves may not always be fully aware of what it is that they want or need. Clinical decision-making can only be as sound and logical as the quality of information made available to the decision-maker. Herein lies the challenge both for assessment and treatment planning when the patient is less than forthcoming, deceptive, confabulating, confused, denying, demented, delirious, malingering, ashamed, scared, alexithymic, misinformed, or otherwise less than a full-fledged participant in their own care.

A YOU SHOULD BELIEVE EVERYTHING PATIENTS TELL YOU – RIGHT?

There are a variety of circumstances where skepticism deserves its place when deciphering the clinical meaning and relevance of a patient's clinical presentation. A useful starting point may be differentiating whether doubt about the patient's narrative derives from intentional versus unintentional obfuscation. *Unintentional* distortions may occur when patients are ill-informed, embarrassed, delirious, demented, psychotic, developmentally disabled, or otherwise cognitively impaired. *Intentional* distortions – such as deliberately concealing information, manipulating facts, or downplaying pertinent details, call into question a more pervasive and perhaps fraudulent quality about the patient's entire presentation. "What do they *really* want?" becomes the skeptical clinician's refrain.

> **Tip**
>
> The words, "I get the feeling there's something you're not telling me," asked in a neutral tone, is not a bad probing question to elicit information that someone might prefer to conceal. As an "I" statement it is more disarming than accusatory; it invites rather than demands a reply; and there is always *something* unsaid that makes this a kind of a projective question based on the patient's response.

Perhaps the most classical examples of intentionally deceptive patient communications in psychiatry come from scenarios that involve malingering or factitious (i.e., consciously manufactured) disorders. Linked with both constructs is the notion of **secondary gain** – that is, the material benefits that derive from having a mental health condition, such as avoiding some financial, social, occupational, or legal responsibility or accountability, procuring controlled substances or other desired medications, or accessing financial, social, or other rewards that incentivize the sick role. In forensic psychiatry, it has been suggested that lying is a more cognitively demanding task than truth-telling, meaning that deception often involves longer time or more hesitancy when answering questions.

> **Tip**
>
> It is often assumed that nonverbal cues such as halting speech, gaze avoidance, or failure to spontaneously elaborate are tip-offs to deceptive communication, but empirical studies fail to identify any reliable behavioral indicators to detect lying (Vrij et al., 2019).

Liars tend to have more trouble remembering consistent details, avoiding contradictions, and maintaining a narrative when asked questions that involve a high cognitive load (such as, inquiring about the timing of onset of symptoms, or recalling events in reverse chronological order, or responding to unexpected questions such as how they feel about their symptoms (Walczyk et al., 2018)). When judging the likely veracity of information being presented, clinicians are equally interested in the *form* with which patients communicate (fluency, consistency, perseveration and repetition, demandingness, self-reflection) as well as content – making the assessment somewhat analogous to judging the presence of intact reality testing. Behavioral and nonverbal clues can sometimes corroborate judging truthful from fictitious communications (Ekman and O'Sullivan, 1991) but in themselves are not necessarily reliable indicators of deception.

Fact

Contrary to what one might expect, "professional lie catchers" such as law enforcement personnel, judges, and customs officers are not necessarily more accurate than untrained individuals in telling when someone is lying (Ekman and O'Sullivan, 1991).

Some authors have focused on the plausibility of information that patients present as a key factor in recognizing false information or a hidden agenda. A formal rating scale known as the Structured Interview of Reported Symptoms (SIRS) captures a number of elements such as rare symptom combinations, improbable and absurd symptoms, blatant versus subtle symptoms, selective reporting of symptoms, and discrepancies between observable signs and self-reported symptoms. A related measure, the Structured Inventory of Malingered Symptomatology (SIMS), quantifies the over-reporting of symptoms, or recognition of atypical or implausible symptoms, using a standardized cut-off score of $\geq$14 summed from a set of five subscales that each contain 15 items (Smith and Burger, 1997). While the SIMS has been used in studies intended to differentiate groups such as individuals with psychogenic from electrical seizures (e.g., Benge et al., 2012) the rather low sensitivity of the SIMS has limited its broader use.

Much the way clinicians step back with puzzlement and curiosity if a constellation of signs and symptoms do not hang together, or when reported side effects defy physiological explanations, so too does the absence of key elements in a patient's narrative – or disproportionate focus on a particular complaint – prompt skepticism about whether a clinical narrative can be taken at face value. Inconsistencies and contradictions in a narrative signal the need for clarification. Boxes 3.1 and 3.2, respectively, consider instances in which a narrative is purposefully invented in the service of some external benefit (as in malingering) and instances in which true symptoms may be present but are amplified, embellished, or otherwise distorted for reasons other than a consciously held ulterior motive.

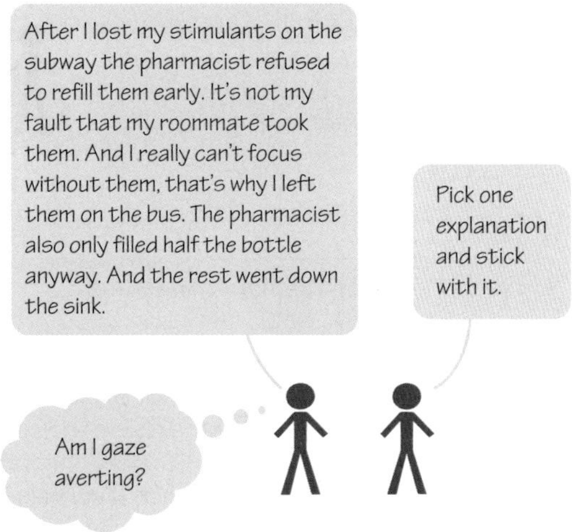

Box 3.1

Are there reliable ways to detect malingering?

Malingering involves the conscious fabrication of symptoms motivated by an external incentive (secondary gain). The concept also includes patients who deliberately or grossly exaggerate actual symptoms in order to achieve a goal other than symptom relief (sometimes called **partial malingering**). Symptoms, and their impact, are often rare or even preposterous. Related concepts are **dissimulation** (minimizing or consciously downplaying actual symptoms for purposes of secondary gain) and **false imputation** (purposefully attributing symptoms to an unrelated cause, as when knowingly blaming pain from a previous injury on a recent accident) (Resnick, 1997). Key to the assessment of malingering involves identifying the presence of secondary gain – such as exemption from an obligation, procuring a financial, work, domestic, legal, or social benefit, or other societal accommodations that are afforded by the sick role. Tip-offs include:

- symptoms that are unlikely or highly amplified
- endorsing numerous or highly exaggerated symptoms that evoke disproportionate, extreme levels of "unbearable" severity
- demonstrating an exaggerated and overestimated struggle to perform simple efforts, trying to convey globally incapacitation
- in alleged psychosis, the *absence of a formal thought disorder* is sometimes considered suggestive of malingering (although disorganized thought processes are absent in delusional disorder). True delusions typically have a more insidious than abrupt onset

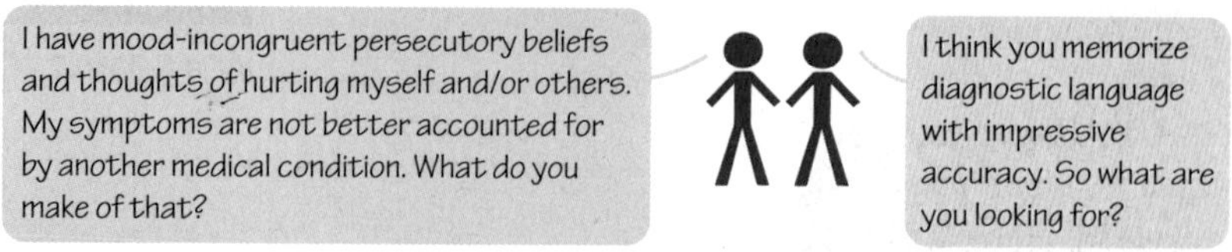

Box 3.2

When patients embellish symptoms

Separate from the business of identifying patients who fabricate symptoms altogether is the matter of patients who may have genuine psychiatric or physical problems but exploit their severity and allege extreme levels of distress that may be in the service of procuring some material or emotional gain. Such may be the case in patients with certain personality disorders, substance use disorders, impulse control disorders, or antisocial traits. Common examples include patients who present to psychiatric emergency departments seeking admission because they claim to have thoughts of hurting themselves when, in fact, they may not be genuinely struggling with urges to act imminently on such thoughts; or patients specifically seeking controlled substances for complaints of anxiety or insomnia who become sullen or uninterested when only noncontrolled substance options are presented. Sussing out such presentations is often delicate and tricky. No clinician wants to minimize the genuine suffering of a serious mental illness; but, on the other hand, it can be hard to know what drives patients who press forward in a demanding and urgent way with a clear intended goal in mind – such as procuring a controlled substance, obtaining shelter, finding respite from a contentious environment, or presenting with a somewhat martyred stance of victimization and suffering inflicted by some blameworthy outside person or entity with whom they may have some grievance.

Asking open-ended rather than leading questions can sometimes shed light on hidden agendas – such as, "What *might* you do if you went home from the emergency department tonight?" (rather than, "Do you think you might hurt yourself if you went home?") or "If your clonazepam dose was not increased, what do you think would happen?" When patients indicate that the main consequence they would expect, if their entreaties did not lead to their desired result, would be to experience intense distress, our decision-making likely goes down a different pathway (e.g., addressing poor distress tolerance; see Section I, below).

What about times when there is more behind a patient's stated narrative than even the patient may realize, and iterative pharmacotherapy approaches alone may prove to be ineffectual? Consider the example of Clinical Vignette 3.1.

Clinical Vignette 3.1

Sam was a 41-year-old burly, multi-tattooed military veteran who had not served in combat but sought treatment for persistent depressed mood and irritability. He and his wife both observed that he had a low frustration tolerance and would rapidly escalate toward verbal aggression, mainly with his wife, when he felt provoked by seemingly small interpersonal transgressions. Apart from dysthymic disorder, he did not meet formal diagnostic criteria for any other psychiatric condition, but was conceptualized as having problems with "anger management" or excessive interpersonal sensitivity and treated with a variety of selective serotonin reuptake inhibitors, mood stabilizers, and second-generation antipsychotic medications with little efficacy. Within a few months after entering psychodynamic psychotherapy it emerged that Sam had a clandestine gay lifestyle involving promiscuous sex with men about which he vehemently chastised himself. He disparaged himself for being attracted to men and struggled to conceal all of the above from his wife, whom he believed had "no clue" about his real identity. This revelation took his treatment in a different, nonpharmacological direction as the driving force behind his previously inexplicable anger toward his wife took on a new context and therapeutic direction.

B COLLATERAL INPUT FROM FAMILY MEMBERS IS USUALLY ACCURATE – RIGHT?

Clinical distortions are not solely confined to the patient's self-report. In families where the interpersonal dynamics may be complex, family members or caregivers may sometimes have either their own agenda or an axe to grind when conveying their observations about their loved one's behavior. In particular, unsavory or objectionable behaviors (i.e., aggression, substance use, externalizing rather than internalizing symptoms) may be prime candidates for citable forms of psychopathology in need of intervention if for no other reason than to restore peace and order within the home. From the perspective of understanding family systems, it can also be important to recognize instances in which the dynamics sometimes may be such that meaningful change or improvement in the so-called identified patient may disrupt an established equilibrium that could be met with less enthusiasm than one might have expected, as depicted in Clinical Vignette 3.2.

Tip

In family systems theory, the "identified patient" is construed as the individual who seeks treatment as a kind of ambassador or representative (or, scapegoat) on behalf of a broader level of dysfunction within the family unit.

Clinical Vignette 3.2

Richard was a 47-year-old man with longstanding major depression who had assumed a passive stance in his relationship with Laura, his 48-year-old second wife of 8 years. Laura had brought him to several consultants over the years, each of whom had suggested various pharmacological changes that either were rejected, never implemented, or never received adequate trials. The most recent consultant advised hospitalization and electroconvulsive therapy (ECT) which Richard and his wife eventually agreed to after much hesitation. Richard's condition improved dramatically. Much less depressed, he began to "lobby" his wife for more independence to spend time with his own friends and with the two young adult children from his first marriage with whom he had maintained only superficial contact. Laura began to express concern that Richard was having a "strange reaction" to the ECT, was becoming more contrary to her in daily interactions, and decided that he must actually have bipolar disorder and now needed antimanic medications to remedy the obvious adverse effects of ECT.

ECT can certainly cause mood destabilization and induce mania, but how reliably can or should we assume that that was the case for Richard, based mainly on his wife's objections to his newfound self-assertion and subsequent change in the established dynamic of their relationship? Entertaining Laura's hypothesis means assessing Richard for signs of psychomotor acceleration on interview, but if those features are absent, what do we tell Laura? And then, how can and should we gently raise questions about the status of Richard and Laura's relationship, and her interpretation (is that her conclusion or hypothesis?) that his presentation and demeanor after ECT reflected his psychopathology rather than a disruption to the equilibrium state of their marriage?

C FAMILY HISTORY/GENETIC INFORMATION IS USUALLY ACCURATE – RIGHT?

Clinicians routinely query patients about mental health conditions in their family members and often take their responses at face value when building evidence for or against a diagnostic hypothesis, or a possible treatment implication, based on purported facts about any degree of blood relative. The importance clinicians attach to a reported family history must be tempered by the fact that psychiatric disorders are complex traits that do not follow Mendelian genetics (meaning, there is likely no single gene that confers susceptibility to a particular psychiatric disorder, and the features that are heritable are less likely to be categorical diagnoses than dimensional traits (such as impulsivity, aggression, or poor attentional processing)). Even among monozygotic twins, concordance is far less than 100% for major disorders such as schizophrenia (about 33% based on large Danish twin registry data; Hilker et al., 2018) or bipolar disorder (about 33–75%; Kieseppä et al., 2014). How much or how little importance should be placed on family history data when gathering information to support clinical hypotheses? The answer probably depends as much on the accuracy of the information as the possible heritability or familiality of a given trait of interest.

Complex (non-Mendelian) traits likely involve the transmission not necessarily of categorical diagnostic entities so much as dimensional aspects of psychopathology such as psychosis, cognitive rigidity, impulsivity, attentional processing, anhedonia, risk aversion, and other transdiagnostic elements – making it all the more difficult to know with confidence exactly what ailment, if any, may have actually been present in relatives who may not have been carefully and systematically evaluated.

Consider Martha, in Clinical Vignette 3.3.

Clinical Vignette 3.3

Martha was a 42-year-old woman with persistent depression that had not improved with multiple antidepressant trials. During a new consultation, Dr. Chase, a new psychiatrist, was probing for possible other diagnoses besides major depression. Martha volunteered that her grandmother had been "institutionalized" for many years during the 1960s and diagnosed with schizophrenia. Her brother also once made a suicide attempt. The evaluator speculated that her grandmother may in fact have had bipolar disorder, because "in the 1960s many people who actually had bipolar disorder were misdiagnosed as having schizophrenia" and that "suicide is more common in bipolar than unipolar disorder, and tends to run in families."

We applaud Dr. Chase's determination for exploring possible missed conditions that could account for multiple antidepressant nonresponses (including bipolar disorder) and also admire his inquiry into family history to help generate further diagnostic hypotheses. However, our admiration diminishes when his adherence to evidence-based fact-finding vanishes. His inference is pure speculation based on no actual clinical data about Grandma. It is true, prior to about 1980 there may have been a tendency to overdiagnose schizophrenia over bipolar disorder (then known as manic-depressive illness), although that information alone does not categorically render pre-1980 diagnoses of schizophrenia fallacious. Permit us a brief historical excursion: mainly two studies shed light on this potential for diagnostic bias. The first was an interesting experiment from an era before diagnostic operational criteria were codified, in which several videotaped patient interviews were shown to several hundred British and American psychiatrists (Kendell et al., 1971). Several of the tapes found that American psychiatrist-raters were more prone to diagnose schizophrenia than their British counterparts. After the third edition of the Diagnostic and Statistical Manual of Mental Disorders (DSM-III; American Psychiatric Association, 1980) narrowed the operational criteria by which to define schizophrenia, and broadened the diagnostic criteria for affective disorders, a survey of hospital discharges from six US-based institutions found a threefold decrease in diagnoses of schizophrenia and a fourfold increase in affective disorder diagnoses from 1972 to 1988 (Stoll et al., 1993).

Back to the veracity of patient-reported family histories. In actuality, eliciting and affirming a true family history of any psychiatric disorder is a rather time-intensive and sometimes dicey undertaking. In formal psychiatric genetics studies, a sometimes onerously long semi-structured interview developed by investigators from the National Institute of Mental Health Genetics Initiative called the Diagnostic Interview for Genetic Studies (DIGS) is often undertaken (Nurnberger et al., 1994). As its authors note, "the DIGS provides more details regarding the phenomenology of mood disorders and schizophrenia than many other available instruments" (Nurnberger et al., 1994, p. 850) and "the time required to conduct the interview may vary considerably, from 30 minutes for an unaffected subject to 4 hours for a patient with complex symptoms" (median interview time = 2½ hours) (Nurnberger et al., 1994, p.851). This represents a vast difference from the typical practice of clinicians in the nonresearch world who may ask a patient in the space of just a few minutes whether "anyone in your family has had similar problems to yours, or other kinds of mental health problems."

Interviews such as the DIGS require formal training and achievement of inter-rater reliability. While it is far from feasible to envision nonresearch clinicians adopting so formal an approach to assessing family histories as this, we would suggest that the veracity of such information can neither be taken for granted nor relied upon as factual from only a cursory assessment. Practitioners must bear these limitations in mind when placing stock in "corroborative" diagnostic information based on *the* family history. We would also point out that the relevance of family history data tends to undergo a dilutional effect as one moves from first- to second- or later-generation relatives of a proband. News that great-great uncle Harry was institutionalized for much of his life and underwent ECT in the 1950s does not necessarily tell us much about what is most likely going on for his remote descendants.

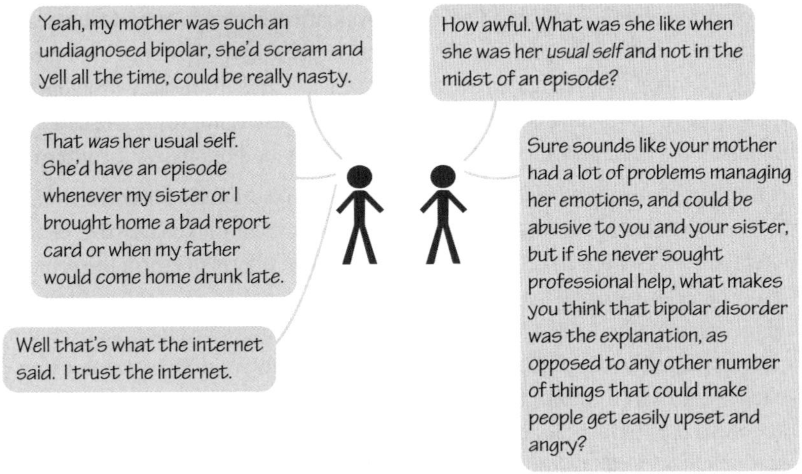

D SUBSTANCE USE SLEUTHING

Before we get much farther into the world of skeptical clinical assessment, let us turn now to the impact of substance use, and the fine line that often exists between substance use and substance use *disorders*. Perhaps foremost, such disorders often cry out for concealment. For many reasons, patients often downplay, disavow, deflect, or otherwise minimize the extent to which problems related to substance use constitute problems in their own right. Cross-sectional surveys suggest that at least 10–15% of psychotherapy patients lie to their therapists about substance misuse (Farber, 2020). Among patients identified on the basis of a substance use disorder diagnosis, deliberate deception is often considered to be a part of the disease of addiction itself – partly based on assumptions about shame and guilt, as well as the premise that lying becomes a protective strategy against any threat to continuing an active addiction.

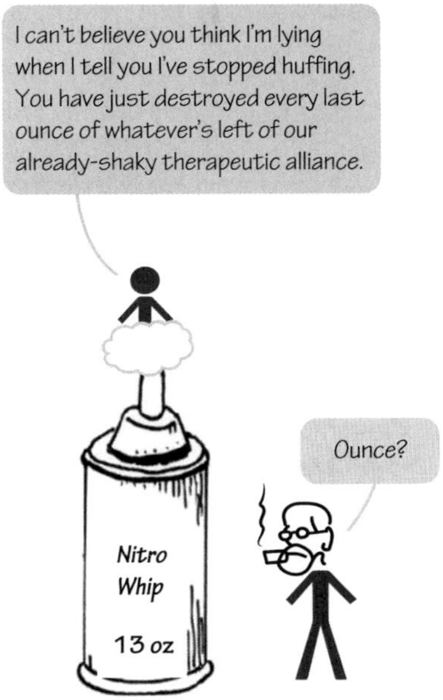

When forming hypotheses about psychopathology and appropriate treatments, even seasoned clinicians can be fooled by under-recognized substance use disorders and their impact on both symptom presentations and pharmacotherapy efficacy. Part of the evaluative challenge often involves uncertainty about when psychiatric symptoms may lead to substance use as a manifestation of a problem *other than substance use itself* as the core problem (as when one presumes that alcohol or other substance use is not really a problem unto itself but rather an attempt to self-medicate a mood or anxiety disorder).

Another challenge when assessing substance use disorders is the entire notion of **confrontation** and a kind of enmity or prosecutorial quality that could potentially ensue between clinician and patient when efforts to affirm the presence of substance use become tantamount to extracting a confession. If the therapeutic alliance is fundamentally a partnership, deception around substance use becomes a dance that at various points may involve tip-toeing, to avoid accusations, or collusion, with its minimization. Such tip-toeing can alternate with what often becomes a partnerless cat-and-mouse game of pursuit for "the truth" about the extent and psychiatric ramifications of excessive alcohol or psychoactive substance use. Stigma about substance use is often cited as one of the factors that often contributes to oblique communication with practitioners around factual aspects of the disorder. Patients may expect that even practitioners might respond to shared information with moralistic or "judgy" responses or lecture-style diatribes about potential adverse consequences of continued use, which may serve only to amplify feelings of alienation. More detail on this appears in Box 3.3.

Box 3.3

Stigma, shame, and distorted clinical narratives

Perceived stigma about mental illnesses in general, and substance use disorders in particular, can contribute more than a little to the ways in which patients reveal information. Patients have little inclination to speak candidly about their thoughts, feelings, and behaviors if they expect their candor to be met with judgments about their ongoing engagement with substances. Moreover, ramifications of candid communication might include jeopardizing their employment, child custody, breach of privacy, or confidentiality; incurring fear of legal repercussions or being perceived as untrustworthy; or a reluctance or refusal on the part of the clinician to see the patient as a whole individual, as opposed to "just an addict" (with no further attention paid to other aspects of mental health such as depression, anxiety, or trauma).

When the specter of substance use disorders seems to be salient, preemptive communication strategies on the part of the clinician might usefully include asking patients questions that are framed in a conditional context: "If you *were* to tell me that you were using a lot of drugs or alcohol, what do you think my reaction would be?", "What do you think would happen?", or "Do you think that you have to downplay how much alcohol or other substances you might use, or else I might not take your other concerns seriously?"

Clinical assessment that involves substance use can be especially challenging because of the ways in which psychoactive substances can mimic primary psychopathology, and patients themselves may hold a vested interest in convincing others that their "real" problem is an underlying (and possibly easier-to-treat) psychiatric condition other than substance use as a primary disorder. Sorting out chronologies between substance use and the emergence of psychiatric symptoms also poses a challenge, particularly because it is often difficult to identify clear and sustained periods of abstinence during which primary psychiatric symptoms can be assessed without the contaminating effects of psychoactive substances (Goldberg et al., 2008).

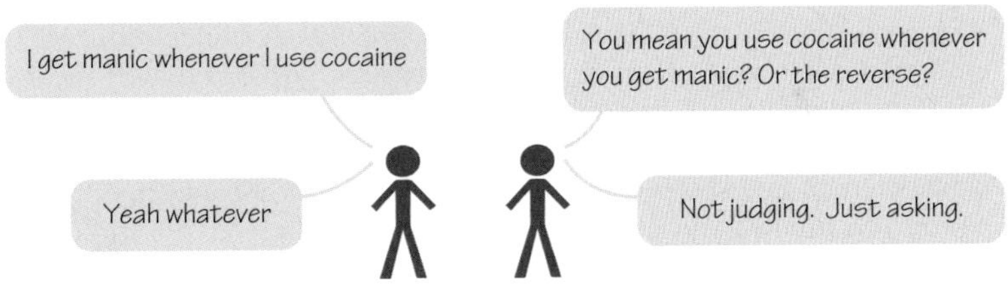

Issues of substance use often strike at the core (or highlight the battle) of trust between clinicians, who want to believe what patients tell them, and patients, who want their concerns to be taken seriously. Patients may even become expert at deceiving themselves about the impact of drugs or alcohol and convince themselves that problems may not exist when contaminating effects simply cannot be ruled out. Sometimes, the only way all parties can know with confidence what the objective reality and extent of substance use actually is requires obtaining drug toxicology testing in one form or another. Consider the case of Janet in Clinical Vignette 3.4.

Clinical Vignette 3.4

Janet was a 27-year-old single graduate student, with no prior psychiatric history, who was hospitalized for a psychotic mania several days after ingesting "copious amounts" of psilocybin. She had a history of depression that had not improved with several traditional antidepressants and, intrigued by the emerging literature on psychedelics to treat depression, independently procured and consumed psychedelic mushrooms. Following an initial barrage of intense sensory experiences (stating "I can feel every individual water droplet in a bath, and taste every molecule in food"), she became sleepless, disinhibited, and reckless (feeling she had divine energy to understand the plight of the homeless, she began visiting random homeless people and offering up her possessions). She claimed to be taking the aripiprazole 10 mg/day that was begun in the hospital, although she said she felt it was unnecessary. During telemedicine visits, her psychiatrist would ask if she felt either restless or stiff in her arms or legs, hoping that adverse effects might corroborate her medication adherence, but to no avail. Over the next few months, she continued to express a heightened preoccupation with sensory experiences alongside euphoric mood and verbose speech. Whenever her psychiatrist would remark that she seemed high, she adamantly insisted she had not reused hallucinogens, although she spoke fondly of their mind-opening powers. Given the short half-life of psilocybin (about 1 hour), her psychiatrist was obliged to diagnose bipolar disorder potentially "unmasked" or precipitated by the psychedelic exposure, rather than a protracted substance-induced mood disorder. However, when her psychiatrist suggested they measure both a serum aripiprazole level to affirm her medication adherence, as well as a hair follicle test to affirm the absence of continued hallucinogen ingestions over the past few months, she proclaimed she was deeply offended by the lack of trust and fired her psychiatrist.

Is there any workaround for assessing Janet's condition and the suspected roles of both medication nonadherence and iffy abstinence from psychotomimetics? With a still-intact therapeutic alliance, one could try appealing to Janet's (heightened) capacity for empathy: "Put yourself in my shoes, Janet. You come across high as a kite and floating on a psychedelic cloud. And you really found your excursion into the world of hallucinogens to be intriguing and pleasurable. Should we really diagnose your current condition as bipolar mania if there is even a chance that substances could be contributing? How could we know for sure unless we test?"

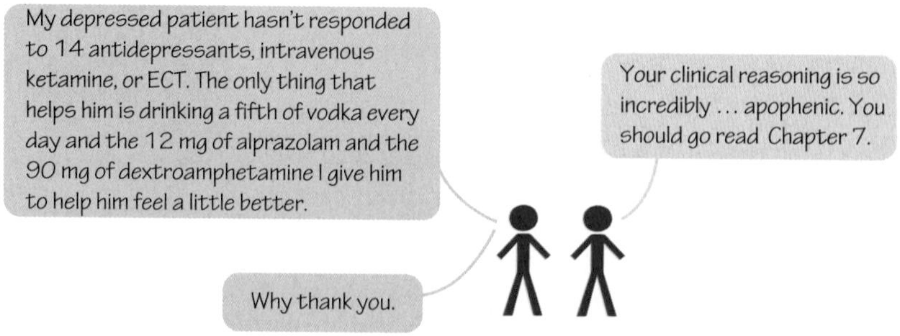

E ANOSOGNOSIA

Thus far we have mainly addressed instances in which clinical assessment and decision-making can become clouded by issues of deliberate patient subterfuge or the presence of ulterior motives for seeking care. Let us now turn to situations in which patients may struggle to give an accurate portrayal of their difficulties through no misinterpretive fault of their own but, rather, due to limitations in their ability to communicate, or otherwise convey, factually accurate information. The pinnacle of such challenges involves loss of insight, or anosognosia – that is, the inability to appreciate the presence or nature of a medical ailment. Such lack of insight could sometimes represent sheer denial (as might occur when a middle-aged overweight man who runs up a flight of stairs begins to experience crushing substernal chest pain), or it could alternatively represent a frank neuropsychological deficit.

F ALEXITHYMIA

Literally, the inability to identify and then put one's feelings into words, alexithymia is perhaps an underappreciated contributor to factually inaccurate, vague, or otherwise puzzling narratives from patients. Patients who score high on measures of alexithymia have been shown in some studies to over-report psychiatric symptoms for reasons unrelated to external incentives or questions about possible malingering (Merckelbach et al., 2018). Moreover, closely linked with alexithymia is the realm of somatization (now known formally as somatic symptom disorder) and the concept that individuals may be more prone to develop medically unexplained physical symptoms when they have trouble labeling their emotions and using language to express emotional discomfort or distress. However, critics of this neo-psychoanalytic perspective argue that it remains more of a theoretical than empirically demonstrated association (Kooiman, 1989).

G PSYCHOSIS

By definition, psychosis involves impaired reality testing, often in ways that the patient cannot discriminate or recognize as deviating from objective reality. Herein lie obvious instances in which the objective validity of reported complaints cannot necessarily be taken at face value, particularly in the context of somatic delusions, somatic hallucinations, or bizarre perceptual abnormalities. The presence of a formal thought disorder (including rigidity of thinking and difficulty in set-shifting) may help guide clinicians toward the need for a more critical analysis of subjective complaints, if the implausibility of content alone is not a sufficient indicator. If patients with psychosis cannot discern certain aspects of objective reality, can they accurately recognize when their perceptions are aberrant – rather like knowing if one is awake or dreaming? For more on this, see Box 3.4

Box 3.4

Can patients with psychosis live simultaneously in reality and nonreality?

Psychiatrist Eugen Bleuler, who developed the modern construct of schizophrenia, coined the phrase "double bookkeeping" to describe the experience of patients' simultaneous awareness of psychotic experiences while remaining cognizant of social norms and likely responses to revealing ideas and perceptions that may seem peculiar to other people. A patient's ability to simultaneously recognize psychotic phenomena occurring alongside objective reality as a kind of duality is relatively rare – as opposed to the ability to exercise intact social judgment when anticipating the responses of other people to ideas that they may find to be unusual (non-normative) or strange.

H LYING ABOUT SUICIDE

Assessment and treatment planning around suicidal thoughts, statements, or behaviors is in many ways its own phenomenon fraught with complexities and pitfalls. In no small part, patients who harbor thoughts of suicide may cautiously want or need to test the reaction of any clinician who evaluates them. Will the clinician display signs of panic and fall behind a litany of rote assessment questions about intent, planning, possible need for hospitalization, and the ever-unpopular charade of having the patient "contract for safety"? Alternatively, will the clinician sidestep the logistics surrounding suicidal statements and instead query the affect, or the meaning, behind their utterances (such as, asking psychologically exploratory questions about anger, or what the person thinks it would accomplish if they were to act on suicidal thoughts)? Will the clinician interpret suicidal statements as shorthand for the need to alter a pharmacotherapy regimen, on the grounds that the sheer presence of suicidal thinking provides de facto evidence that whatever medications are now being prescribed must not be doing a very good job? Up to 70% of psychotherapy patients who have suicidal thoughts report that they avoid speaking freely about them, most often for fear of repercussions such as the imposition of involuntary hospitalization (and, less often, based on shame or embarrassment) (Blanchard and Farber, 2020).

One tactic to help disarm the potential volatility of discussions about suicidality – and the patient's experience of suicidal thoughts as adversely impacting clinical decision-making – is to normalize the experience, or at least normatize it. "Many people who describe the kinds of feelings you have might find themselves thinking about death or suicide. Do you?" A follow-up question can pose things from the more hypothetical or conditional stance: "If you *were* having suicidal thoughts, what would be your biggest concerns about how

I might react to them?" Or one might even try reframing things from a more historical that-was-then and this-is-now perspective, such as: "Was there ever a time in the past when you did find yourself thinking about suicide, or even acting on those thoughts? What happened?" While asking explicit questions about suicidal thoughts is a standard approach in risk assessment, doing so does beg the question of whether someone who truly had suicidal intent would be likely to conceal rather than reveal that information. Clinicians ask such questions not simply for the face-value content of responses they receive, but also for assessing the form of response. Do patients hesitate and stumble or elaborate freely on the topic? Do they seem nonplussed by questions about suicide or do they seem at all stunned, as if their cover has been blown and their efforts to conceal a well-kept secret have been thrown to the winds. "Iffy" responses to questions about suicide also invite clarification and further probing, as when a patient who is asked about suicidal thoughts says, "Not really," simply "I would never *do* that" (a separate question), or if they ask the evaluator to reframe or clarify their questions in a more precise manner (e.g., "You mean, do I think about suicide *now*, or ever?" or "What do you mean by suicide – like, intentionally?").

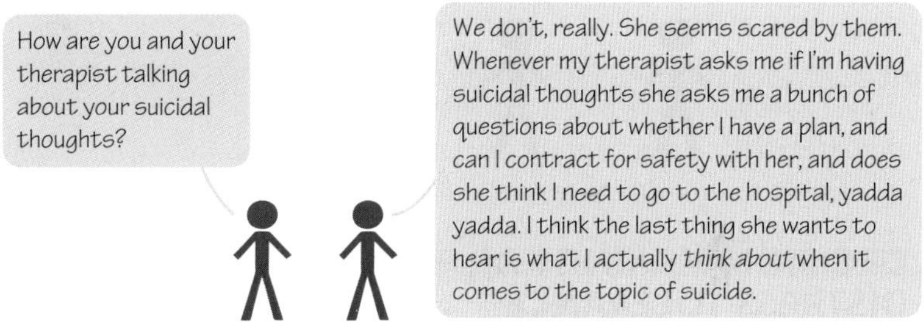

Clinical decision-making for patients who have suicidal thoughts can be a complex and multifaceted endeavor. How one interprets suicidal communication depends in part on how well one knows the patient, the quality of the therapeutic alliance, and the context in which suicidal thoughts arise. When suicidal content is raised by the patient, it can be useful to clarify if they are invoking the concept of suicide literally or figuratively. The phrase, "I'm so upset I could kill myself" might well have literal face value, but what if it was more an expression of exasperation or hyperbole than a declaration of intent? The pronouncement "I'm so hungry I could eat a horse" does not usually elicit follow-up questions about homicidal intent toward equines, or inquiries about concrete plans for logistics about the meal. There is obviously no sure-fire method for predicting suicidal behavior but, from among the multitude of risk factors traditionally rattled off, particular attention is worth noting in connection with the features summarized in Box 3.5. In Chapter 5 (Section J), we further discuss decision-making around the management of chronic versus acute suicidal ideation.

Box 3.5

Suicide risk factors of particular importance in decision-making

- There have been one (or more) previous suicide attempts
- Any previous suicide attempts involving high risk of lethality
- There exists a psychiatric disorder with known elevated risk for suicidal behavior (notably, substance use disorders, major depression, bipolar disorder, and schizophrenia or other psychotic disorders)
- Intense feelings of distress and hopelessness about the ability to solve problems that may feel insurmountable
- Skepticism that treatment – or anything else, for that matter – can help

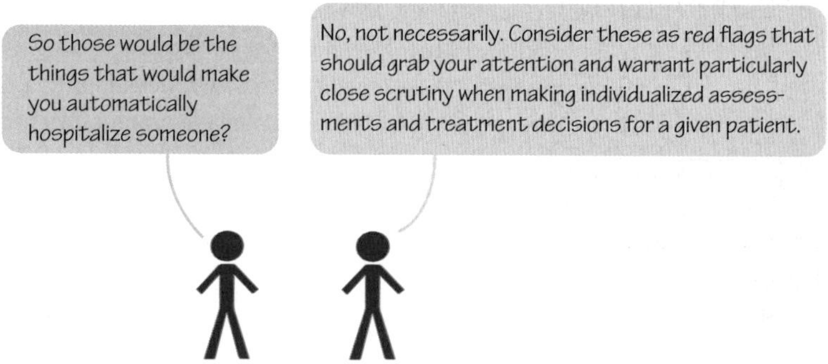

I DECISION-MAKING FOR PATIENTS WITH POOR DISTRESS TOLERANCE

As alluded to in Box 3.2, patients with poor distress tolerance skills sometimes convey a sense of urgency and demandingness for clinicians to "do" something tangible in order to alleviate their sense of inner turmoil. Overwhelming distress coupled with poor coping skills never brings out the best in anyone, but depending on factors such as temperament and personality structure, patients succumbing to what DSM-5 (American Psychiatric Association, 2013) calls the "anxious distress" course specifier may appear regressed, primitive, helpless, desperate, or less than capable to participate meaningfully in efforts to help them manage how they feel. From the standpoint of decision-making, clinicians might sometimes "react" rather than "respond" to high distress entreaties in ways that may be influenced more by emotions than reason. To assuage distress (either the patient's or the clinician's), practitioners might sometimes feel emotionally compelled to do things they may not necessarily feel are entirely appropriate. Seasoned RIME managers or educators (see Chapter 1, Section M) would think twice before doing the things described in Box 3.6.

Box 3.6

Dubious decisions made by clinicians in response to patients' poor distress tolerance

- Prescribe controlled substances, or more than reasonable doses of controlled substances, or for longer periods than they may think are appropriate
- Change the dosing or basic structure of a medication regimen without undertaking a more thorough decision-making process to determine if fundamental changes are actually warranted (see Section K on "blips" below)
- Order laboratory or other medical tests that may not be clinically relevant or necessary
- Underappreciate when treatment nonadherence or medication discontinuation may be the proximal cause of immediate distress
- Agree to requests for entitlements (attestations for disability, work or jury duty exemptions) in order mainly to allay distress rather than affirm the presence of true incapacitation
- Suggest making emergency calls or emergency department visits that conflate "urgency" with "emergency" – particularly in the absence of safety concerns or the presumed need for a higher level of care
- Fail to identify a possible source and cogent management plan for a transient crisis
- Fail to identify a patient's poor distress tolerance as a potentially broader problem of its own that requires a thoughtful treatment plan rather than an immediate definitive solution
- Forgo suggesting that a sooner appointment may be the most appropriate way to evaluate and manage an urgent-distress situation

As we further contemplate factors that can color a clinical presentation, let us now turn to the perceived adverse effects of medications and, in particular, the fascinating yet often-underappreciated phenomena associated with the nocebo effect.

J PARADOXICAL DRUG REACTIONS AND THE NOCEBO PHENOMENON

Clinical reasoning and decision-making can be especially difficult when patients report negative experiences after taking a medication or other product that leads them to conclude a worsening in their mental state which may defy physiological rules. The nocebo effect describes adverse events that occur from taking a placebo or pharmacodynamically inert substance. Patients who report suspected nocebo effects (such as improbable side effects) pose a unique challenge to the therapeutic relationship because they often have a conclusion ("I am being harmed") rather than a hypothesis ("Something does not feel right – could it be a result of my medication?"). Consequently, efforts to invoke logical reasoning, rules of physiology, or anything that challenges the veracity of the patient's experience runs the risk of quashing empathy, curtailing further data-gathering, and putting a damper on the forward momentum of treatment, as illustrated in Clinical Vignette 3.5.

Clinical Vignette 3.5

Annette was a 64-year-old widow with persistent depressive disorder (previously termed dysthymia), who had taken numerous medications for depression over many years, often resulting in diverse side effects, and had ultimately "settled" on a regimen of fluoxetine 60 mg/day plus buspirone 60 mg/day. On the advice of her primary care doctor, she began taking vitamin D 2,000 IU daily to treat a low serum level (16 ng/ml) and called her psychiatrist to insist that her depressed mood worsened the day after she began taking it. She stopped the next day and felt her mood was better. Resumption after a few days again led to a worsening of depressed mood. She insisted that her "on/off/on" exposure was proof-positive that vitamin D was exacerbating her depression and was at a loss about what to do.

What *to* do for Annette? Just for the sake of completeness, a quick MedLine check on "vitamin D" and "depression" was found to yield over 1,600 publications, and a brief perusal of the titles and abstracts found none reporting an induction or worsening of depression in response to the administration of vitamin D. Telling Annette that her causal inference is simply wrong would be invalidating, unempathic, and likely of no value to her problems. (It is fairly unlikely that Annette would breathe a sigh of relief and express thanks for the information that her worsening depression is not explainable by the one thing she has grabbed on to as a plausible hypothesis for how she is feeling.) Consider the options described in Box 3.7 for addressing Annette's concerns.

Box 3.7

Possible ways to approach Annette's concerns

- One could invoke *medical humility*: "The brain is complex and works in ways we still only understand poorly – anything, really, is possible." That response would be empathic, but not terribly useful in terms of what Annette should do next
- We could invite *watchful waiting*, along the lines of encouraging Annette to be patient and ride out the way she is feeling as a way to affirm whether her hypothesis is accurate. One could make analogies

Box 3.7 (cont.)

to the stock market – a bad day or two is not reflexively a signal to sell off one's portfolio or make rash decisions. There is some appeal to this approach in that it sidesteps any questioning of Annette's reality testing and instead invites a rather collaborative approach to gathering more information that addresses her concerns – validating her apprehension without either stoking or dismissing them. It also gently imposes on Annette a period of reflective delay, during which time her trepidations may spontaneously recede or intensify, depending on the driving force behind them

- We could also ask Annette if she has a preference in her own mind as to what her wishes are. In other words, does she know what she would like to do, and is she essentially asking for medical permission to follow through? An important point of distinction here is recognizing the difference between a patient who truly does not know what to do (and who might then actually be factually relieved and reassured if told of the low probability that her hypothesis is correct – like someone who feels a lump in their skin and is truly relieved to hear it is not cancer), as opposed to a patient who has already made up their mind that their hypothesis is correct. In the latter case, they may not so much be asking the opinion of a professional so much as seeking affirmation that their beliefs and inferences will be taken seriously

The simplest approach in Annette's case may be a combination of medical humility and deference to patient autonomy. One might truthfully acknowledge the unusualness of Annette's experience, reassure her factually that vitamin D supplementation is not known to cause depression, but acknowledge that nobody can dispute that she feels the way she feels after taking it. Perhaps it would spare everyone's narcissism to contemplate whether she might be having some kind of peculiar reaction to an inactive excipient; and then ask if she has a preference in mind as to what she would like to do before offering up one's own suggestions. This approach strives to impart to Annette more of an internal locus of control, while reinforcing the notion that her safety and fundamental well-being are not in jeopardy.

Tip

When in doubt about what to do by way of choosing from among intervention options, make an empathic observation about the patient's experience. ("You have been through an awful ordeal. It must take every ounce of energy for you to persevere.") Doing so can help clarify what they think they need and may help to eventually reveal what it is they actually do need.

Unfortunately, in actuality, Annette responded to the above intervention in a more pushy and rather paranoid–demanding style, exhorting the psychiatrist to "think harder – you can figure this out" and going on to express her annoyance that she is sacrificing her mood in order to take a vitamin that she has been told she needs. Sometimes there is just no winning! It would probably be pointless to further insist on our counter-hypothesis behind the veil of scientific plausibility, or (worse) to call into question Annette's reality testing. Where would that lead? Annette surely would in no way be relieved to know that her psychiatrist thinks she is verging on the delusional, although her response does supply useful data in that realm. There is also seldom if ever anything to be gained by disputing the point of view of someone who has a fixed belief. Though she is demanding something more thoughtful from her psychiatrist about her unusual experience, there is little more one can do on that front than to convey that her concerns are being taken seriously (e.g., "I conducted a review of the online medical literature and can tell you there are no published cases of vitamin D-induced depression") followed by acquiescence. Her medical victimhood is on the line but it probably cannot be called out as such in any way that would likely be psychologically useful to her.

At this point, one must yield. There is no room for dialogue or negotiation. Annette could be a one-of-a-kind case. Her experience defies explanation, but the one certainty she articulates is her unwavering belief in her hypothesis. The only viable initial solution then becomes stopping the vitamin D and observing. Is that collusion with magical thinking? In a way, yes, very much so. Does it carry a cost? Likely not in terms of her bone mineral density, at least in the short term. Why not lobby her to *increase* the vitamin D on the grounds that low vitamin D levels could cause her depression? Because she will not believe that if it is contrary to her own personal experience. Watchful waiting off the vitamin D now becomes a critical next step in the assessment and longer-term decision-making process. In no small part, we are keen to know how her quasi-paranoid belief-conviction evolves before we go on to propose adding an atypical antipsychotic drug that possesses antidepressant properties. In the absence of more fulminant psychosis or escalating severity of depression, the course over time becomes an essential piece in solving this puzzle.

K BLIPS VERSUS TRENDS

A related concept to the value of longitudinal course and one-off complaints, such as Annette's, involves the distinction between a possibly fleeting occurrence (a "blip") versus an enduring trend. Decision-making, whether in medicine or the stock market, generally fares better when relying on solidly recognizable trends over time, and invites caution when an observation point could be an outlier. Seldom does the patient herself offer the observation, "I am feeling badly but it's only been for a few days, so I don't know if that establishes enough of a consistent pattern that warrants a change in my treatment plan." One useful strategy for newly reported nonhazardous symptoms or potential adverse drug effects (that are not obvious emergencies) is to gather longitudinal data. Recording the persistence versus transience of a phenomenon over time provides invaluable information about timing, potential proximal causes (in relation to parsing iatrogenic from noniatrogenic factors, such as for Annette), and patterns over time. Engaging patients in the process of tracking symptoms over time also helps to facilitate the process of shared decision-making, as discussed more in Chapter 4.

L MOTIVATIONAL INTERVIEWING

Motivational interviewing involves the effort to raise a patient's awareness of their own goals and priorities and the ways in which their actions may be contradictory to achieving those objectives. Its intended purpose as a therapeutic tool in itself is to prompt "change talk" from the patient – that is, language geared toward making modifications to habits, routines, or other behaviors that are at cross-purposes with someone's stated intended goals. It becomes a powerful tool for identifying contradictory or conflictual points in a narrative or set of engrained behaviors or routines ("You say you want to feel more awake in the morning but you are reluctant to try my suggestion of lowering the dose of your sleeping medication").

Table 3.1 presents core concepts captured within motivational interviewing aimed to evoke language from a patient that directs them more toward making changes in their thinking and actions that are more consistent with their stated goals. Clarifying a patient's own goals is an essential ingredient for their participation in shared decision-making (see Chapter 4) as well as a core influence on medical decision-making processes in general.

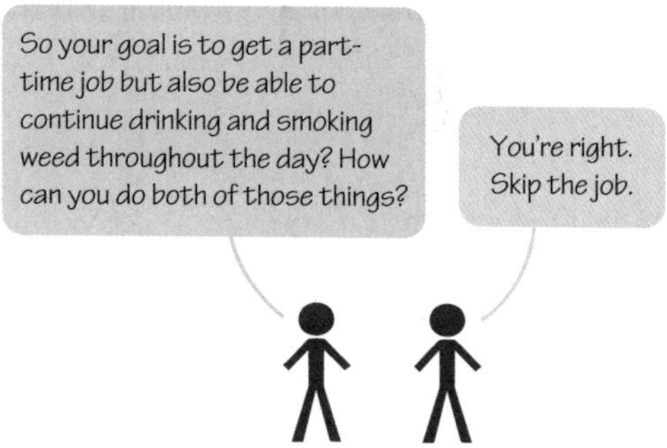

A significant potential obstacle for inspiring someone to change their circumstances (whether that means their daily activities, the focus of their psychotherapy, or their medication regimen) involves challenging their comfort level with the familiarity of the status quo – or, said differently, finding a way to convert an objective problem from being ego-syntonic to ego-dystonic. As clinicians impose clinical reasoning processes with an eye toward problem-solving and decision-making, humility does at some point demand taking into account the ways in which an individual (or a family system) may have established accommodations to the problems being presented. Are the presenting

Table 3.1 Core concepts in motivational interviewing

Preparatory change talk			
Component	**Description**	**Prompts**	**Examples**
Desire	Wanting to cause a change to happen	"What would you wish was different?"	Waking up earlier; being able to redirect intrusive thoughts; having more energy
Ability	Recognizing the ability to change; how could change occur?	"Which of these options seems most feasible for you?"	Try out a new behavioral technique; discuss the pros and cons of a medication change
Reason	What are reasons for change? What would change accomplish?	"Why would you want the status quo to be different?"	Exercise before work; schedule an informational interview; look up job postings; call or email a friend
Need	Why is change important, and what would happen without it?	"How important is this to you?"	Lose 5 pounds; go to bed earlier; buy a pill box to organize medicines
Implementing Change Talk			
Commitment	What do you intend to do?	"I have decided that I will do the following ..."	I will get the lab tests I have put off getting; I will go to a 12-step meeting
Activation	What are you now willing to do?	"I am ready to ..."	I am ready to begin tapering a benzodiazepine dose as planned
Taking Steps	What have you actually done?	"I have already laid this groundwork ..."	Record a mood chart for 2 weeks before next appointment

problems accepted with quiet resignation or protested because of their disruption to functioning or emotional well-being? How would change jeopardize an established (albeit complaint-filled) system of operations? If compensatory mechanisms have long been in place to accommodate the expectations associated with the status quo, a shake-up will likely do more than just lower someone's ratings on a measurement scale of symptoms. When are the forces of perpetuation stronger than the forces of change?

Ⓜ PARADOXICAL INJUNCTIONS

A kind of flip side to motivational interviewing is the old psychoanalytic concept of paradoxical injunctions (popularly regarded as "reverse psychology") among efforts to motivate change behavior. Paradoxical injunctions involve calling attention to symptoms or problems that the patient identifies as unpleasant or unwanted and then proposing ways to amplify the problem, giving patients sole agency to decide if their wish for change exceeds the desire to maintain the status quo.

As summarized in Table 3.2, paradoxical injunctions take the form of interventions that are either *compliance-based* (where the patient is expected to

Table 3.2 Forms of paradoxical injunction

Subtype	Description	Example
Compliance-based interventions		
Reframing	Relabeling something problematic as being positive or favorable.	Suggesting that the value of depression renders someone very sensitive to other people's needs.
Symptom prescription	Identifying a problem or symptom and encouraging the patient to "take control" of the symptom by actively pursuing it.	"You say you and your partner fight all the time. Let's see what happens if you schedule a planned hour each day to have a fight. Be sure not to miss." "You struggle with anxiety. Schedule an hour a day where your task is to feel anxious. Come prepared with a list of things that evoke anxiety."
Defiance-based interventions		
Restraining strategies	Prohibit the patient from taking any steps to change a problem.	"I want you to keep drinking the exact same quantity of alcohol each day. No more nor less. Do not try to cut down. Do not let yourself fall behind."
Positioning	Exaggerating a patient's negative appraisal of themself or a situation.	Pointing out that things could get worse, anticipating that death or suicide may be right around the corner; negating an obvious positive attribute ("You're right, it's probably just a fluke that you got that job after preparing so hard for the interview").

comply with the recommendation, usually most successful in people who tend not to resist interpersonal influence) or *defiance-based* (where the expectation is that the patient will defy, or do the opposite of, what the clinician proposes). Unlike motivational interviewing techniques, where overt efforts are made to prompt change, deploying a paradoxical injunction makes no overt effort to persuade the patient but, rather, invites the patient to persuade themself.

Using paradoxical injunctions, unlike motivational interviewing, a clinician might align with and even magnify a patient's ambivalence, rather than counter with intellectual rationales for change. They might warn the patient of hazards associated with change, or even point out the possible benefits of their current situation. The goal is to provoke change by creating some sense of cognitive dissonance on an emotional level, as opposed to trying to engage desire to change on more strictly intellectual or logical grounds. For example:

- "You haven't started the new antidepressant medicine that we discussed after we went over the pros and cons of making a change. So … what do you like about the status quo of feeling depressed?"
- For the patient who will not take necessary risks outside of their comfort zone because they are convinced they fail at everything, one might propose making a list of true efforts that are guaranteed to fail and then devoting designated time to pursuing guaranteed failures in order to empirically test their hypothesis. For example: "Whatever you do, don't study for your exam, otherwise you'll risk not failing it. And be sure to show up to take it, otherwise you'd fail by forfeiting rather than by truly failing."

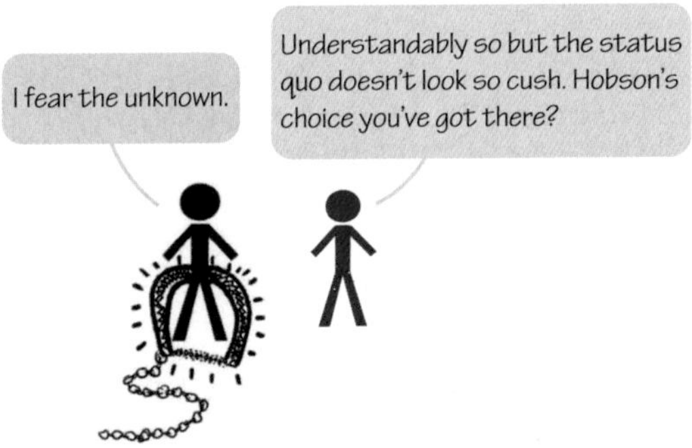

- Following a train of thought to its logical (or illogical) conclusion sometimes incorporates elements of paradox. For example, consider Clinical Vignette 3.6

Clinical Vignette 3.6

James was a 31-year-old recently divorced man whose job was terminated due to company layoffs. He brought himself to the emergency department, distraught and feeling suicidal, after his estranged wife, who had been his primary emotional support, blocked his calls and refused further contact with him. He had not followed through on several previous referrals to outpatient treatment and had made a serious suicidal gesture about 6 months earlier for which no intervention occurred. After speaking at length with the psychiatry on-call resident in the emergency department and agreeing to voluntary admission, he changed his mind and "just want[s] to go home." The resident offered James the following response:

> "Let me make sure I've got this straight. You are home alone all day, ruminating about suicide with no structure or plan to change your routine. You told me you are unsure about what you might do if you continue staying at home like this and when you felt like this once before you ended up writing a suicide note and trying to hang yourself. So, you *courageously* brought yourself to the emergency room tonight for help because you said you were afraid that could happen again, and now that I've agreed with you that coming in to the hospital could be helpful you've changed your mind and want to go back to the suicide-ridden home environment that you so heroically extricated yourself from because … so you can … so you can … why is that again? Help me understand the logic."

From the standpoint of decision-making, deploying techniques such as those described above can be applied to just about any clinical situation, whether pharmacological, behavioral, or otherwise, to better refine an understanding of the nature of an underlying ailment and devise the most appropriate biopsychosocial treatment plan.

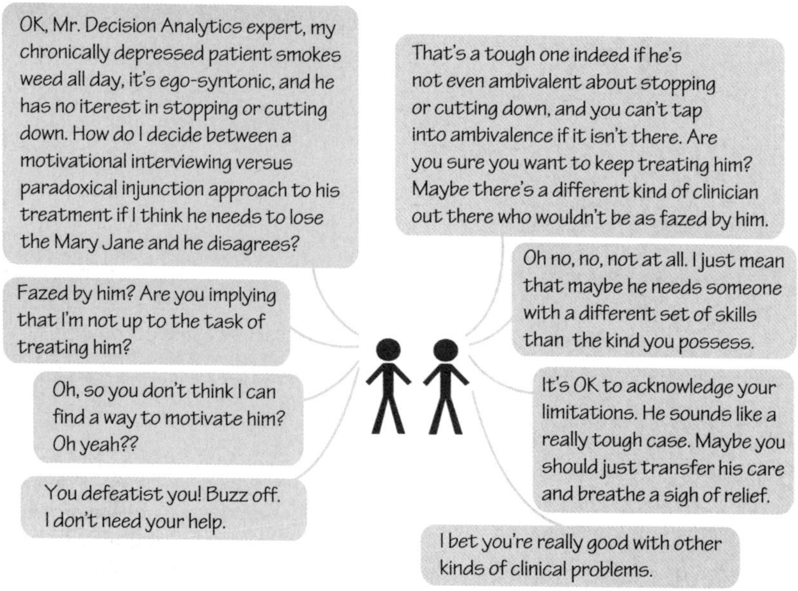

TAKE-HOME POINTS

- Recognize clinical situations in which there is a high likelihood for pertinent factual information to become hidden, reframed, disavowed, or otherwise distorted in ways that can significantly influence clinical assessment and decision-making
- Reliance on collateral historians can often be helpful as part of a clinical assessment, but remain mindful of the potential for collateral historians to bring with them their own biases and perceptions that may also add to a sense of distortion as much as clarity
- Differentiate instances in which patients may consciously fabricate, embellish, or otherwise distort their problems or internal experiences from circumstances in which they may provide inaccurate information due to neuropsychological or other inherent deficits in their capacity to relate factually correct information
- Malingering patients tend to present excessive and often implausible symptoms; nonverbal cues have limited value in efforts to differentiate truthful from deceptive communication
- Patients with substance use disorders may lie about the magnitude of their use due to reasons involving shame, guilt, a wish to protect and maintain their use, and fears that their broader mental health concerns may not be taken seriously
- Alexithymia is a known cause for the over-reporting of psychiatric symptoms that is unrelated to malingering, but may not necessarily be linked as closely to the development of medically unexplained physical symptoms as was once thought

References

American Psychiatric Association. Diagnostic and Statistical Manual of Mental Disorders, 3rd edition. Washington, DC: American Psychiatric Association, 1980

American Psychiatric Association. Diagnostic and Statistical Manual of Mental Disorders, 5th edition. Washington, DC: American Psychiatric Association, 2013

Benge JF, Wisdom NM, Collins RL, et al. Diagnostic utility of the Structured Inventory of Malingered Symptomatology for identifying psychogenic non-epileptic events. Epilepsy Behav 2012; 24: 439–444

Blanchard M, Farber BA. "It is never OK to talk about suicide": Patients' reasons for concealing suicidal ideation in psychotherapy. Psychother Res 2020; 30: 124–136

Ekman P, O'Sullivan MO. Who can catch a liar? Am Psychol 1991; 46: 913–920

Farber BA. Client deception about substance use: Research findings and a case study. J Clin Psychol 2020; 76: 277–285

Goldberg JF, Garno JL, Callahan AM, et al. Overdiagnosis of bipolar disorder among substance use disorder inpatients with mood instability. J Clin Psychiatry 2008; 69: 1751–1757

Hilker R, Helenius D, Fagerlund B, et al. Heritability of schizophrenia and schizophrenia spectrum based on the nationwide Danish Twin Register. Biol Psychiatry 2018; 83: 492–498

Kendell RE, Cooper JE, Gourlay J, et al. Diagnostic criteria of American and British psychiatrists. Arch Gen Psychiatry 1971; 25: 123–130

Kieseppä T, Partonen T, Haukka J, et al. High concordance of bipolar I disorder in a nationwide sample of twins. Am J Psychiatry 2014; 161: 1814–1821

Kooiman CG. The status of alexithymia as a risk factor in medically unexplained physical symptoms. Compr Psychiatry 1989; 39: 152–159

Merckelbach H, Prins C, Boskovic C, et al. Alexithymia as a potential source of symptom over-reporting: An exploratory study in forensic patients and non-forensic participants. Scand J Psychol 2018; 49: 192–197

Nurnberger JI, Blehar MC, Kaufmann CA, et al. Diagnostic Interview for Genetic Studies (DIGS): Rationale, unique features, and training. Arch Gen Psychiatry 1994; 51: 849–859

Resnick PJ. Malingering of posttraumatic stress disorders. In Rogers R (ed.), Clinical Assessment of Malingering and Deception, 2nd edition. New York: Guilford Press, 1997, pp. 130–152

Smith GP, Burger GK. Detection of malingering: Validation of the Structured Inventory of the Malingered Sympomatology (SIMS). J Acad Psychiatry Law 1997; 25: 183–189

Stoll AL, Tohen M, Baldessarini RJ, et al. Shifts in diagnostic frequency of schizophrenia and major affective disorders at six North American psychiatric hospitals, 1972–1988. Am J Psychiatry 1993; 150: 1668–1673

Vrij A, Hartwig M, Granhag PA. Reading lies: Non-verbal communication and deception. Ann Rev Psychol 2019; 70: 294–317

Walczyk JJ, Sewell N, DiBenedetto NB. A review of approaches to detecting malingering in forensic contexts and promising cognitive load-inducing lie detection techniques. Front Psychiatry 2018; 9: 700

4 Shared Decision-Making

LEARNING OBJECTIVES

- ☐ Define shared decision-making and describe its use in the setting of psychiatric treatment planning
- ☐ Recognize the potential for therapeutic mishaps when clinicians and patients differ in their therapeutic objectives or unspoken agendas in the negotiation process of shared decision-making
- ☐ Discuss logistical issues when attempting to engage patients with psychosis, diminished capacity, or major cognitive deficits in the process of shared clinical decision-making

Thus far we have discussed how clinicians are the primary if not sole evaluators and decision-makers when it comes to devising treatment recommendations. Shared decision-making (SDM) is a not-so-new but increasingly recognized form of patient-centered care in which a patient and their clinician actively collaborate to determine which treatment options are most consistent with the patient's own values, priorities and goals. As described originally by Charles et al. (1997) and later expanded on by Elwyn et al. (2012), an SDM model first involves **introducing choice** followed by **describing options** (sometimes using patient decision-support tools – such as charts, graphs, brochures, interactive websites, or audiovisual materials) followed by helping patients **explore their preferences** in order to make the best decisions *for them*. Greater focus is placed on the patient's own narrative and personal experience as influencing treatment decisions, rather than on general diagnostic issues or outcomes.

A WHY SHARED DECISION-MAKING?

SDM has gained enormous attention within organized medicine and public policy-making, as reflected by endorsements of its wide adoption by the Institute of Medicine and the United States Preventative Task Force (United States President's Commission, 1982; Berwick, 2002) as well as the establishment of the Patient Centered Outcomes Research Institute (Emanuel and Pearson, 2012). SDM did not arise from mental healthcare specifically, but from general healthcare more broadly – although it quickly becomes apparent that decisions involving the assessment and management of psychiatric conditions incur risks involving diminished patient insight and/or compromised decisional capacity, even beyond "capacity" in the technical sense. For instance, a severely depressed patient may think that suicide represents their best option but their preference is unlikely to be endorsed if the clinician is the ultimate arbiter. (On the other hand, an SDM approach might invite a "pro–con" analysis of suicide as a patient preference, and prompt exploration of the patient's reasoning and openness to alternative conclusions. This really then becomes an instance of cognitive reframing. In fact, one might argue that the process of any cognitively oriented psychotherapy itself involves efforts to identify faulty reasoning or negative assumptions and guide patients toward alternative attitudes and less-biased conclusions.)

Several historical forces led to the rise of SDM. One has involved what some authors have called efforts to achieve "emancipation" from older models of paternalistic medicine in which it is assumed that clinicians are the best if not sole experts about a health problem and therefore are the ones most capable of devising a remedy. This view holds that patients' own preferences, fears, opinions, and objectives are secondary to the goal of identifying "the best" treatment by some objective standard. The movement toward SDM grew not simply from perceptions that patients are the ultimate custodians of their own treatment, but more from a need to overthrow the perceived oppressive mantle of control over patient autonomy and individualism.

A second driving force has involved the hypothesis that better clinical outcomes might result if patients became more active stakeholders in decision-making processes around their own care; this means inviting the patient to grapple more directly with the risk–benefit questions that clinicians have traditionally undertaken fairly independently, and borne primary responsibility for the consequences. Consider as an example Clinical Vignette 4.1.

Clinical Vignette 4.1

Dr. Singh believes that electroconvulsive therapy (ECT) is necessary to treat a severe and otherwise multi-drug-resistant depression experienced by her patient Henry. She states that its potential benefits make it the unrivaled preferred option. But if Henry is insistent on instead trying an eighth antidepressant medication, his preference might be dismissed if Dr. Singh disagrees. In a traditional decisional model, Dr. Singh may feel that Henry is making a terrible choice and, if she feels strongly enough, she might even refuse to continue to treat Henry unless he agrees with her recommendation. Henry is also free to seek a second opinion or otherwise search for another clinician who may be more inclined to tell him what he wants to hear. By contrast, an SDM approach would encourage a dialogue rather than a dispute over the preferred course of action. SDM would not only pursue clarification of Henry's reluctance to accept what Dr. Singh favors as a necessary intervention but, moreover, place Henry's concerns and preferences on an equal footing to those of Dr. Singh.

As noted above, SDM invites the sharing of risks. Perhaps Dr. Singh is most concerned that without ECT Henry might die from suicide or malnutrition; or she might feel that she has no other intervention to offer him that has a compelling likelihood for managing his problem. Henry might be most concerned about the risk for cognitive side effects associated with ECT, or his decision-making may be colored by expectancy biases from things he read about ECT online. Henry might also be more comfortable living with his risk for suicide than is Dr. Singh. SDM would bring a pro–con decision-analytic process to the forefront of identifying next steps.

B BASIC TENETS OF SHARED DECISION-MAKING

A number of features describe clinician behavior in the course of SDM (Makoul and Clayman, 2006), as outlined in Box 4.1.

Box 4.1

Clinician behaviors in shared decision-making

- Define/explain the healthcare problem
- Present options
- Discuss benefits/risks/costs
- Clarify patient values/preferences
- Discuss patient ability/self-efficacy
- Present what is known/make recommendations
- Clarify the patient's understanding
- Make or explicitly defer a decision

The above steps are largely self-evident, but it can be useful to lay the process out for the patient, either explicitly or implicitly, if for no other reason than to reinforce that discrete steps exist in the decision-making process and to clarify where and when each participant's input matters most, so there is less mystery about how conclusions are ultimately reached. It can also be helpful to point out that decision-making is a process that often requires revision based on the results of a first pass-through discussion. Symptoms (or side effects) can change over time, unforeseen events can occur, and any good plan needs to involve flexibility and openness to revision as circumstances may dictate.

In the case of psychopharmacological treatment, it also can be helpful when presenting options and discussing benefits to forecast some expectation about time courses for judging improvement. Clinicians need not hedge behind general statements about unpredictability or merely encourage patients to be patient when they ask how long it will take until they might feel better. Evidence-based medicine allows us to share with patients a few likely "rules" about treatment time course without necessarily guaranteeing efficacy. It is useful to define for the patient the concept of an "adequate" trial for judging response, and enlist them not as guinea pigs but as co-collaborators in a clinical trial, aware of the relevant parameters (time, dose, assessment methods) and inviting their questions and observations along the way. Other general concepts from evidence-based medicine that are worthy of sharing with a patient/co-collaborator are summarized in Box 4.2.

Box 4.2

Points clinicians might share about forecasting pharmacotherapy outcomes

- The time course for judging response may not really begin until an adequate threshold dose of a medication is reached; and reaching an adequate threshold dose may depend in part on dosing titrations that are in place to optimize safety by minimizing side effects (e.g., in the case of initiation of lamotrigine and the risk of cutaneous reactions).
- Know the time course for side effects that may be likely to emerge before efficacy becomes apparent - and what to do about them, if anything.
- Clarify what measurement tools are being used to judge efficacy (see Chapter 6).
- Indicate that judgments about "response" or "remission" often take 4–6 weeks with many if not most psychiatric medicines, assuming an adequate dose and proper adherence to the regimen.
- Oftentimes, some inkling of improvement should be visible by week 2. Seeing at least a 20% reduction in symptoms according to whatever rating scale is being used is often taken as a harbinger of a subsequent eventual likelihood for response in the case of major depression (Papakostas et al., 2006), bipolar depression (Kemp et al., 2011), schizophrenia (Leucht et al., 2007; Samara et al., 2015), panic disorder (Pollack et al., 2002), and generalized anxiety disorder (Rynn et al., 2006). Absence of any glimmer of improvement by week 2 sometimes prompts the need to alter the plan, either by modifying a medication dose, adding an adjunctive therapy, or otherwise making some alteration to the original plan that was outlined.
- Recognize that longstanding, chronic conditions often take longer to improve.
- Conditions in which there are two or more distinct psychiatric ailments present (i.e., comorbidities) tend to slow down the time course for judging improvement and generally pose a more challenging set of treatment problems than when only one disorder is present.

C THE IMPACT OF SHARED DECISION-MAKING ON CLINICAL OUTCOMES

Enthusiasm about SDM tends to revolve heavily around its ethical appeal and subjective impressions about the virtues of greater patient involvement in treatment planning. There is relatively little literature assessing the impact of SDM on clinical outcomes – and, within that sparse literature, there is some divergence of findings based on patients' versus clinicians' or other observers' perspectives. For example, a meta-analysis of 39 published SDM trials found that ratings of patient satisfaction, quality of life, and affective–cognitive patient-reported outcomes (e.g., concerns about illness, anxiety after seeking a consultation) were significantly better in patients who participated in SDM, but objective measures (e.g., medication adherence) or symptom-based outcomes were not significantly different in SDM versus other treatment groups (Shay et al., 2015).

The use of decision aids in themselves has been shown to have a positive effect on treatment outcomes (Stacey et al., 2011), but their use is not strictly tied to SDM and it is unclear whether their value for the SDM process itself necessarily extends beyond general psychoeducational purposes.

D COLLABORATIVE DECISION-MAKING IN ITERATIVE PSYCHOPHARMACOLOGY: IDENTIFYING PATIENT PREFERENCES

One fundamental issue regarding treatment decisions, over which patients and practitioners may have differing perspectives, is the notion of what we might call "definitive" versus "iterative" treatment approaches. Some patients may think about psychopharmacotherapy with an assumption that, after establishing a clear diagnosis, a clear treatment pathway seamlessly follows and there is little reason to expect much need for modification or changes in a treatment plan once it has been established. Some clinicians may think that certain laboratory tests can provide shortcuts to finding which medication is most effective – such as measuring serum or urine neurotransmitter levels (which are rather esoteric and not considered to be established biomarkers of drug response) or pharmacogenetic testing (which mainly tells about drug tolerability and metabolic efficiency of a given drug, rather than relative efficacy of one medication versus another). A true SDM dialogue would involve the clinician addressing patient preferences but also dispelling myths or correcting scientific misinformation that may contribute to a patient's preferences. Such discussions can sometimes strike at the heart of basic trust in the provider and their knowledge base if a contest arises between the validity of medical information a patient might present versus the clinician's agreement or disagreement.

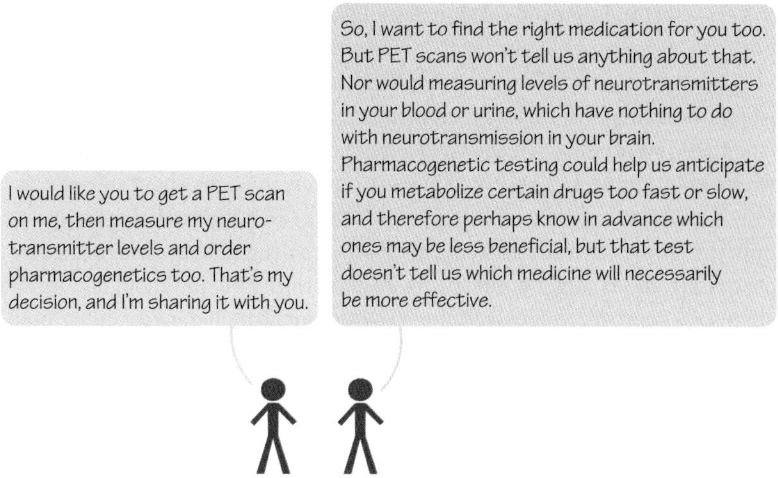

Interchanges that pit the clinician's versus the patient's scientific understanding can become a delicate matter that requires interpersonal attunement, empathy, and sensitivity on the part of the clinician in order not to dismiss the patient's perspective – particularly in the face of disputed information or unproven hypotheses – or to incur an adversarial stance from either side.

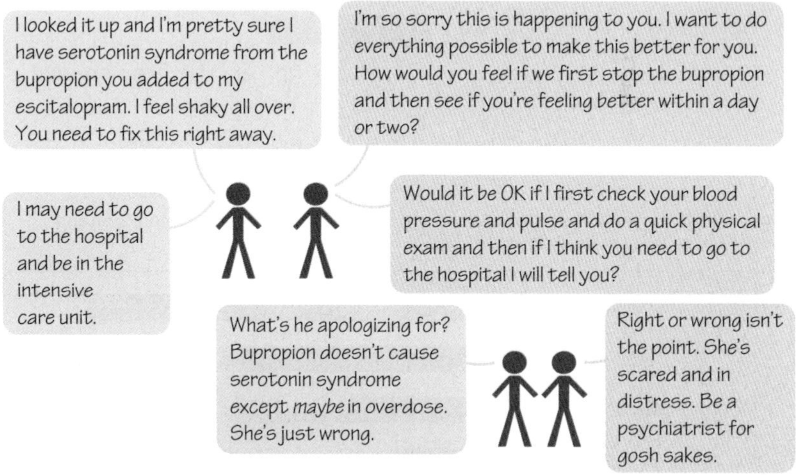

E DEFINING PATIENT AND PRACTITIONER GOALS

What do patients prioritize when defining their own treatment goals, and how do their priorities compare with those of mental health practitioners? Surveys of patients with major depressive disorder show that most prioritize *functional recovery* – that is, improved role functioning across work, social, and home life domains – as much if not even more than symptom reduction (Zimmerman et al., 2008). A 2016 online survey of individuals with major depressive (unipolar) disorder or bipolar disorder queried factors that patients themselves identified as being most important when choosing a treatment (Figure 4.1) or when changing medications (Figure 4.2). As noted in these figures, concerns about side effects were the main consideration for treatment choice (identified as being most important by over two-thirds of all patients), with drug efficacy (as reflected by how quickly effects might occur) being the top priority in only about one-third of patients. By contrast, when asked about reasons for changing medications, both patients with bipolar and unipolar disorder accorded similar importance to the presence of side effects as well as lack of efficacy.

Figure 4.1 Patient-reported "important factors when considering a treatment": survey of the Depression and Bipolar Support Alliance (Rosenblat et al., 2018)

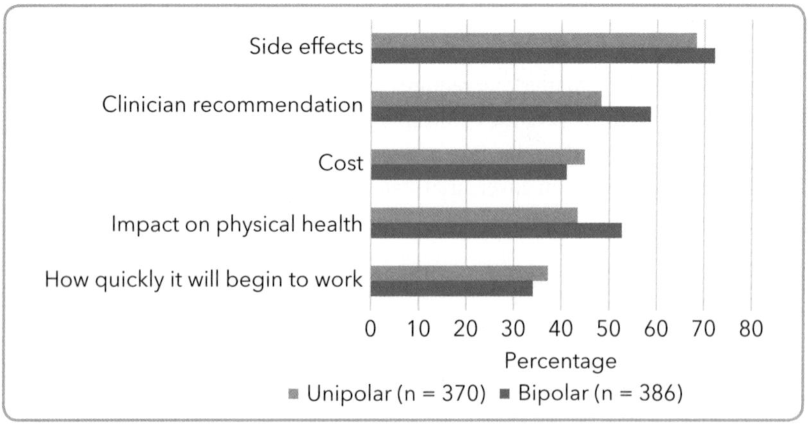

Figure 4.2 Most common reasons for changing medications: survey of the Depression and Bipolar Support Alliance (Rosenblat et al., 2018)

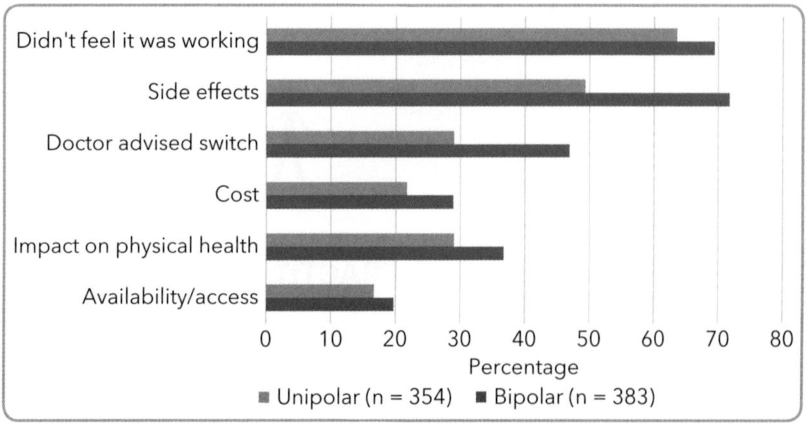

Let us take one more clinical example of a collaborative SDM model in which the clinician strives to help the patient decide what their own preference is for next steps in the treatment process, when choosing from among several viable options. Consider Clinical Vignette 4.2.

Clinical Vignette 4.2

Claude was a 37-year-old man with bipolar II disorder involving depression polarity-proneness, who had been well maintained for about 6 months on a regimen of lurasidone 20 mg/day plus lamotrigine 200 mg/day. He self-reduced his lurasidone to 10 mg/day about 3 months earlier due to concerns about long-term effects of dopamine-blocking drugs. He then began to notice emerging sleeplessness without fatigue, higher energy than usual with some impulsive spending (purchasing some high-end musical equipment on a whim that stretched his budget), coupled with feelings of despair, hopelessness, and passive suicidal thoughts. To address what his psychiatrist, Dr. Parsimonia, called a hypomanic episode with mixed features, he was presented with three options: (a) raise the lurasidone back to 20 mg/day, (b) augment with lithium, or (c) augment with divalproex – having never previously taken either of the latter two. Dr. Parsimonia presented these all as viable options to Claude, noting that while resuming the higher dose of lurasidone might be a swift remedy, if Claude's preference was to avoid higher dosing of a dopamine-blocker then that option garners less enthusiasm. She then asked if Claude philosophically preferred to "work with the existing materials" (i.e., raise the lurasidone dose) rather than add an additional medicine. Claude then asked about raising his dose of lamotrigine as an option, to which Dr. Parsominia said he could try that, but lamotrigine has no known efficacy for hypomanic symptoms, making it a less compelling option. Claude was intrigued by the idea of adding lithium to find out if he had a lithium-responsive bipolar subtype, and preferred to think of raising lurasidone as a viable back-up plan.

F SHARED RISK-TAKING

The potential for any drug (even placebos) to cause adverse effects is ever present. The dialogue between the clinician and the patient for discussing risks versus benefits with viable medication options can easily become lopsided. Clinicians might sometimes find themselves favoring or agreeing to medication options that have small effect sizes or a low likelihood of benefit if they think such options pose a lesser risk for adverse effects, without necessarily making clear to patients that such an approach runs the risk of failing to meaningfully improve symptoms. They may skirt a discussion of side effects altogether, or defer a discussion until acute symptoms improve but then neglect to revisit the question of discussing side effects for fear of inspiring nonadherence. Or they may find themselves trying to persuade, cajole, minimize, or otherwise assuage patient concerns about the possibility of undesirable drug effects in efforts to prioritize efficacy over tolerability. For their part, patients may feel they are being placed in a passive role with little choice other than to acquiesce. Like any informed consent process, the key challenge for shared risk-taking is to assure that patients understand the need for treatment, the viable options for treatment, the risks of treatment, and the risks of forgoing treatment. In an SDM model, clinicians can certainly frame their recommendations based on their own appraisal of the above, and invite questions from the patient in order to help them decide how they wish to proceed. This approach becomes especially important when it makes clear that – in the absence of involuntary treatment or the imposition of medications that are court-ordered over patient objection – the decision to assume risk is a matter of patient choice. This is an important framing of the problem because it makes the decision-making process bilateral.

G CAPACITY TO MAKE AN INFORMED DECISION

Formal assessment of decisional capacity, as classically described in the literature by Appelbaum and Grisso (1988), involves four core components described in Box 4.3.

Box 4.3

Core tenets of intact decisional capacity

- The ability to communicate a choice
- The ability to understand relevant information
- The ability to appreciate the current situation and its consequences
- The ability to manipulate information rationally

Several points regarding decisional capacity bear on how patients might engage in an SDM process. Decisional capacity can fluctuate over time and may be preserved in some matters but not others (e.g., the capacity to agree to a blood test versus the capacity to consent to a major procedure such as ECT). Impaired cognitive ability (such as impaired comprehension or information processing, and executive dysfunction) would expectably affect decision-making skills, although some studies report that frank cognitive impairment accounts for no more than 25% of the variance in explaining medical decisional capacity (Jeste and Saks, 2006). Cognitive problems that involve impaired memory or organizational skills also can lead to poor treatment adherence, which, in turn, can impede someone's ability to participate meaningfully in treatment decisions, especially if they disavow or are unaware of their own cognitive deficits. (Consider the dementia patient who regularly forgets to take prescribed medications but claims their adherence is intact, and refuses to allow supervised medication administration.)

The criterion of "manipulating information rationally" does not explicitly address the issue of *reasonableness* when making choices, and we would suggest that this component often becomes a major sticking point when undertaking an SDM model with patients who have severe levels of psychopathology, such as the suicidally intent depressed patient who wants to argue for his own death as a rational existential solution to life problems; or the patient with schizophrenia who will not take pills because she is convinced they are poison, as discussed more in Section N below.

Consider this delicate scenario: a patient has diminished decisional capacity by virtue of severe psychopathology, but the available viable treatment options are limited; and suppose the patient insists on a patient-centered, SDM approach, rejects the clinician's recommendations, has no psychiatric advanced directive or family/significant others who can assist in the decision-making process, and the severity of disability from the psychopathology does not quite rise to the level of warranting involuntary treatment. This was the unfortunate dilemma faced by Al and his psychiatrist, Dr. Coercitiva, in Clinical Vignette 4.3.

Clinical Vignette 4.3

Al was a 72-year-old widower living alone with longstanding bipolar I disorder, having had several hospitalizations in the remote past and now with increasingly limited treatment options. Now taking divalproex 1,500 mg/day (with a serum valproate level of 84 mcg/dL), he was symptomatically manic, euphoric, provocative, spending excessively on "deals" at trinket stores, and not sleeping, but he claimed to feel the best he had ever felt in his life. Previously having a mediocre response to lithium, the development of stage 3b chronic kidney disease (estimated glomerular filtration rate of 36 mL/min/1.73 m^2) further diminished his candidacy for its resumption, which he in any case refused as an option. Carbamazepine previously was unhelpful. He did not want to undergo ECT, which he had received many years earlier and felt that it caused him permanent memory problems. He had significant tardive dyskinesia from previous antipsychotic medication use that was poorly responsive to a vesicular monoamine transporter type 2 inhibitor and offered this as his reason for refusing any adjunctive antipsychotics, including clozapine. He refused voluntary hospitalization and was not considered gravely impaired or unsafe to the point that merited involuntary admission. Although Al had a longstanding treatment relationship with his psychiatrist, Dr. Coercitiva, he bristled when Dr. Coercitiva suggested to Al that the grandiosity of his mania was interfering with his ability to make a reasonable decision that was consistent with good self-care.

Al's problems are complicated pharmacologically as well as from an SDM perspective. One issue involves his difference of opinion with Dr. Coercitiva about the presence and severity of his current symptoms and the need for treatment. (Dr. Coercitiva judges Al as lacking in insight, while Al (who savors the concept of SDM) insists that he knows more about his own condition than Dr. Coercitiva possibly ever could.) How does SDM engage patients who lack insight and there is no leverage available from family members or significant others? In fact, suppose there comes a time when Al's mania resolves and he were to then rebuke Dr. Coercitiva for not having "done more" to somehow strongarm him into treatment in order to save him from himself?

A second issue involves the reality that Al has no obvious excellent treatment options; all involve consequential risks that he has stated his preference against.

A third component is that, while he is symptomatic, there is no basis at the moment to pursue treatment over his objection. Our dilemma at present is not to decide what treatment is "best" for Al; there likely is no "best" option, only relative pros and cons. Our dilemma, rather, is to figure out how to pursue a decision-making process either *with* Al or *on behalf of* Al. Perhaps the task would be easier if Dr. Coercitiva felt there was an obvious, far-and-away best option for Al to pursue, analogous to Dr. Singh in Clinical Vignette 4.1 trying to knock some sense into Henry about agreeing with her recommendation for ECT. There being no such luck for Al – even if paternalistic medicine tried to grab the upper hand, it has nothing special to offer – there is a stalemate, if not an outright standoff, about how to proceed. All that Dr. Coercitiva can do is to stick to his guns, offering his opinion about the available options and their pros and cons as best he can articulate them, while simultaneously trying to maintain a dialogue with Al. This pharmacological standoff might start to feel like a hostage negotiation situation, where Dr. Coercitiva might hope that, if he just waits long enough, Al will accede. That is not really true to the spirit of SDM, though. Should Dr. Coercitiva wait around hoping that Al will at some point have an epiphany of insight that allows him to overcome his denial, and let the treatment proceed? Or will Dr. Coercitiva eventually succumb to fatigue from "waiting" for Al to see the light?

The biggest SDM challenge in this case may rest with Dr. Coercitiva, who struggles to see Al's point of view beyond the most superficial level, as he judges Al's refusal to accept his recommendations as the byproduct of his illness, which makes Dr. Coercitiva think that SDM in this case is at best a charade. Dr. Coercitiva quietly wishes that Al's condition would deteriorate to the point that a phone call to emergency services could be made and the process of involuntary treatment could begin, unimpeded by Al's stubborn objections. That might happen, which would indeed change the decision-making paradigm; SDM only works when the patient is not so gravely ill that involuntary treatment becomes a life-saving moral obligation. That clearly has not yet happened, and may or may not down the road. In the meanwhile, Dr. Coercitiva hunkers down for a long road ahead.

H WHEN PATIENTS MAKE FAULTY INFERENCES

What happens when patients draw wrong conclusions about medication effects, or have erroneous expectancy biases that influence their participation in decision-making, but they may not be so receptive to "clarifications" that feel like challenges to their autonomy? (We saw shades of this for Annette in Chapter 3, Clinical Vignette 3.5.) Consider the patient with frank psychosis who misidentifies their paranoia as "anxiety" and lobbies for benzodiazepines over antipsychotic medication; or the patient with psychosis whose symptoms persist despite taking an antipsychotic medication and they deduce that the drug has then caused their symptoms rather than failed to ameliorate them; or the manic patient who insists they are depressed and balks at the idea of accepting anything other than an antidepressant medication; or the patient whose social anxiety disrupts their attentional processing when speaking publicly and wrongly infers they must have attention deficit–hyperactivity disorder. SDM offers an opportunity for patients to present their symptoms alongside their own hypotheses about what they think may be wrong, but one would hope that they would prefer the clinician to bring to bear their expertise in making sense of the problem, rather than simply endorsing the patient's conclusions.

How does one handle SDM when patients propose ideas or make suggestions about their own care that strike the clinician as eccentric, irrelevant, or misguided, though not necessarily hazardous? One might indulge suggestions that are farfetched but benign, but where does one draw the line in deciding how far to go? We describe such a scenario in Clinical Vignette 4.4.

Clinical Vignette 4.4

Zoë, a 31-year-old yoga instructor, who had been diagnosed with chronic fatigue syndrome and something she called "thalamic burnout," was thrilled to make the acquaintance of Dr. Newage, whose reputation for engaging patients in SDM was unsurpassed. To her first appointment, she brought with her a large stack of information downloaded from the internet on the use of a wide range of nutraceutical products. She asked Dr. Newage to research each of the products she had found and provide her with a summary of his opinions at their next meeting, which she would then review with him, and then decide if she was comfortable proceeding with him as her doctor.

An immediate dilemma for Zoë and Dr. Newage is not so much the medical advisability and safety of the concoction of pills she has interest in but, more pressingly, the gauntlet she has asked Dr. Newage to run on her behalf in order to satisfy her criteria for his acceptability as her next physician. There is nothing "shared" about her unilateral decision-making, nor does she seem particularly interested in Dr. Newage's genuine opinion about the ideas and products she is presenting to him, other than testing his willingness to accede to her demands. Dr. Newage may be quite in favor of SDM as a general principle, but may be less than pleased about the prospect of a collaboration with Zoë on her own terms … which he is free to decline to accept if her terms run counter to his own conceptualization of SDM.

I INAPPROPRIATE REQUESTS

Yet another realm in which SDM becomes a shaky proposition involves the handling of medically inappropriate requests – especially if the inappropriateness of the request itself strikes at the core of the very psychopathology for which the patient is seeking treatment, such as Randy in Clinical Vignette 4.5.

Clinical Vignette 4.5

Randy was a 27-year-old woman with dysthymic disorder and anorexia nervosa. She had significant distorted perceptions about her body image: at a height of 5′4″ and a weight of 105 pounds, her body mass index (BMI) was 18 and her ideal body weight was 121 pounds. She felt that she was grossly overweight and at one point was treated with aripiprazole augmentation of fluvoxamine in an effort to counter the intensity of her body dysmorphia. Randy gained 8 pounds over 4 months' time on this regimen but was reluctant to discontinue either drug because she felt "calmer" with the pairing. She lobbied for antidote strategies to counteract iatrogenic weight gain but after 3 months on metformin 1,000 mg twice daily her weight neither increased nor decreased. Her prescriber viewed this as an utter success because she both felt a clinical improvement and her weight gain no longer persisted. Randy viewed the 8-pound weight gain as making a bad problem worse, and lobbied for more aggressive weight-loss strategies, including lisdexamfetamine as well as semaglutide (noting, of the latter, "*Everybody's* on Ozempic®, why can't I be too?"). She was miffed when her prescriber disagreed with her position, noting that her request was really a perpetuation of her body dysmorphic symptoms and desire for an unrealistically low body weight, and was medically inappropriate. Randy decided to pursue treatment elsewhere because of the refusal to acquiesce to her request.

J WHEN CLINICIANS MAKE FAULTY INFERENCES

Patients are not the only ones susceptible to drawing wrong conclusions about the effects of a medication or other psychiatric intervention, or misinterpreting information from the literature or other sources. Perhaps the most vivid instance in this respect is when the clinician believes more strongly than the patient that a medication is delivering a substantial benefit, or is fundamentally necessary (disease-modifying?) despite substantial doubt on the patient's part. What might you do if Dolores, in Clinical Vignette 4.6, came to you for a second opinion?

Clinical Vignette 4.6

Dolores was a 45-year-old human resources administrator with bipolar II disorder who had been maintained on lithium 900 mg/day plus quetiapine 300 mg/day and lamotrigine 200 mg/day for several years. She continued to experience symptoms of depression as well as sedation and weight gain and was generally unhappy with her treatment regimen. Her psychiatrist, Dr. Strontium, pointed out that because Dolores's mother had lithium-responsive bipolar disorder, she had a "genetically responsive" form of the illness which would make it "irresponsible" for him to agree to her request to stop it. He also told her that because lithium is neuroprotective, her brain might shrink without it. Dr. Strontium also is philosophically opposed to using antidepressants in patients with bipolar disorder because "they make patients manic." A stickler for evidence-based medicine, Dr. Strontium also told Dolores that there is synergy for bipolar depression when combining lamotrigine with lithium (citing van der Loos et al., 2009) or with quetiapine (citing Geddes et al., 2016) and that quetiapine itself has the most extensive database with five randomized trials for bipolar depression, including in patients with bipolar II disorder.

Well, a counter-stickler response to Dr. Strontium might be to point out that lumateperone has efficacy data (even in conjunction with lithium) for bipolar II depression, with a substantial effect size in that subgroup (Cohen's $d = 0.81$) (Calabrese et al., 2021), thus representing at least one viable alternative to quetiapine. But the bigger-picture issue at play in this situation is less about which alternative pharmacotherapy might be best for Dolores than the faulty decision-making that Dr. Strontium brings to the SDM table. It is true that lithium responsivity may "breed true" in bipolar pedigrees, based on data showing about a two-thirds concordance of response in first-degree relatives (Grof et al., 2002). While this can be a helpful variable in deciding whether or not lithium may be a useful intervention for someone with bipolar disorder, Dr. Strontium seems to wrongly infer that the possible familiality of lithium response is more definitive than it is, and perhaps assumes that its benefits are somehow evident even if Dolores remains symptomatic and is clearly unaware of them. There is not much flexibility in how Dr. Strontium otherwise admirably seeks to apply the literature to provide evidence-based care; when something *should* work, but in Dolores' case does not, he appears inflexible about modifying the treatment plan, wielding a rather rigid and concrete stance behind the guise of the known clinical trials literature.

Examples of other instances in which the clinician might proffer wrong conclusions about the effects of medications are summarized in Box 4.4.

Box 4.4

Practitioner blunders, or less-than-elegant clinical maneuvers

- Retaining a particular antidepressant medication within a treatment regimen when the patient remains significantly depressed, and there is no clear evidence that the retained antidepressant has delivered a benefit; or, if a previous benefit has been lost, failing to alter the dose or augment the antidepressant in efforts to recapture its previous effect
- Leaving a subtherapeutic dose of a medication unchanged for someone who reports ongoing symptoms, and there is no obvious contraindication to a dosing change or other modification of the treatment regimen
- Using a medication for purposes that have no demonstrated efficacy, or when published clinical trials are predominantly negative (e.g., lamotrigine in acute mania, aripiprazole for acute bipolar depression)
- Not offering options to manage an otherwise manageable side effect (such as benign tremor with a beta blocker, or weight-loss strategies for iatrogenic weight gain)

K ULTIMATUMS

At the opposite end of the SDM spectrum lies the use of ultimatums. Issuing ultimatums, or non-negotiable demands, is among the most complex and treatment-threatening transactions that can occur between a clinician and patient. Patients sometimes issue ultimatums, which are really demands, or requests framed with insistence, but ultimately it is the clinician who decides what they feel is medically appropriate and are comfortable doing. A patient who demands an increased dose of a scheduled substance, insists that the prescriber make up for a shortfall of a drug that they lost, or demands a prescription that the prescriber may feel is inappropriate, has little recourse apart from seeking treatment elsewhere if they are adamant and their demands go unmet. Demands tend to highlight breakdowns in the fundamental communication process between clinician and patient, and in that sense become the antithesis of SDM, when an insistent stance leaves no room for an evaluative process of the concerns raised by either party.

When does a practitioner declare that, unless the patient follows their instructions, the treatment alliance becomes untenable? Some examples of conceivable ultimatums appear in Box 4.5.

Box 4.5

Examples of psychiatric ultimatums

- Demands to obtain drug toxicology screens as a part of a substance use disorder program
- Demands to refrain from using or requesting (or otherwise obtaining) controlled substances
- Following and abiding by a behavioral contract (e.g., in the setting of conduct disorder)
- Keeping scheduled appointments in the absence of medical emergencies
- Agreeing to use a medication only as prescribed, share it with no one else, and be responsible for not losing any pills
- Obtaining safety laboratory tests (e.g., renal function tests in a patient taking lithium) or else risk having a medication stopped

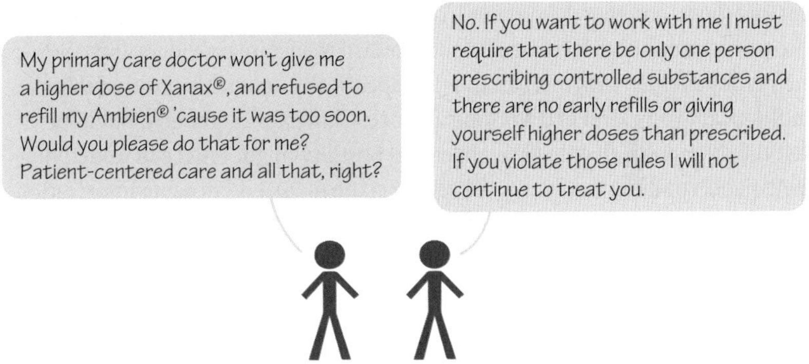

There is an axiom that the clinician cannot work harder than the patient when behavioral change is an objective of a psychiatric treatment plan. If a behavioral plan involves, say, following a sleep hygiene regimen with a regular time to wake up, followed by structured daytime activity that may involve agreed-upon tasks (e.g., time devoted to job-searching, attending support group meetings, doing household chores), it falls on the patient to follow through. If the patient does not, a clinician's ultimatums tend to do little by way of motivating behavioral change. Ultimatums may come from other stakeholders, such as family members, who may impose consequences (such as loss of financial support) unless the patient follows through on target behaviors (such as attending classes or job-hunting). From the clinician's standpoint, if the patient faces adverse consequences for not following through on expectations, SDM would entail exploring their reasons for not holding up their part of a bargain, and clarifying what they think will happen if they renege on agreed-upon behaviors. Schwartz (1990) notes that when a clinician does issue an ultimatum – as is true for life in general – its impact has little value and credibility becomes lost if there is no follow-through on ramifications; ultimatums in general limit a practitioner's future responses to a patient.

Ultimatums can also come from other stakeholders in a patient's life, such as employers, child welfare agencies, or the criminal justice system. While many patients who enter treatment for substance use disorders report that they did so because of ultimatums issued to them by family members, employers, or other third parties (Weisner et al., 2010), there is remarkably little empirical research tracking outcomes for recovery in the aftermath of coerced (e.g., "interventions") versus noncoerced treatment initiation. Studies of community samples have shown no differences in substance use patterns following coerced versus noncoerced substance use disorder treatment (Pilarinos et al., 2020).

L ANGER AND HOSTILITY

Patients who display overt anger and hostility, particularly at the clinicians treating them, are poor candidates to engage in a collaborative treatment model. Those who mount an adversarial stance toward their care providers alienate their allies and place themselves in a therapeutically untenable position that is antithetical to any kind of a working alliance. Clinicians might hold out hope that the differential diagnosis of anger and hostility might reflect an underlying remediable condition such as psychosis or acute mania, or an acute intoxication state, for which appropriate treatment (sometimes administered over the patient's objections) might ultimately remedy the aggression and render an otherwise unreasonable patient more amenable to collaboration. Call it giving someone the benefit of the doubt, and a psychiatrist's innate effort to try to attribute antagonistic behavior to some more benign and remediable psychiatric cause. Families themselves often contend with similar dilemmas, bringing hostile loved ones to treatment with hope that a "fixable" solution for menacing or oppositional behavior can occur through some diagnostic and pharmacological transformative process. More often than not, however, it becomes virtually impossible to establish a working therapeutic alliance once aggression escalates to the point of verbal abuse or threats toward the clinician. Threats, in turn, bring about a different kind of (often abrupt) endpoint to an existing treatment plan. Consider the examples in Vignettes 4.7 and 4.8.

Clinical Vignette 4.7

Delia was a 47-year-old woman with paranoid personality disorder, who had been maintained on quetiapine 200 mg/day with modest benefit. An apparent misunderstanding about the date of a next medication refill with her pharmacist resulted in her being told she was seeking her next prescription too early. She became enraged, accused the pharmacist of committing fraud, and then threatened to call the police. She left multiple telephone messages for her psychiatrist accusing him of malpractice and being "complicit." Delia had declined previous suggestions to increase her dose of quetiapine when she had expressed rage over perceived mistreatment by coworkers, telling her psychiatrist that more medications would not "right the wrongs" others were committing against her.

Her psychiatrist could find no way to ally with her rage and paranoia, engage willingness to increase the dose of her quetiapine, or consider a different antipsychotic medication in the service of trying to reduce her distress. Her global mistrust continued unabated and, as it engulfed her psychiatrist as an identified adversary, she was left in utter emotional isolation.

Clinical Vignette 4.8

Peggy was a 42-year-old single woman diagnosed with chronic depression, whose interpersonal relationships were marked by chaos and instability, emotional volatility, angry outbursts of disproportionate intensity, primitive splitting, and the projection of accusations that others deliberately meant to mistreat or otherwise take advantage of her whenever they could. On one occasion she insisted that her pharmacy had never received a refill prescription for the benzodiazepine she had long taken and angrily accused her psychiatrist of "messing up" by not properly calling in her correct prescription. Choice words followed from Peggy after the psychiatrist showed her documentation of the sent prescriptions, followed by threats of legal retribution for alleged professional misconduct that she said caused her excessive emotional pain and suffering.

M SHARED DECISION-MAKING AS MOTIVATIONAL INTERVIEWING

Patients think they know what they want. Do they really? Are they sure? What happens when their actions contradict stated desires and intentions? Here we enter the realm of motivational interviewing, the mechanics of which are discussed in Chapter 3, Section L, vis-à-vis the SDM process. Part of the SDM role of the clinician is to help patients accurately identify their own needs and preferences, which they may not even be fully aware of.

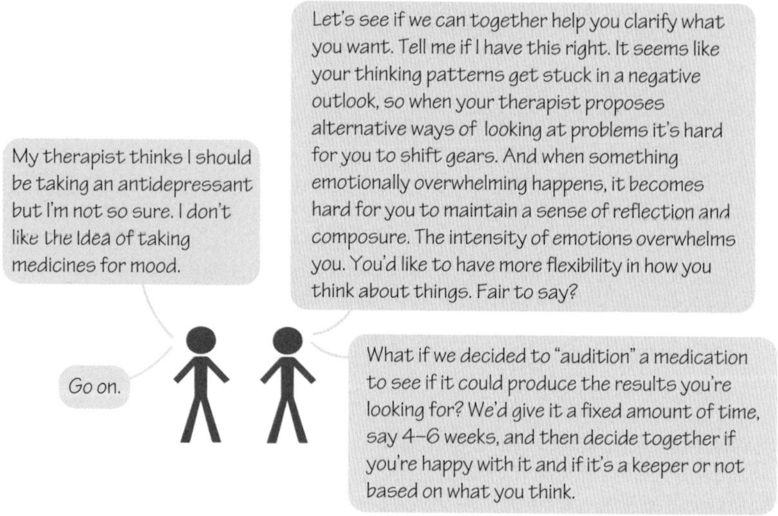

A motivational interviewing approach to SDM involves explicitly offering to the patient a process of helping them articulate their treatment goals, noting at the outset that sometimes patients may not even be fully aware of them. A patient who is mainly concerned about possible side effects may be disavowing the relative importance of alleviating anxiety, insomnia, depression, or other symptoms that ostensibly prompted their efforts to seek treatment. Ambivalence about embarking on a particular treatment path may hold only partial awareness for some patients, who might even benefit from being told that they may still be in a "precontemplative" stage and not quite ready to pursue a formal treatment program. Some may present with obvious contradictions between stated goals and behaviors (such as a track record of poor medication adherence despite a stated desire to achieve better symptom management via pharmacotherapy). Open-ended questions and reflective listening can help patients transition from *focusing* (that is, identifying their change target) to *evoking* (that is, promoting change talk from the patient by concretely identifying strategies to achieve their stated goals). Gently pointing out discrepancies between stated goals and actual behaviors may help prompt change talk.

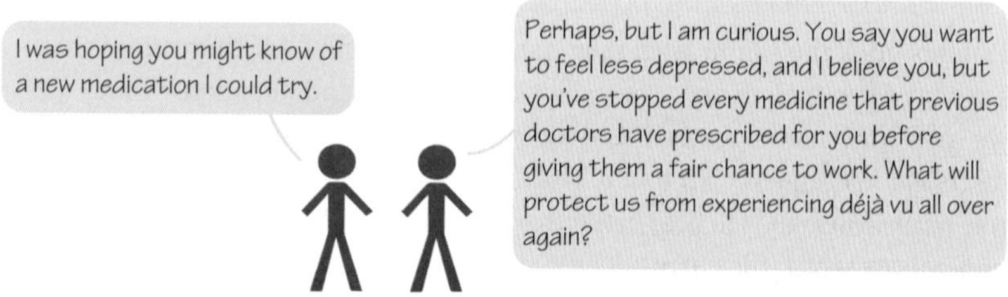

N PSYCHOSIS

One might anticipate that patients with psychosis, poor insight, and impaired reality testing would be especially difficult to engage in SDM. Particularly in the case of individuals with paranoid or persecutory beliefs, a stance of mistrust can turn medical decision-making into a more adversarial than collaborative process. Let us first consider what patients with psychotic disorders themselves say about their involvement in treatment decisions. In one study of 122 inpatients with schizophrenia, an expressed desire for SDM was noted in those who were younger and had negative attitudes about pharmacotherapy (Hamann et al., 2005). Other recognized correlates of a preference for SDM in schizophrenia patients include poor treatment satisfaction, negative attitudes toward medication, better perceived decision-making skills, and higher education (Hamann et al., 2011a). Clinicians, for their part, report that they perceive schizophrenia patients who engage in SDM to be more skeptical of treatment and more "difficult" (Hamann et al., 2011b), posing challenges on both sides of the SDM table.

Sensing a theme? Perhaps not surprisingly, the utility of SDM in the setting of psychosis may bear not so much on the pursuit of a collaborative endeavor but, rather, as a poised response to distrust and an expectancy bias of authoritarian coercion. The catch phrase "make no decisions about me without me" takes on a different tenor when the focus shifts from a desire for inclusivity or an effort toward destigmatization and instead becomes a battle cry for self-protection against perceived exploitation and downright assault.

An SDM approach then becomes not much different from the clinical stance one might take when addressing delusional content, and its affective overtones, in the interview setting. Some pointers for this are summarized in Box 4.6.

Box 4.6

Clinical strategies to engage patients with psychosis in shared decision-making

- Gauge cognitive flexibility versus rigidity - that is, a person's ability to see more than one side of an issue - preferably by assaying relatively neutral or more impersonal content
- Inquire about past experiences in which the patient may have felt that their wishes went unheard, or worse, were deliberately overridden. Express genuine curiosity to understand their perspective about why that may have been the case. It may be helpful not to ask if their prior stance was reasonable or unreasonable, in hindsight, but rather, if anything about *how they presented their point of view* could have been perceived by others as less than reasonable
- Acknowledge the intrinsic importance of trust in the relationship between a clinician and patient; ask if the patient is aware of anything the clinician can say or do that would help to build a greater sense of trust
- Align with the affect

The last point in Box 4.6 cannot be overstated, and there is no such thing as being overly empathic. Steer clear of inciting a debate over the content or objective reality of someone's concerns, particularly in the setting of cognitive rigidity. In fact, the clinician has no way to know past facts. For all we know, who's to say the last doctor *wasn't* trying to poison the patient, or may have been less than competent? The intent is not so much to validate or invalidate the *events* so much as the *concerns* – and to recognize how the patient interprets events; what may appear as a previous clinician's obliviousness or seemingly callous disregard for drug side effects may very well feel like abject indifference about inflicting suffering. One can certainly align with a sense of outrage, or mistrust, or an appreciation for the need for caution in future interactions with clinicians.

Declaring "You can't trust doctors" is not so much a proclamation of fact as a lamentation of the patient's plight, as this may very well be the predicament they find themselves in. Do they wish they could trust doctors more, or is their distrust more resolute and entrenched? What would greater trust require? In the case of inviting an SDM approach to medical decision-making, an open stance can help. "You have not known me long, how are you supposed to know whether you can trust what I say or decide if what I'm advising is right for you?" Put the patient to work in sketching out a roadmap for collaboration.

Lastly, SDM requires particular tact on the part of the clinician when addressing treatment requests that spring from delusional content and grossly impaired reality testing. What is the best response to a schizophrenia patient who requests a stem-cell transplant in order to rid their body of implanted eavesdropping devices? This is a tough job if SDM is taken to mean a factual discussion of treatment options. Maintaining a stance of neutral curiosity never hurts ("What makes you think that, do you know?"). The clinician could also express their honest concern that the procedure a patient is requesting is, in their opinion, unlikely to be helpful and could be harmful – although that leaves the psychosis itself unaddressed, and the patient may well press onward or look elsewhere to satisfy their agenda. One could try to appeal to the partnership aspect of SDM by expressing concern for the patient's welfare, assuming both parties agree that psychosis could be operative (e.g., "we know you have a condition in which your brain may sometimes play tricks on you – I would not be doing my job by ignoring that fact. How do we know that's not happening right now?"). And finally, since SDM in no way means that the clinician becomes a passive entity dispensing requested medications or anything else on demand, one might remind the patient of the partnership involved in any good treatment alliance: "You rely on my knowledge and ability to let you know when I see that you are symptomatic. I've promised to tell you my opinions. What should we do if you don't like hearing what I think?"

O TREATMENT OVER OBJECTION

It is hard to imagine collaborative decision-making when patients may be retained in a treatment facility against their will, or are being prescribed medications over objection. However, there are ways to invite collaboration and provide patients with some greater sense of agency over what happens to them even if, fundamentally, they register their disagreement with the need for treatment.

One such opportunity is inviting the patient to choose from among viable medication options, such as a preference for oral versus injectable medications in the setting of agitation, or otherwise finding ways to present them with options over which they can exert some sense of control, whenever possible (Garriga et al., 2016). Longitudinally, patients who previously have experienced treatment over objection may be particularly good candidates to develop a psychiatric advanced directive (PAD; Murray and Wortzel, 2019) that enables them to articulate their preferences and wishes regarding future treatment decisions in the event that their future symptoms might render them less than fully capable of participating as equal partners in decisional processes. PADs are further described in Box 4.7.

Box 4.7

Psychiatric advance directives

PADs involve a series of expressed wishes and preferences usually developed by a patient and their clinician with regard to medications and other treatments, involvement (or exclusion) of family members or significant others, and mental health facilities that they consider to be acceptable options. For example, a patient might indicate that they do not wish to undergo ECT if that were raised as a future treatment option. They might indicate that they would prefer to receive a long-acting injectable antipsychotic if they became nonadherent to oral antipsychotic medication. They might designate a sibling to arbitrate in the event they become suspicious of their spouse's intentions toward them. A guiding premise, similar to nonpsychiatric medical advance directives, is the patient's declaration of their wishes made at a time when their ability to express a preference and demonstrate intact decisional capacity is not in question. Notably, in the United States, PADs are not legally enforceable in most jurisdictions and unfortunately may be overridden by inpatient providers, leaving the patient feeling betrayed if they generate a PAD that is ignored. Such instances also run the risk of casting the outpatient clinician as the patient's advocate against an inpatient team, engendering a split that may very well prove to be therapeutically counterproductive all around.

P INFORMATION SHARING: TRANSLATING FROM THE BENCH TO THE BEDSIDE

How can a clinician best communicate to a patient the essential information they need about a proposed treatment in order to make an informed decision? While every decision involves a risk–benefit analysis, let us first say more about benefit. How do we explain "benefit" as a tangible entity to patients in language that is accessible and meaningful? We would propose that there are several aspects, no different than how clinicians communicate as colleagues when discussing relative treatment benefits and risks in professional discussions. The key parameters involve statistical significance, data from large-scale replication trials, effect sizes, as well as the clinician's own impressions (for example, judging from anecdotal experience whether a generic drug formulation may be less effective than a branded formulation). (Those of you who read ahead to Chapter 7 will recognize the latter of these concepts as hypothesis-generating observations, which we will also call post hoc because they occur in hindsight after a treatment decision has been made and implemented.) In order to ensure that patients possess necessary factual information to participate meaningfully in an SDM dialogue, clinicians might present their portion of the dialogue in segments, as depicted in Box 4.8A–D.

Box 4.8A

Fostering a shared decision-making dialogue: Part I

"Let me describe for you some useful ways to think about, and evaluate, the treatment options we should consider for the problems you are having. There are a number of different types of medicines that can be helpful for addressing the kinds of mood and anxiety and thinking symptoms you have described. I want you to be informed about the choices you have so I should first ask you, do you prefer if I give you a little, a medium amount, or a lot of detailed information about how the different medicine options work?"

Box 4.8B

Fostering a shared decision-making dialogue: Part II

"Here's what I would consider a medium amount of detail. Nowadays, we think that when medicines can help symptoms it is because the brain circuits that process information around mood, thinking, and behavior are not running as efficiently as they should. The science leads us to think that effective medicines work by turning on genes in the brain that help nerve cells form stronger connections in order to transmit signals better – kind of like making a 3G phone network into a 5G network. So, they don't really change who you are as a person, so much as they make the communication systems in our brains work more efficiently. Does that make sense?"

Box 4.8C

Fostering a shared decision-making dialogue: Part III

"So, medicines that are known to treat the kinds of symptoms you're describing can vary in how reliably they work better than a sugar pill – meaning, the results they produce are not random or due to chance, but due to a real effect of the medicine. That's called statistical significance, when we say one drug produces a "significant" benefit. Second, medicines obviously also can vary in how potent they are. Two drugs could both work better than a placebo, but one might have a bigger effect than another. That's called the effect size, or its clinical meaningfulness. There are actually numerical formulas for expressing these things. The third consideration is how extensive the research is. Are there only a few studies – or many – to support our expectations that a medicine will have an effect that is both statistically significant and clinically meaningful? Stop me if I've said anything confusing so far."

Box 4.8D

Fostering a shared decision-making dialogue: Part IV

"The fourth and final part that we want to consider is the possibility of side effects. Nearly every medicine can have possible side effects, which sometimes are minor or fleeting and other times could be more annoying or even medically concerning. We always think about the risk–benefit ratio when choosing a medicine. This will be especially important in SDM because, on the one hand, you wouldn't want to pick a drug that's ineffective just because it has few if any side effects, while on the other hand, if there are any side effects, they ought to be manageable, safe, and certainly be outweighed by the benefits. Does that all make sense?"

Q NOW THAT I'M WELL CAN I STOP MY TREATMENT?

At various points in this book, we allude to uncertainties about pharmacological endpoints and the parameters that influence decisions about when to stop a particular treatment, or all treatment altogether. Largely, for recurrent or chronic conditions involving mood or anxiety, as we have noted, treatments tend to be more disease-managing than disease-modifying, placing the patient who wishes to halt treatment at risk of relapse or recurrence. When treatments for chronic or recurrent conditions are only disease-managing, virtually all patients will eventually relapse, and there are no excellent predictors for anticipating who will remain well off medications long term – even when "good prognosis" features such as late age at onset, abrupt onset, and absence of comorbidities are evident. Here, we wish to turn our attention to the SDM dialogue that might occur with patients who raise the prospect of tapering off or stopping a treatment in the face of those inescapable unknowns. We would frame the discussion along the lines of informed consent, with efforts to assure that a patient possesses as much information as possible in order to help them make the best decisions for their unique situation.

R WHEN DECEPTION AND MANIPULATION SERVE A THERAPEUTIC FUNCTION

There are times when clinicians may seek to capitalize on the power of suggestion, a possible placebo effect, a paradoxical injunction, or another manipulative technique in order to achieve a therapeutic benefit (see Chapter 3, Section M) – especially for conditions in which pharmacodynamic efficacy alone may be modest. High expectancy of response is a known mediator of treatment outcome in major depression (Rutherford et al., 2017), but this is not likely information that, when shared explicitly with a patient, will necessarily facilitate placebo responsivity. How does one broach the concept of SDM when deliberate deception becomes a necessary element of beneficent care? One would not ask permission to violate the patient's autonomy on the grounds of a possible therapeutic benefit, although some authors offer an ethical justification to support clinical deception when it is performed in order to benefit the patient, as opposed to the deceiver (Gold and Lichtenberg, 2014). The impact of a paradoxical injunction goes nowhere if the clinician tells the patient that part of the treatment will involve making observations or recommendations with the hope that the patient will do the opposite of what is suggested. On the other hand, there have been open trials of placebo in major depressive disorder in which patients are told at the outset that they will be receiving a substance that has no active medicine in it, with response rates rivaling those of active antidepressant medications (Kelley et al., 2012).

Manipulation around expectancy bias can also potentially leverage pharmacotherapy response. Consider Clinical Vignette 4.9.

Clinical Vignette 4.9

Stacy was a 37-year-old woman with persistent depressive disorder whose condition had failed to improve after multiple trials of selective serotonin reuptake inhibitors (SSRIs), adjunctive second-generation antidepressant medications, and adjunctive stimulants. She was now taking dextromethorphan-bupropion plus lamotrigine without noticeable benefit, and previously had no benefit from intranasal esketamine, pramipexole, or olanzapine-fluoxetine combination. She was embroiled in a difficult long-distance divorce from an emotionally abusive husband, living with her parents, unemployed, and generally finding it hard to experience a sense of influence over most aspects of her life. She found her involvement in cognitive therapy to be equally unhelpful. When her psychiatrist, Dr. Disperata, proposed as next steps either a monoamine oxidase inhibitor, transcranial magnetic stimulation, or ECT, the prospect of each frightened her and left her feeling "unfixable." At one point she asked about trying either bupropion or escitalopram, stating that friends had told her personal success stories with each. Dr. Disperata fought the urge to remind her that she already tried bupropion unsuccessfully in the form of dextromethorphan-bupropion (at least, 210 mg/day's worth) and that escitalopram would be a random choice with no database in treatment-resistant depression. Instead, Dr. Disperata declared that each was a very reasonable idea, confessing that he himself had not thought of either, marveled at the extent of Stacy's friends' success, and said it was certainly worth a try, and in fact, why not try both together. Stacy was amazed and exhilarated by the idea of combining both and eagerly embarked.

So, did this pharmacotherapy decision work? Permit us to say that the actual outcome was less important than the manipulation Dr. Disperata undertook. After multiple unsuccessful treatment trials in major depression, the probability of anything working becomes quite low (see Chapter 9, Section D), and because Stacy was less than eager to agree to Dr. Disperata's suggested options, why not meet her where she is at? Stacy experiences the world as an incessant external locus of control. Does that element in itself contribute to her depression and its unyielding persistence, as suggested by the literature (e.g., Wiersma et al., 2011)? Dr. Disperata sought not so much to test the hypothesis that bupropion–escitalopram might be a pharmacodynamic superpower but, rather, that an intervention aimed to restore to Stacy some measure of having an internal locus of control with regard to how she feels in life might translate to some benefit. And even if this particular intervention, which was her own idea, failed to improve her condition, the very fact that she could experience her own sense of influence over what happens to her might engage her to consider other, perhaps more pharmacodynamically impactful, options in the future, especially if she was the one to propose their undertaking.

Tip

The construct of locus of control (LOC) derives from social learning theory and involves expectancies that one's fate is determined either by one's own behaviors and abilities (internal LOC) or by pure fate, chance, or luck (external LOC).

In our view, the role for deliberate and beneficent deception in clinical care remains underexplored in studies of SDM, and may pose an instance in which utter "transparency" about the intended manipulation could be countertherapeutic and therefore potentially undermining of a patient's stated desire for symptom relief. Consider the example in Clinical Vignette 4.10.

Clinical Vignette 4.10

Ellen was a 27-year-old woman with obsessive-compulsive disorder, an unspecified anxiety disorder, and an intense fear of swallowing that was previously diagnosed as pseudodysphagia by an otolaryngologist. She reported varied intolerable adverse effects from small doses of SSRIs, including lowest possible doses of benzodiazepines, gabapentin, or compounded liquid formulations of ultra-low dose SSRIs. She found no relief from cognitive-behavioral therapy and complained of "laryngeal dystonia" when given the lowest possible doses of several second-generation antipsychotic medications. Her new psychiatrist, Dr. Devoro, deferred any treatment recommendations after an initial visit until he could properly research her unusual condition. On a second visit he reported that he had extensively searched the medical literature and consulted with several specialists who suggested that saline nasal spray used three times daily might solve the problem by "reactivating the ciliated epithelium" that normally lines the esophagus during development. He cautioned that she might experience a choking sensation, which was an indication that the process was working. He proposed they meet weekly to review her progress and record in a notebook the results of anything she tried to swallow. After several days she called to ask if increasing the frequency to four times daily might make the treatment work better and Dr. Devoro reluctantly agreed. As she continued to meet with him regularly, she found herself "forgetting" to use the nasal spray and saying little about her problems swallowing unless asked directly.

S SHARED DECISION-MAKING WHEN ONE PARTY HAS AN AGENDA

Shared decision-making presumes an equal partnership in which joint solutions are explored for commonly held goals. That process can quickly go awry when the goals are not so common, when there is not a shared appreciation of treatment risks and benefits, when subterfuge enters the picture, or when the therapeutic relationship turns adversarial. Let us take as an example of the potential hazards to a treatment dyad posed by the use of controlled substances, as shown in Clinical Vignette 4.11.

Clinical Vignette 4.11

Debra was a 28-year-old woman with persistent depressive disorder, borderline personality disorder, and anxiety. She had been taking lorazepam 0.5 mg/day in addition to a succession of monoaminergic antidepressant medications without success, and recently had begun adjunctive intranasal esketamine without apparent benefit after the first six insufflations. She called her psychiatrist, Dr. Endorf, to request an early refill of her lorazepam stating that she had run out of it about 10 days too soon because she was taking more than prescribed and the pharmacist was unwilling to provide her with an early refill. A similar occurrence had happened a few months earlier and Dr. Endorf at that time agreed to "make up" for the "shortfall" this one time, but told her she could not continue to take more than the prescribed quantity of a controlled substance. Dr. Endorf now told her he would not refill the lorazepam but would work with her to find an alternative noncontrolled substance for her anxiety. She was deeply upset by that decision, threatened that if she now had a withdrawal seizure it would be Dr. Endorf's fault, and refused to discuss noncontrolled substance alternative anxiolytic medication options.

Scenarios such as Debra's are probably not so rare. From the standpoint of SDM, they make collaboration a more difficult undertaking because as the interaction unfolds it reveals different goals on the part of the prescriber and the patient. Debra also conveys a demanding and overtly adversarial stance toward Dr. Endorf, further undermining any hope of a collaborative undertaking. Debra may very well have a bona fide anxiety disorder that merits treatment, but her inability or unwillingness to follow directions about the safe use of a controlled substance shifts the decision-making process toward a more unilateral effort. Were they to disagree about what constitutes "safe use," SDM also suffers when Dr. Endorf invokes an authoritative stance, or makes reference to other potential ramifications he might incur (such as jeopardizing his license) if he disagreed with her position but still yielded to her request.

For her part, Debra is now mainly lobbying to take more lorazepam as her apparent greater priority over finding an alternative anxiolytic treatment. For his part, Dr. Endorf is now forced into the position of refusing to accede to her wishes, confronting or at least managing her belligerence, and setting aside at least for now their joint effort to alleviate anxiety. When he tries to redirect their focus to the mutual goal of finding a safer alternative potential remedy, she is unengaged, frankly oppositional, and somewhat menacing. Situations such as this one are best dealt with by foreseeing their inevitability and averting them before they occur, to the extent clinicians sense the likelihood of such outcomes. Did Dr. Endorf err the first time he agreed to "make up for the shortfall" of lorazepam? Would a firmer stance then have been better? Or establishing a more explicit verbal if not written contract in which mutually acceptable terms regarding the use of benzodiazepines were established? Some might think that such extreme measures take their own toll on collaborative/SDM work with patients, since they draw attention to a basic sense of mistrust. Did Dr. Endorf skate on thin ice by prescribing benzodiazepines in the first place, in light of the literature casting doubt on the wisdom of using long-term benzodiazepines in patients with borderline personality disorder (Ripoll, 2013)? Or was he perhaps imagining that in an SDM model there would somehow be fewer risks for the playing out of dynamics around power struggles?

Having an *agenda* can also enter the picture when family members or significant others have strongly held concerns or objections about their loved one's behavior or decision-making that the patient themself may not necessarily share. It then sometimes falls to the clinician to play the juror in deciding whose narrative seems more plausible and corresponds to their own perception and interpretation of the symptoms or problems being presented. Clinical Vignette 3.1 in Chapter 3 presents circumstances that bear on this dilemma.

T WHEN PATIENTS JUST WANT TO BE TOLD WHAT TO DO

As progressively appealing as it may seem to invite patients routinely to participate in the decision-making process, there are times when some patients may be uninterested in assuming a collaborative role. Some may feel uncomfortable being asked to "share" responsibility for medical decisions, or feel that the responsibility for exercising medical expertise resides with the clinician alone. Some patients who are invited to offer their opinion on a preferred course of action may feel as perplexed as a surgical patient who was invited to express their preference about the best approach for debulking a vascularized tumor. There is indeed sometimes a fine line between having an expert provide sufficient relevant information about the pros and cons (and evidence base) for (or against) various treatment options and asking patients to make their own technical decisions about complex medical circumstances.

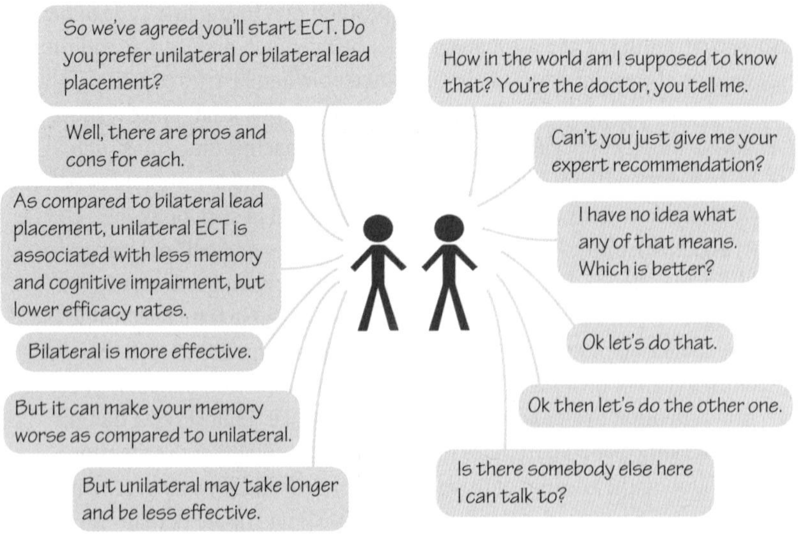

TAKE-HOME POINTS

- The process of shared decision-making strives to accord equal priority to patients' preferences and active role in choosing from among viable treatment options. It should represent a collaborative endeavor between clinician and patient in which each brings their expertise about the clinical condition, and the patient, respectively, to the discussion table
- In SDM, mental health professionals are tasked with providing patients with scientific information about their condition and its appropriate treatments
- Gauge individual patients' degree of interest in playing an active role in treatment decisions, as well as the level of detail with which they prefer to have treatment options and rationales explained to them
- Present risk-benefit analyses of treatment options matter of factly as a necessary component of all treatment decisions, and invite patients to present their own views and priorities when gauging a fair balance
- Patients with diminished decisional capacity, loss of insight or anosognosia, cognitive deficits, or psychosis, may very well be able to play a more limited role in SDM but efforts to engage patients' own preferences and priorities remain an essential component of fostering a sense of patients' agency and autonomy to the extent possible
- Patients with impaired decisional capacity or those receiving treatment over objection may later benefit from developing psychiatric advance directives to articulate their preferences and treatment wishes for purposes of guiding future psychiatric treatment
- SDM has been shown to increase patients' subjective satisfaction in healthcare interactions but studies have not, thus far, demonstrated a significant impact on treatment adherence or other aspects of clinical outcome

References

Appelbaum PS, Grisso T. Assessing patients' capacities to consent to treatment. N Engl J Med 1988; 318: 1635–1638

Berwick DM. A user's manual for the IOM's 'Quality Chasm' report. Health Aff (Millwood) 2002; 21: 80–90

Calabrese JR, Durgam S, Satlin A, et al. Efficacy and safety of lumateperone for major depressive episodes associated with bipolar I or bipolar II disorder: A phase 3 randomized placebo-controlled trial. Am J Psychiatry 2021; 178: 1098–1106

Charles C, Gafni A, Whelan T. Shared decision-making in the medical encounter: What does it mean? (Or it takes at least two to tango). Soc Sci Med 1997; 44: 651–661

Elwyn G, Frosch D, Thomson R, et al. Shared decision making: A model for clinical practice. J Gen Intern Med 2012; 27: 1361–1367

Emanuel EJ, Pearson SD. Physician autonomy and health care reform. JAMA 2012; 307: 367–368

Garriga M, Pacchiarotti I, Kasper S, et al. Assessment and management of agitation in psychiatry. World J Biol Psychiatry 2016; 17: 86–128

Geddes JR, Gardiner A, Rendell J, et al. Comparative evaluation of quetiapine plus lamotrigine combination versus quetiapine monotherapy (and folic acid versus placebo) in bipolar depression (CEQUEL): A 2 × 2 factorial randomised trial. Lancet Psychiatry 2016; 3: 31–39

Gold A, Lichtenberg P. The moral case for the clinical placebo. J Med Ethics 2014; 40: 219–224

Grof P, Duffy A, Cavazzoni P, et al. Is response to prophylactic lithium a familial trait? J Clin Psychiatry 2002; 63: 942–947

Hamann J, Cohen R, Leucht S, et al. Do patients with schizophrenia wish to be involved in decisions about their medical treatment? Am J Psychiatry 2005; 162: 2382–2384

Hamann J, Mendel R, Reiter S, et al. Why do some patients with schizophrenia want to be engaged in medical decision making and others do not? J Clin Psychiatry 2011a; 72: 1636–1543

Hamann J, Mendel R, Meier A, et al. "How to speak to your psychiatrist": Shared decision-making training for inpatients with schizophrenia. Psych Serv 2011b; 62: 1218–1221

Jeste DV, Saks E. Decisional capacity in mental illness and substance use disorders: Empirical database and policy implications. Behav Sci Law 2006; 24: 607–628

Kelley JM, Kaptchuk TJ, Cusin C, et al. Open label placebo for major depressive disorder: A pilot randomized controlled trial. Psychother Psychosom 2012; 81: 312–314

Kemp DE, Ganocy SJ, Brecher M, et al. Clinical value of early partial symptomatic improvement in the prediction of response and remission during short-term treatment trials in 3369 subjects with bipolar I or II depression. J Affect Disord 2011; 130: 171–179

Leucht S, Busch R, Kissling W, et al. Early prediction of antipsychotic nonresponse among patients with schizophrenia. J Clin Psychiatry 2007; 68: 352–360

Makoul G, Clayman ML. An integrative model of shared decision making in medical encounters. Patient Educ Couns 2006; 60: 301–312

Murray H, Wortzel HS. Psychiatric advance directives: Origins, benefits, challenges, and future directions. J Psychiatr Pract 2019; 25: 303–307

Papakostas GI, Perlis RH, Scalia MJ, et al. A meta-analysis of early sustained response rates between antidepressants and placebo for the treatment of major depressive disorder. J Clin Psychopharmacol 2006; 26: 56–60

Pilarinos A, Barker B, Nosova E, et al. Coercion into addiction treatment and subsequent substance use patterns among people who use illicit drugs in Vancouver, Canada. Addiction 2020; 115: 97–106

Pollack MH, Rappaport MH, Fayyad R, et al. Early improvement predicts endpoint remission status in sertraline and placebo treatments of panic disorder. J Psychiatr Res 2002; 36: 229–236

Ripoll L. Psychopharmacologic treatment of borderline personality disorder. Dialogues Clin Neurosci 2013; 15: 213–224

Rosenblat JD, Simon GE, Sachs GS, et al. Factors that impact treatment decisions: Results from an online survey of individuals with bipolar and unipolar depression. Prim Care Companion CNS Disord 2018; 20: 18m02340

Rutherford BR, Wall MM, Brown PJ, et al. Patient expectancy as a mediator of placebo effects in antidepressant clinical trials. Am J Psychiatry 2017; 174: 135–142

Rynn M, Khalid-Kahn S, Garcia-Espana JF, et al. Early response and 8-week treatment outcome in GAD. Depress Anxiety 2006; 23: 461–465

Samara MT, Leucht C, Leeflang MM, et al. Early improvement as a predictor of later response to antipsychotics in schizophrenia: A diagnostic test review. Am J Psychiatry 2015; 172: 617–629

Schwartz RS. The use of ultimatums in psychiatric care. Hosp Comm Psychiatry 1990; 41: 1242–1245

Shay LA, Lafata JE. Where is the evidence? A systematic review of shared decision making and patient outcomes. Med Decis Making 2015; 35: 114–131

Stacey D, Bennett CL, Barry MJ, et al. Decision aids for people facing health treatment or screening decisions. Cochrane Database Syst Rev 2011; 10: CD001431

United States President's Commission. Making Health Care Decisions: A Report on the Ethical and Legal Implications of Informed Consent in the Patient-Practitioner Relationship. Washington DC: President's Commission for the Study of Ethical Problems in Medicine and Biomedical and Behavioral Research, 1982

van der Loos MLM, Mulder PGH, Hartong GThM, et al. Efficacy and safety of lamotrigine as add-on treatment to lithium in bipolar depression: A multicenter, double-blind, placebo-controlled trial. J Clin Psychiatry 2009; 70: 223–231

Weisner C, Hinman A, Lu Y, et al. Addiction treatment ultimatums and US health reform: A case study. Nordik Alkohol Nark 2010; 27: 685–698

Wiersma JE, van Oppen P, van Schaik DJF, et al. Psychological characteristics of chronic depression: A longitudinal cohort study. J Clin Psychiatry 2011; 72: 288–294

Zimmerman M, McGlinchey JB, Posternak MA, et al. Remission in depressed outpatients: More than just symptom resolution? J Psychiatr Res 2008; 42: 797–801

5 Deciding on Appropriate Treatment Modalities: Medication, Psychotherapy, Hospitalization, and Other Levels of Care

LEARNING OBJECTIVES

- ☐ Identify the indications for pharmacotherapy, psychotherapy, and their combination
- ☐ Recognize pharmacological and other treatment endpoints and factors that impact decisions on indefinite versus time-limited interventions
- ☐ Recognize how to match levels of treatment care and intensity with a presenting clinical condition and its vicissitudes over time
- ☐ Understand the unique role of psychotherapeutic interventions when making clinical decisions and formulating treatment plans

Deciding when psychiatric medications or other types of treatments are indicated – and defining precise targets and goals of treatment – is perhaps the most fundamental of all undertakings in clinical psychiatry. As with all medical treatments, clinicians and patients should both have a clear and explicit understanding of what they expect medications, psychotherapy, or other interventions, to do. Medicines do not fix bad relationships or resolve existential dilemmas, but they can equip people with more intact capabilities to solve problems through better concentration and executive functioning, or improve someone's capacity to negotiate stresses with less bias and influence from distorted beliefs or intense emotions. Pharmacotherapy is somewhat analogous to eyeglasses when it comes to driving a car; glasses do not confer driving skills but they can help minimize visual obstructions and improve how the brain processes information in ways that might otherwise prevent someone from making the fullest use of their knowledge about the rules of the road. Psychotherapy constitutes driving lessons.

A DISEASE-MODIFYING VERSUS DISEASE-MANAGING TREATMENTS

Treatment goals ideally should align between clinicians and patients. As noted in Chapter 4, patients' concerns often focus more on psychosocial functioning and interpersonal effectiveness, while clinicians tend to pay more attention to symptom reduction and basic safety and welfare. In one sense, mental health treatments could be dichotomized as either **disease-modifying** or

disease-managing interventions. The former category strives to ameliorate symptoms in the service of eliminating or at least suppressing the outward expression of a medical disorder. Examples of therapies meant to be disease-modifying, or potentially "curative," in nonpsychiatric medical practice include antibiotics to eradicate an infection or antineoplastic therapy aimed to render someone cancer-free. Disease-management models aim to palliate, minimize the impact of symptoms, or suppress the progression of an underlying condition without necessarily eliminating it. Examples here would include antiretroviral therapy for HIV, vesicular monoamine transporter type 2 inhibitors for tardive dyskinesia, pro-cholinergic drugs for dementia, or carbidopa–levodopa for Parkinson's disease. In these instances, stopping the therapy almost inevitably invites the return of symptoms. Decisions about psychiatric treatments, whether pharmacological, psychosocial, or otherwise, are often guided (explicitly or implicitly) by the clinician's intentions and expectations about rendering disease-modifying versus disease-managing remedies.

Tip

The word "palliative" derives from the Latin word *palliare*, meaning, to cloak.

Identifying the goals of treatment, beyond making categorical diagnoses, might involve highlighting key symptoms that can be targeted by specific interventions. Insomnia, anxiety, fatigue, inattention, or suicidal behavior are examples of specific symptoms that sometimes merit uncoupling from a broader overarching diagnosis to represent independent therapeutic objectives, particularly in more treatment-resistant presentations of a given psychiatric disorder. In palliative models of psychiatry, one may at times need to acknowledge that only limited inroads can be made to leverage conditions such as highly treatment-resistant depression, negative symptom schizophrenia, or major cognitive disorders. Reformulating more modest goals of treatment, such as an individual symptom-reduction approach, can be a useful way to minimize demoralization or maintain a sense of hope when disease-modification approaches may not be so feasible.

B SITUATIONAL SITUATIONS AND RECOGNIZING A DIATHESIS

Clinicians and patients alike often question whether symptoms that arise within the context of a particular psychosocial stress warrant pharmacotherapy on the grounds that they may be "situational." Perhaps the two most compelling responses to such questions are: (a) Are the operationally defining features of a pharmacologically responsive psychiatric disorder present (skip ahead to Section D in this chapter)? and (2) Does the "situational" context in which symptoms arise point to an underlying biological predisposition or vulnerability to psychopathology? Stressful situations in and of themselves do not impart inevitable psychopathology, and in fact often yield information about a person's capacity for resilience (that is, the ability to withstand stress without its triggering a psychiatric ailment). Horrific events, or instances of abuse, do not necessarily or automatically cause posttraumatic stress disorder (PTSD) in all trauma survivors unless there exists some biological predisposition or diathesis (see Box 5.1). Factors such as resilience, adaptive coping skills, and strong social supports are known protectants against PTSD (Weisaeth, 1998), and to the contrary, could lead to posttraumatic growth. Grief is a normal emotional response to loss but it can morph into clinical depression if its normal on-and-off waves and sense of loss give way to persistent despair, anhedonia, vegetative signs, feelings of worthlessness, and suicidal thinking.

Box 5.1

The diathesis-stress model in psychiatry

The diathesis-stress model for understanding mental illness refers to the presence of some biological predisposition for psychopathology that becomes activated or evoked in response to a particular kind of environmental stressor. While the etiology of mental illnesses remains unknown and largely speculative, the concept of a recognizable diathesis (e.g., a strong family history for a particular condition) may be a factor that is accorded greater importance in deciding on appropriate psychiatric interventions, particularly when the elements of psychopathology for a given individual are not manifested as a variation on the theme of a recognizable disorder (e.g., highly recurrent depression in someone with a strong family history of bipolar disorder).

Does situational context matter when reasoning through clinical information and making treatment decisions? Of course, but more so as a descriptive than etiological element in understanding the nature of a clinical problem. If someone ran up a flight of stairs and collapsed with a heart attack, nobody would refrain from starting resuscitation measures on the grounds that the heart attack was situationally provoked. Angina can occur spontaneously at rest (i.e., unstable angina) or only upon exertion – making the environment a precipitant rather than a cause. Some people develop shortness of breath and wheezing spontaneously while, for others, asthma is only inducible with exercise, during a respiratory infection (i.e., reactive airway disease), or in response to ragweed in those with the biological vulnerability to hay fever. One would not avoid using a beta-agonist inhaler for "situational" versus spontaneous asthma, or antiemetics if vomiting was situationally provoked by food poisoning.

A useful tenet when making decisions about the appropriateness of pharmacotherapy is to determine whether a medication-responsive condition is recognizably present. That is not so simplistic as it sounds. One of the first steps in clinical assessment is to determine if the "criteria" for a treatment-responsive condition are present (as discussed in Chapter 1, Section C) – in which case, situational context per se may be no more than a nuance. A broken leg is a broken leg is a broken leg regardless of whether it occurred because someone fell, they were pushed, or a spontaneous stress fracture occurred. Orthopedists do not differentially apply leg casts in the clumsy versus the nonclumsy. But, once the limb has been properly tended to, interest can usefully turn to why someone may be prone to falling, or knocking into objects. At that point, the follow-up to casting rightfully involves some exploration of predisposing factors, for which additional clinical decisions and recommendations turn their focus to context and situation. Bob's vulnerability to broken legs may come from his poor vision in a cluttered house, while Mary's may come from osteoporosis coupled with gait instability due to her Parkinson's disease, and poor Ed may have bone cancer without knowing it until he incurs a spontaneous fracture. They all get their legs casted, but then follow different clinical trajectories in order to address their unique underlying predisposing circumstances. Consider the idea that psychotherapy may be the appropriate intervention for someone who has fallen many times and wants to learn how to negotiate treacherous environments more successfully in order to emerge unscathed. More on this a bit later.

Let us consider the example in Clinical Vignette 5.1.

Clinical Vignette 5.1

Arthur was a 51-year-old finance manager with no prior psychiatric history, who became severely depressed and withdrawn after his job was terminated. Nonresponse to escitalopram 20 mg/day was followed by a switch to desvenlafaxine 100 mg/day with adjunctive aripiprazole 5 mg/day as prescribed by his internist, which in turn led to referral to a psychiatrist, Dr. VanderGraaf. The psychiatrist was impressed with a marked degree of apathy and poor relatedness, an unkempt appearance, and a communication style that involved frequent heavy sighs and "I don't know" responses to many questions, with little spontaneous elaboration and an increased latency of response to most questions. Arthur often shifted in his seat and would wring his hands and grimace. Although he denied suicidal thoughts, he expressed deep-seated hopelessness about his future, which Dr. VanderGraaf could not dispel. Arthur wondered aloud if he was being punished for having done something wrong in his life.

Arthur's brother, a social worker, suggested that the desvenlafaxine dose be increased. Arthur's cousin, who works as a pharmaceutical representative for cardiovascular products, asked why he could not just take psychedelic mushrooms. His sister, a yoga instructor, advised that he adopt a healthier lifestyle and have his neurotransmitter levels checked by a holistic doctor. His nephew, a premedical college student, said that psychopharmacology is a trial-and-error process and his uncle just needed to keep trying additional antidepressants until the right one "clicks." The family, and Arthur, were shocked and dismayed when Dr. VanderGraaf advised electroconvulsive therapy (ECT) as "far and away" the treatment of choice. Are you?

Dr. VanderGraaf's mental status description of Arthur portrays someone with agitated depression and possible psychotic features, given the intensity of Arthur's feelings of despair, hopelessness, and belief-conviction around ideas that he is being punished. Decisions about treatment options in the aftermath of nonresponse to two monoaminergic antidepressant trials with low-dose second-generation antipsychotic augmentation place Arthur not only in the category of treatment-resistant depression but, moreover, treatment-resistant depression within a peculiar context. Consider the parameters that enter into the clinical reasoning and decision-making process shown in Table 5.1.

Table 5.1 Decision-making parameters for Arthur

Clinical feature	Treatment implications
Excellent premorbid functioning	Associated with good prognosis and treatment response
First lifetime episode	Looking good!
Good treatment adherence	Arthur is the proverbial boy scout
Absence of comorbid psychiatric or substance use disorders	Still a boy scout
Bipolar diathesis?	Never been manic or hypomanic
Occult medical etiologies?	Euthyroid, normal labs, no exotic travel, no head trauma, rashes, exposures, tick bites, paresthesias, funky autoimmune issues
Late age at onset	Arthur should be better by now
Abrupt onset	Arthur has even more reason to have gotten better by now
Likely presence of emerging psychotic process	Ding-ding-ding! Unrecognized delusional thinking is a common explanation for poor initial treatment response in depression and its presence is missed in at least one-quarter of cases (Rothschild et al., 2008). It carries some sense of particular urgency inasmuch as psychosis confers about a 1.4-fold increased risk for suicide attempts or completions (Huang et al., 2018), and that risk may not be well communicated or obvious.

Beyond the above prognostic characteristics, however, let us explore a little further why Dr. VanderGraaf identified ECT not just as one of several viable treatment options, but rather as the "far and away" most compelling option. The tell-tale signs here would not lie in Arthur's rating scale score for depression, or just in the history of a good-prognosis first-episode patient having an unexpectedly protracted course. The answer lies in what Dr. VanderGraaf saw in the mental status exam: motor agitation; lack of fluency; absence of reciprocal affective connection; perhaps rigid thinking or difficulty shifting sets; and a somewhat guarded degree of spontaneous communication about his internal experience, which appears to involve guilty delusions. The composite of these features paints a picture of a type of depressive illness process that is unique and cries out for an urgent and high-yield intervention.

Now, suppose Arthur did not have likely psychotic or agitated features, but was just persistently depressed despite the prognostic factors in Table 5.1 that tell us he *ought to* have gotten better by now. Rumor has it a famous psychopharmacologist once quipped that a "psychopharmacologist" is a prescriber who uses higher medication doses than everyone else. Would ECT still be "the" preferred treatment? Maybe, maybe not. What credence, if any, belongs to Arthur's brother's suggestion about simply raising his dose of desvenlafaxine?

In this case, as it turns out, not much. For more on that point, skip ahead to Chapter 7, Table 7.2.

C WHEN IS PHARMACOTHERAPY INDICATED?

In mood disorders, treatment guidelines tend to be explicit in recommending clinical indications for pharmacotherapy, for example the American Psychiatric Association practice guideline for the treatment of major depressive disorder (Gelenberg et al., 2010) advocate the use of antidepressant medication for "mild-to-moderate major depressive disorder and definitely should be provided for those with severe major depressive disorder" (p. 17), and the British Association for Psychopharmacology guidelines for the treatment of depression recommend antidepressant medications as "first line treatment for moderate and severe major depression in adults irrespective of environmental factors and depression symptom profile" (Cleare et al., 2015). Antimanic therapy is widely regarded as a necessity to treat bipolar mania or hypomania, and, for bipolar depression, second-generation antipsychotic medications that have antidepressant efficacy are cornerstone therapies (i.e., lurasidone, cariprazine, lumateperone, quetiapine, or olanzapine–fluoxetine combination). Cyclothymia – where neither the highs or the lows are extensive enough to constitute full syndromes – involves a less well-established role for pharmacotherapy.

Antipsychotic therapy is standardly indicated for the treatment of psychotic disorders (schizophrenia, schizoaffective disorder, psychotic mood disorders) but may be less efficacious in variants such as delusional disorder

(González-Rodriguez et al., 2020) or paranoid or schizotypal personality disorders. In more straightforward psychotic disorders such as schizophrenia, in the absence of known treatment resistance, the confidence intervals overlap among most traditional antipsychotic medications (Huhn et al., 2019), meaning that decisional choices from among existing agents probably have more to do with differences in tolerability or idiosyncratic responses seen for a given individual for no particularly identifiable reason. Interestingly, one single-site feasibility-based randomized trial of cognitive–behavioral therapy (CBT; 26 sessions over 6 months) versus antipsychotic medication versus their combination for early-episode psychosis found comparable study retention among groups and no significant differences in positive and negative symptoms over 1 year among CBT-only versus antipsychotic-only recipients (Morrison et al., 2018).

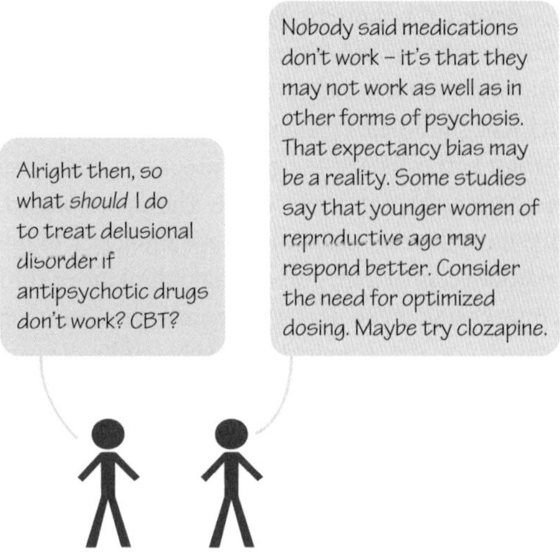

In the case of anxiety disorders, broadly speaking, formal indications for pharmacotherapy relative to other treatment modalities (such as a cognitively based therapy) are not as well established. Practice guidelines often identify patient preference as being an important guiding criterion when making treatment recommendations. For example, in the case of panic disorder, the American Psychiatric Association practice guideline advises that "pharmacotherapy (usually with an SSRI [selective serotonin reuptake inhibitor] or SNRI [serotonin–norepinephrine reuptake inhibitor]) is recommended for patients who prefer this modality or who do not have sufficient time or other resources to engage in psychosocial treatments" and that "combined [treatment modalities] should be considered for patients who have failed to respond to standard monotherapies" (Stein et al., 2010, pp. 11–12).

D ARE ALL MENTAL HEALTH CONDITIONS PHARMACOLOGICALLY RESPONSIVE?

The short answer to the above question is, empirically, nobody could possibly know for sure – but it is helpful to know which conditions, or target symptoms, are more or less likely to be influenced by pharmacological versus psychosocial interventions. From among the 265 diagnoses listed in the DSM-5TR (American

Psychiatric Association, 2022), only a small fraction have been formally studied in clinical pharmacotherapy trials. It should also be noted that the threshold for judging a clinically meaningful pharmacological impact, the magnitude of improvement that defines a "response," often varies across disorders, often with remarkably low expectations. For example, while "response" is generally defined in major depression or bipolar disorder by at least a 50% reduction in measured symptoms, "response" is more often defined by an improvement of only at least 35% in obsessive–compulsive disorder (OCD; Mataix-Cols et al., 2016), ≥30% in PTSD (Varker et al., 2020), and ≥20% in schizophrenia (Leucht, 2014).

From among the major psychiatric disorders for which randomized pharmacotherapy trials exist, a handful of caveats about the role for pharmacotherapy can be drawn, as summarized in Box 5.2.

Box 5.2

Limitations of pharmacotherapy across psychiatric conditions

- In anxiety disorders, panic disorder appears significantly more responsive to CBT than to pharmacotherapy (with a medium between-group effect size of $g = 0.50$) (Roshanaei-Moghaddam et al., 2011); for simple phobias, exposure-based behavioral therapies are widely regarded as the treatment of choice, with a much more limited role, if any, for pharmacotherapy (Choy et al., 2007)
- In PTSD, with only two pharmacotherapies carrying US Food and Drug Administration approval (sertraline and paroxetine) and a limited database otherwise, exposure-based or trauma-focused psychotherapies are considered *the* first-line treatments (Forbes et al., 2010)
- In OCD, pharmacotherapy in general may more effectively target obsessions than compulsions; psychotherapy (specifically, CBT) appears more effective than pharmacotherapy, with a medium effect size of $g = 0.64$ (Cuijpers et al., 2013)
- In eating disorders, pharmacotherapy (SSRIs) appears more effective for bulimia than anorexia (Crow, 2019)
- In mood disorders, lithium has been shown to reduce suicidal behaviors but not necessarily influence suicidal ideation
- In severe personality disorders such as borderline personality disorder, pharmacotherapy demonstrates only very limited symptom-targeted utility: antipsychotic medications may help reduce anger ($g = 0.69$) and cognitive-perceptual symptoms ($g = 0.56$); antidepressant medications have little effect on depressed mood but may modestly improve anger ($g = 0.34$) and anxiety ($g = 0.30$); and mood stabilizers exert a more distinct impact on impulsive-behavioral dyscontrol ($g = 1.51$), anger ($g = 1.33$), and anxiety ($g = 0.80$) (Ingehoven et al., 2010). Practice guidelines tend to advise psychotherapy, rather than pharmacotherapy, as the core treatment of borderline personality disorder (Oldham et al., 2001)

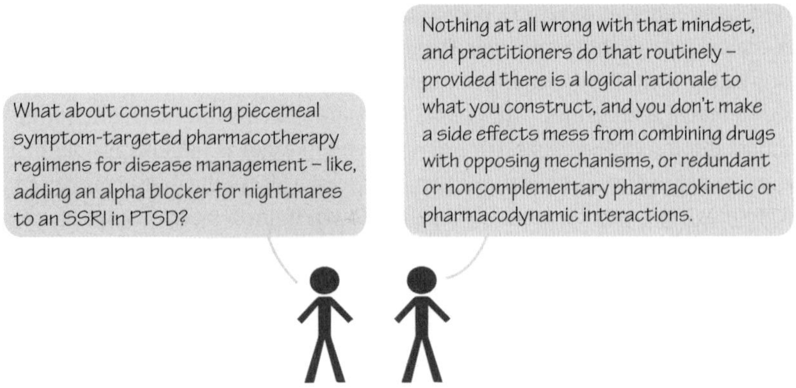

E WHEN IS PSYCHOTHERAPY INDICATED?

It may surprise some readers to learn that the differences in outcomes between pharmacotherapy and structured psychotherapies – at least in the case of depression or anxiety – are not so vast as one might imagine. Patient preference for one modality relative to another has considerable bearing on treatment efficacy (Cuijpers et al., 2021). Collectively for all depressive and anxiety disorders, a meta-analysis of 67 randomized trials involving 5,993 subjects found essentially no significant difference in the magnitude of effect between pharmacotherapy and psychotherapy ($g = 0.02$) (Cuijpers et al., 2013), although pharmacotherapy emerged in that meta-analysis as having a significantly greater effect than psychotherapy for the treatment of dysthymia ($g = 0.30$). In schizophrenia and other primary psychotic disorders, cognitively based therapies yield relatively small effects on core symptoms and functioning (Laws et al., 2018).

Even when the identified main focus of treatment is "medication management" – where visits may be briefer and not as regular and frequent as might occur in a formal psychotherapy – so-called "common factors" behind psychotherapeutic principles (Laska et al., 2014), such as establishing a therapeutic alliance, maintaining empathy, validating a patient's perspective and emotional experience, and setting reasonable expectations, nevertheless often become an integral part of a successful treatment outcome.

Beyond psychoeducation about disease states, psychotherapies address an interpersonal component of how people engage, build resilience, make decisions, and manage stresses. In that respect, treatment decisions to incorporate psychotherapeutic principles, above and beyond pharmacotherapy or psychoeducational counseling, include circumstances such as those listed in Box 5.3.

Box 5.3

Clinical circumstances in which psychotherapy may be uniquely beneficial

- The presence of strong interpersonal factors that bear on the presence of mood or anxiety symptoms
- Resolving issues of psychological conflict or ambiguity
- Dealing with past trauma as it affects the here and now
- A poor capacity to tolerate negative affect states or feelings of distress
- When formal diagnoses are truly ambiguous
- The need to develop enhanced coping strategies for managing life adversities or chronic medical/psychiatric conditions

F WHEN SHOULD PSYCHOTHERAPY BE CONSIDERED AS AN AUGMENTATION TO PHARMACOTHERAPY?

At first glance, one might think that psychotherapy could or should always be considered as a useful adjunctive treatment modality for just about anybody who is taking a psychotropic medication. After all, who would not benefit from talking in depth about their experiences and emotional reactions to stressful life events, particularly if a condition such as depression or anxiety in itself constitutes a life stress above and beyond the occurrence of adverse life circumstances? A more nuanced distinction for purposes of devising a treatment plan may involve the role of implementing a formal psychotherapy program as opposed to borrowing from psychotherapeutic principles in the course of prescribing a treatment that more formally consists of prescribing medications. Consider as an analogy the management of Type II diabetes: a diabetologist would be remiss to simply write prescriptions for oral hypoglycemics or insulinmimetics and tell someone just to go get their laboratory work checked every 6 months, paying no attention to the broader behavioral and lifestyle context in which diabetes exists. What some might call "medical counseling" bears analogy to the psychoeducational component of all psychotherapies.

From an evidence-based standpoint, and perhaps contrary to popular perception, combined pharmacotherapies and psychotherapies may not routinely yield better outcomes than either modality alone. In the case of anxiety disorders, for example, one meta-analysis of 26 randomized trials found no evidence of superiority for combined pharmacotherapy plus psychotherapy over either individual treatment approach (Black, 2006), although other studies present more optimistic findings about combination therapies (Cuijpers et al., 2014). Similarly, for adult attention deficit–hyperactivity disorder (ADHD), short-term (10–12 week) randomized trial data have shown no advantage in symptom improvement for stimulant therapy combined with CBT as compared to stimulant therapy alone (Corbisiero et al., 2018).

Psychotherapeutic interventions may become especially useful for people who grapple with negative affect states or life adversities but for whom the quest for making "the" diagnosis (with implications that "the" right treatment will render a dramatic transformative benefit) may be an unrealistic expectation – as illustrated for Stephanie in Clinical Vignette 5.2.

Clinical Vignette 5.2

Stephanie was a 47-year-old recently divorced self-employed woman, who had previously been diagnosed with dysthymic disorder, an unspecified anxiety disorder, and adult ADHD. She had been treated off and on for many years mainly with SSRIs and benzodiazepines as well as stimulants, with little benefit but no obvious iatrogenic detriment. In the aftermath of a contentious divorce, she found herself increasingly irritable and impatient, snapping at friends and alienating clients. After a new psychiatrist wondered if she might "be bipolar" she was prescribed a succession of second-generation antipsychotic medications, lithium, and lamotrigine with no obvious benefit. Yet another consultant suggested that her symptom profile did not so neatly conform to the diagnosis of bipolar disorder or major depression but noted that her moods reacted strongly to emotionally provocative situations and she had great difficulty coping and maintaining a sense of emotional composure when stressed. She became dismayed that "the right" drug was not being found to help her and began leaving short but frequent phone messages to her psychiatrist reporting that she felt "awful" soon after appointments occurred and new medication plans were discussed, but it was unclear what response she was seeking other than a plea to feel less distressed.

Stephanie is running the risk of accruing an ad infinitum pharmacopoeia coupled with a sense of demoralization that the remedy for her sense of suffering may not lie either in the clinching of a definitive diagnosis or in the form of any pharmaceutical product. The delicate balance for her, particularly after she has experienced little or no relief after multiple appropriate pharmacotherapy efforts targeting dysphoria and mood instability, involves the two-fold task of not altogether abandoning pharmacology as a potentially useful tool but at the same time redirecting her away from overvalued ideas that the solution to her problems will be as easily solved by pharmacology as if her diagnosis was strep throat in need of an antibiotic. When it was suggested to Stephanie that augmenting her pharmacologically oriented treatment with a psychotherapy that could enhance her coping skills – namely, dialectical behavior therapy (DBT) – she bristled and said she was "talked out" from previous therapies and skeptical that "another round" of talk therapy would do much for her, insisting that there "had to be" a right medicine for her.

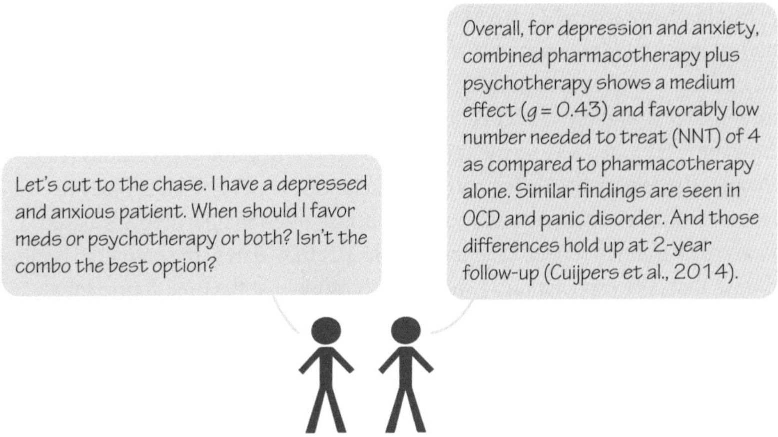

G PSYCHODYNAMICALLY INFORMED PHARMACOTHERAPY

Psychodynamic principles involve recognizing likely motivators for behavior for which patients themselves may not have conscious awareness. In the vintage 1950s psychoanalytic literature, Bibring (1954) identified five basic therapeutic techniques that nowadays still hold value for describing the actions that psychotherapists of all stripes carry out to varying degrees, noted in Box 5.4.

Box 5.4

Basic psychotherapeutic techniques

(a) **Suggestion** - overt statements or recommendations that point out factual realities and forecast the consequences of a course of action (e.g., "If you take this medication, you might feel less sad and worried"); or, advice-giving (e.g., "See what happens if you stop smoking marijuana for a week")

(b) **Abreaction** - an emotional reaction caused by exposure to something that evokes recall of a past emotionally difficult experience (cf. **catharsis**, which pertains to the emotional release of thoughts or feelings that were outside of someone's conscious awareness)

(c) **Manipulation** - statements or actions intended deliberately to prompt a responsive behavior

(d) **Clarification** - reflecting back the essence of a patient's words to affirm that their intended meaning has come across, or resolve any points of confusion or ambiguity

(e) **Interpretation** - offering a hypothesis to explain a psychologically driven reason or meaning behind a thought, feeling, or behavior that may not be obvious

Psychopharmacologists, whether they realize it or not, often have particular interest in (a) and (c), inasmuch as they strive to forecast how someone might feel after taking a medication, exploit placebo effects through suggestibility, minimize nocebo effects, and provide direction and instruction. Elements of manipulation come into play when setting the stage for pharmacodynamic expectations (e.g., "People who experience dissociation with ketamine tend to be more likely to have an antidepressant response"; or, by contrast, offering up a defiance-based paradoxical injunction (see Chapter 3, Table 3.2) that "dares" the patient to improve in ways that defy expectations – such as forecasting that the time course for judging improvement with clozapine could be 6–9 months or even longer (and any improvements that might occur sooner will be imbued with miraculous overtones). Decisions about pharmacotherapy options may yield different results depending on the ways in which suggestion and manipulation are brought into play.

How can clinicians best decide when a formal recommendation for psychotherapy is appropriate? And, for that matter, from the standpoint of theoretical orientations, one might imagine that there should exist a database pointing to the value of one particular modality of psychotherapy over another in the context of certain symptoms. This certainly makes intuitive sense; one would suppose that CBT, for example, would be a logical modality when patients show patterns of thinking that reflect negative biases about their own attributes and their expectations for what happens to them in their worldly interactions. One would think that DBT would be especially relevant for situations in which someone has trouble tolerating frustrations or self-regulating their emotional reactions to situations or interactions with others that cause them to feel intensely upset or distressed. Psychodynamic psychotherapy would presumably hold greatest relevance for situations in which someone wants to better understand the driving forces that lead them to make unsatisfying life decisions, or repeat patterns in their relationship choices or professional strivings that could be self-sabotaging or self-defeating. Trauma-focused therapies such as exposure therapy would make the most sense when the nature of current problems involves elements of autonomic hyperarousal and high emotional reactivity in the traceable aftermath of a discernible, tangible traumatic event. Couples' or family-based psychotherapies would seem logical when the context of problems revolves around discord within relationships such that the relationship itself is the patient.

There are few direct comparative studies of one psychotherapy modality versus another for a given condition. (Perhaps that reflects assumptions that there are enough "common factors" across different psychotherapies to make their comparative efficacies subtle.) Major depression may represent the best-studied such example. One meta-analysis comparing short-term CBT versus interpersonal therapy, involving 7 trials with 741 subjects, found no significant differences in symptom reductions (e.g., using the Hamilton Rating Scale for Depression) (Jakobsen et al., 2012).

Apart from studying changes in affective symptoms per se, little attention has been paid to examining the "fit" between differential psychotherapy modalities and the psychological circumstances or contexts with which patients present for treatment. We offer some initial thoughts to facilitate thinking about differential psychotherapeutic approaches in Table 5.2.

Table 5.2 Examples of psychotherapy modalities and their likely differential indications

Psychotherapy modality	Core tenets	Modality would seem most appropriate when …
Cognitive-behavioral therapy	Identify and challenge distorted beliefs and attitudes	Symptoms involve ideas and beliefs that may reflect biased perceptions of experiences
Dialectical behavior therapy	Learn skills for distress tolerance, emotional self-regulation, mindfulness, and interpersonal effectiveness	Problems exist with modulating emotions, impulses, self-harming behaviors
Interpersonal therapy	Understand how current relationships and social context contribute to symptoms	Managing a significant life change such as the death of a loved one, a role transition (e.g., retirement or job loss, divorce, geographic relocation), relationship conflicts or social isolation
Exposure therapy	A behavioral desensitization approach that involves gradual exposure to the stimuli that evoke anxiety or distress	Eliminating phobias, managing present-day anxiety or autonomic hyperarousal caused by past traumatic experiences
Psychodynamic therapy	Explore unconscious motivations or conflicts that may lead to low satisfaction in work and social endeavors	Experiencing a sense of loss of meaning in life, coming to terms emotionally with anxiety-provoking experiences, seeking to develop more satisfying relationships or work efforts
Acceptance and commitment therapy	Accept, rather than eliminate, negative emotions in favor of behaviors that pursue greater value and meaning	Enhancing psychological flexibility around conditions such as depression, anxiety, OCD, eating disorders
Mindfulness-based cognitive therapy	Draw someone's conscious attention to their thoughts, emotions, and visceral sensations in the present moment without judgments or distractions about their implications or consequences	Managing and tolerating symptoms of depression, anxiety, chronic pain, or other persistent medical problems, improving stress reduction skills

H PSYCHOTHERAPY AS A PREFERRED INTERVENTION WHEN MEDICATIONS PROVE UNHELPFUL

Psychotherapy in and of itself is likely to be as helpful at any point in the overall course of a persistent psychiatric disorder (cf. some medications that may be more efficacious when introduced early rather than late in the illness course, such as lithium for the prevention of recurrences in bipolar disorder (Gelenberg et al., 1989)). While psychotherapy can be used as a first-line treatment in some conditions, and certainly should not be thought of as a measure of desperation or defeat when medications prove unsuccessful, there are a number of psychotherapy modalities that are structured around the management of chronic health and/or mental health conditions, such as mood or anxiety or psychotic disorders that fail to respond to multiple appropriate pharmacotherapy interventions. Skip ahead to Chapter 8, Table 8.4, and Figure 8.5, to obtain more clinical context for scenarios such as this.

Acceptance and commitment therapy, as noted in Table 5.2 and further depicted in Figure 5.1, may particularly lend itself to treatment approaches in which optimal coping and stress relief demand a kind of radical acceptance of life adversities – including the physical and psychological limitations imposed

Figure 5.1 The "hexaflex" model of acceptance and commitment therapy

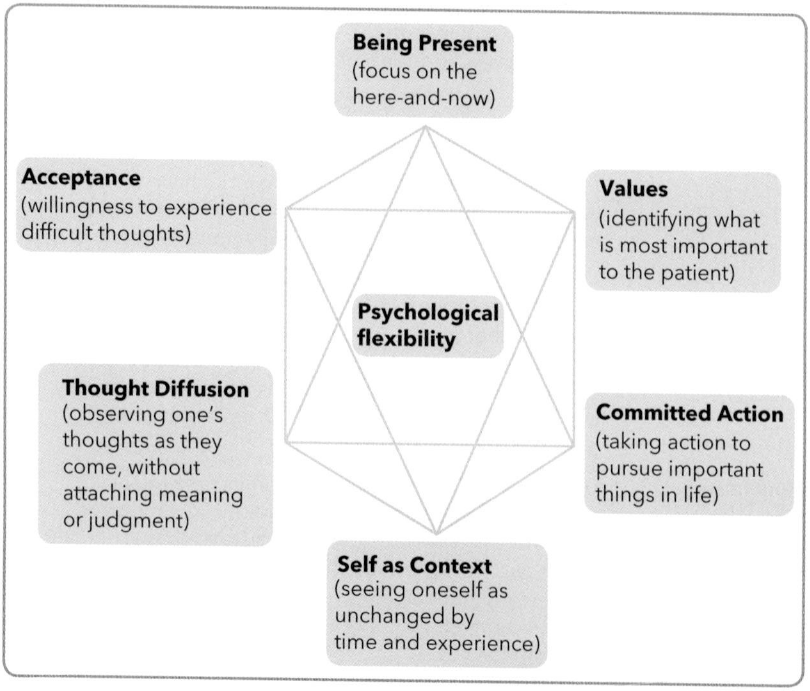

by chronic medical or mental health disorders. A basic premise is that efforts to *eliminate* a particular adversity are not so likely to be successful, and having one's emotional resources consumed on an untenable path becomes counterproductive to any kind of mental health recovery. How does one then learn to effectively live with symptoms that are not so likely to go away, at least any time soon? Integrating acceptance and commitment therapy concepts into pharmacotherapy does not necessarily mean abandoning pharmacological efforts, but it typically does mean relegating pharmacotherapy to a secondary or subsidiary role as the goals of treatment become more starkly revised toward disease management rather than disease modification. The case of Helen in Clinical Vignette 5.3 illustrates these concepts for managing residual symptoms after aggressive pharmacotherapy for major depression.

Clinical Vignette 5.3

Helen was a 43-year-old woman with chronic depression who had had incomplete responses to a large number of adequate and optimized pharmacotherapy trials, including intravenous ketamine, repetitive transcranial magnetic stimulation (TMS), and ECT. Her condition largely improved after the addition of tranylcypromine dosed up to 90 mg/day in conjunction with quetiapine 150 mg at night but she nevertheless had residual initial and middle insomnia. Her sleep problems did not improve with various trials and combinations of "Z"-drugs, benzodiazepines, ramelteon, trazodone, and dual orexin receptor antagonists, all in conjunction with proper sleep hygiene. Tranylcypromine dosing was shifted to predominantly morning administration to minimize its risk for exacerbating insomnia. Higher doses of quetiapine produced daytime lethargy and cognitive dulling without improving sleep continuity. There was no suggestion of sleep apnea, restless legs, or another independent sleep disorder, although the suggestion was made for obtaining an independent sleep study, which she felt would not be helpful. A trial of CBT for insomnia was recommended as one of the "last remaining therapeutic options" to target persistent insomnia. Denise expressed disappointment and dismay that there was not a pill she could take to further improve her sleep problems but said she was "open-minded" about "going for more therapy."

I DECISION-MAKING IN THE SETTING OF SHAKY TREATMENT ADHERENCE

"Adequate" medication adherence is defined by some experts as taking at least 80% of one's medications as properly prescribed. Poor or inconsistent adherence is a ubiquitous problem across most psychiatric disorders for wide-ranging reasons; Box 5.5 cites a number of commonly recognized causes of poor adherence broadly mentioned within the peer-reviewed literature, with varying reasons holding greater or lesser applicability across specific diagnoses.

Box 5.5

Common reasons for poor medication adherence across psychiatric disorders

- Poor drug tolerability
- Feeling one has insufficient information about a disease state to make an informed decision about the need for medications
- Mistrust of the clinician or their knowledge base
- Fear that continued medication use will cause harm
- Unawareness (or lack of interest) in strategies to manage adverse effects
- Complex dosing regimens
- Cost
- Forgetting
- Fear of the need for laboratory monitoring/bloodwork and its potential consequences
- Feeling that medication is unnecessary or no longer needed
- Curiosity about the effects of stopping
- Missing some aspect of how they felt before medications (e.g., hypomania)
- Acting out some sense of defiance in the therapeutic relationship, or another important relationship

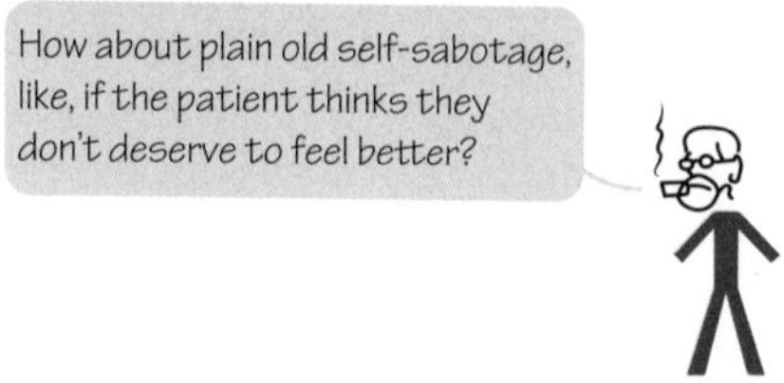

Tip

In the setting of relapse after an initial therapeutic success, assume nonadherence as an explanation until proven otherwise.

When making treatment decisions for patients with historically poor adherence, one could always opt to favor medications with long half lives (e.g., aripiprazole, with a half-life of about 75 hours, or vortioxetine, with a half-life of about 66 hours), or compounds with active metabolites that have long half-lives (e.g., fluoxetine, whose active metabolite norfluoxetine has a half-life of 7–15 days; or cariprazine, whose didesmethylated active metabolite has a half-life of 1–3 weeks). Long-acting injectable antipsychotics offer another pharmacokinetic strategy for managing poor adherence. Therapeutic drug-monitoring, or pill counts, are other obvious concrete strategies for detecting nonadherence. Are there other behavioral or psychotherapeutic strategies for tackling poor adherence? We offer several approaches in Box 5.6.

Box 5.6

Nonpharmacological strategies for managing poor medication adherence

- Normalize and even predict the experience in nonjudgmental, matter-of-fact terms. For example: "Many people miss doses of medication for a variety of reasons. How often would you say that happens to you?"
- Invite the patient to raise any thoughts they might have about stopping a medication as a point of discussion before taking matters into their own hands
- Invite the patient's speculation about what they envision as best- and worst-case outcomes in the coming weeks and months if they opt to forgo medications
- Pose nonadherence as a complex, multideterminate phenomenon unto itself; invite the patient's own speculation about reasons for missing doses
- Engage in a partnership by asking the patient if they are aware of any ways to make it easier for them to take medications more consistently (such as reducing the number of medications or trying to simplify regimens)

Pharmacological decision-making requires an assessment of the patient's ability and willingness to assume the role of a responsible partner – which may be untenable in someone with diminished capacity to participate in their own care at that level. It is a big ask for a dementia patient, or someone with a chronic formal thought disorder, to properly follow a medication regimen, and doing so may even be disingenuous on the part of the clinician if they fail to appreciate the patient's own cognitive or other limitations that preclude their ability to participate on such a level. Engaging a family member of other trusted designee to oversee medication administration or laboratory monitoring may be the only viable alternative. For patients who may be more unwilling than unable to participate responsibly in end-organ monitoring, the challenge may be greater. Patients taking lithium who cannot or will not obtain periodic laboratory work to monitor renal and thyroid function place both themselves and the clinician at risk for a poor outcome, especially if drug dosing is near the higher end of the therapeutic index. A shared decision (and shared risk) approach may be the only way to engage someone in such a collaboration ("We need you to follow up with laboratory work in order to safely take this medicine; otherwise, I won't be able to continue to prescribe it, and the alternative options might not be as effective.") If the preferred agent is one for which viable alternatives exist, it may be easier to sidestep the issue (for example, switching lithium to divalproex, where end-organ monitoring (i.e., hepatic function) may be less critical).

Let us now shift our attention to a few specific clinical scenarios in which clinical decision-making requires a nuanced and delicate appreciation of parameters that impact pharmacotherapy, psychotherapy, and levels of appropriate care.

J MANAGING CHRONIC VERSUS ACUTE SUICIDAL IDEATION

Clinical circumstances that surround longstanding suicidal thoughts are often fundamentally different than those which contribute to the emergence of new or acute suicidal thinking. How so? Longstanding suicidal thoughts in the absence of suicidal behaviors may reflect a stable and even organizing kind of psychological equilibrium state for some people. Empirical studies on chronic suicidal ideation are not extensive but suggest that it may bear some relation to obsessive thinking rather than self-directed aggression (Garakani et al., 2022). Some people may also take a kind of perverse comfort from the presence of suicidal thinking, in that it does represent a last stronghold for maintaining an internal locus of control ("If things ever really got bad enough, I and I alone can always be the one to bring about an ultimate end to a sense of suffering"). While suicidal ideation is often recognized as a precursor to suicidal behaviors (De Leo et al., 2005), chronic stable thoughts are neither synonymous with nor inevitably linked to actions that pose an immediate actual safety risk. Decisions about managing chronic suicidal ideation might therefore usefully focus on whether or not a change has occurred in the existing equilibrium state (i.e., how are the thoughts different in quality or severity as compared to their usual baseline presence? Are new or additional elements present (such as alcohol or substance use) that might increase the probability of acting impulsively on an otherwise stable chronic set of thoughts?)

Acute suicidal ideation, by contrast, is a departure from a stable equilibrium state. It connotes the potential for volatility and, by definition, comes with no track record in a given individual for how they are inclined to manage (that is, not necessarily act upon) ideas about self-destruction. As such, both the assessment and management of new acute suicidal ideation carry a level of urgency and possible emergent decision-making that is often fundamentally different from chronic suicidal ideation.

Longstanding suicidal thoughts without meaningful precedent for someone acting on them invite the opportunity for dialogue, beyond using interview time to conduct sheer safety assessments. Does the person have an idea about what suicide would accomplish? Do they really mean that they want to cause their own death, or are they invoking suicide language as a kind of shorthand communication for other ideas or feelings, such as anger about a situation or rage toward another person in their lives, through indirect expression? Is there a sense of demoralization that could be more directly addressed? Undertreated depression obviously warrants scrupulous consideration in the setting of chronic suicidal thinking, but the strategic approaches to its management may not be confined to (or necessarily even based mainly around) pharmacotherapy rather than psychosocial interventions.

K THE NEED FOR A HIGHER LEVEL OF CARE

A fundamental component of clinical decision-making that is often underappreciated, and not always addressed as explicitly as it perhaps should be, is gauging what level of care is most appropriate for a given patient at a given time for a given psychiatric problem. Sometimes this is patently obvious, as in the need for hospitalization (either voluntary or involuntary) after a serious suicide attempt or when someone is gravely impaired and unable to take care of themselves. Or the role for sober living after time spent in rehab after time spent in acute detoxification from alcohol and sedative–hypnotic use disorder. Other times, shades of gray complicate the decision-making process, or mislead a clinician into thinking that the decision-making process is confined solely to assessing whether psychotropic medications should be begun or altered in an existing regimen. Consider the situation in Clinical Vignette 5.4.

Clinical Vignette 5.4

Tara was a 27-year-old unemployed single woman living with a roommate, who left nursing school a year ago and had carried a diagnosis of recurrent depression since college. She was taking an SNRI plus bupropion and was in a weekly cognitively based psychotherapy. In the context of the break-up of a relationship she experienced a worsening of depression that involved crying spells, hopeless feelings, spending excessive time lying in bed and/or sleeping, and reduced attention to her physical self-care (not bathing or brushing her teeth for a week) but adamantly denied suicidal thoughts or other kinds of serious threats to her physical well-being. A decision was made to increase the dose of her existing medication. Now what?

Should Tara continue as is in her weekly psychotherapy? Should the therapist be consulted about increasing the frequency of visits at Tara's discretion? Or should some mental health homework projects be devised to engage her between appointments? Should she go find a break-up support group? Should she be told to go to the emergency room if she starts to feel suicidal, in the belief that she would follow through with that suggestion? She has little structure in her day – does that mean her medication adjustments should occur more frequently or aggressively? Probably not; but what if she does not or cannot follow through on the suggestion to impose more structure in her day and increase her physical activity level (that is, *behavioral activation*, in the parlance of CBT)? When should Tara's psychiatrist suggest they next meet, or should he leave that decision up to Tara as an expression validating her autonomy?

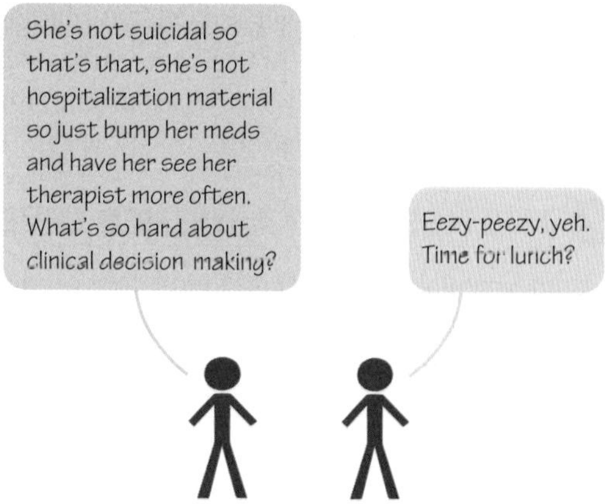

A pertinent element in Tara's case is that she is being treated by a team (her psychiatrist and her nonpsychiatrist psychotherapist) rather than by an individual. How much, and how often, if at all, should they be conferring about her, both at present and as a more general rule? Consider that if Tara's therapist meets with Tara and then calls the psychiatrist to "report" on the appointment, the transaction can be viewed rather delicately on different levels: in one sense, their communication can be beneficial to assure that both clinicians are equally informed about circumstances, or technical details, which involve risk for the welfare of their mutual patient (analogous to the surgeon communicating with the anesthesiologist); another level is to coordinate roles and responsibilities and avoid duplication of efforts, and assure that each party has the same intel and the heard stories align; but, on another level, delegating Tara's therapist to be her agent as the person to communicate with the psychiatrist about her status also places Tara in a passive and possibly infantilized role. Is Tara not able to share pertinent information herself directly with her psychiatrist? And, if not, is that because Tara is so impaired or distorted in her perception of things that the therapist does not, or should not, trust the reliability of Tara's direct communication (for instance, if Tara might be psychotic; or steeped in denial about her condition; or prone to minimization in ways that may not be so transparent)? We think she is cognitively intact enough to convey her own narrative fairly accurately. Is Tara's therapist falling into a trap of enactment as her rescuer, tacitly communicating that Tara is incapable of relaying information as part of her own self-care, and instead having the therapist do Tara's bidding for her when the content of her plight more rightfully falls under Tara's own jurisdiction?

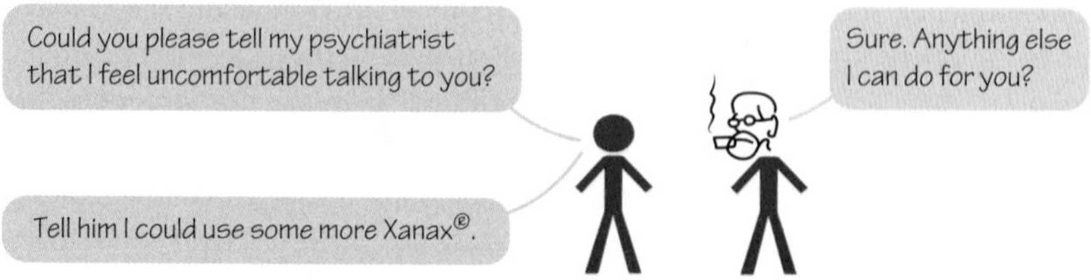

Critical in the decision-making process in scenarios such as this is knowing how synchronous or asynchronous both clinicians are in their assessment of Tara's situation with respect to the fundamental nature of the problem, its urgency, how best to respond to urgency, how to assess and manage shared risk, and how roles in the treatment plan become delegated. Splitting becomes a real risk if the team is uncoordinated in the choreography of its joint movements.

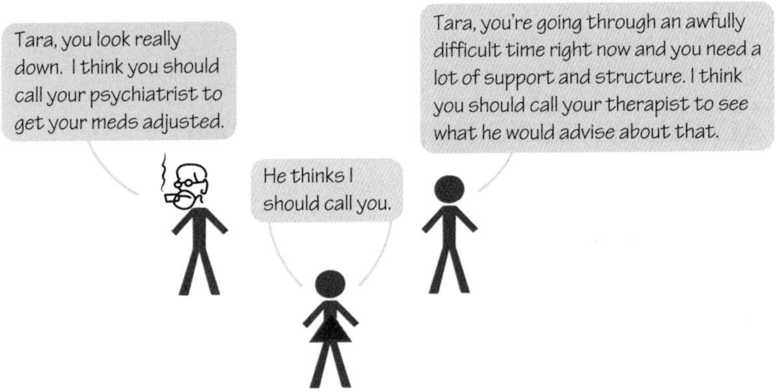

Clinical Vignette 5.4 Continued

Five days after seeing her psychiatrist, Tara failed to keep an appointment with her therapist and did not respond to phone calls or text messages from her therapist. The therapist had no emergency contact information for Tara so she called Tara's psychiatrist, who in turn tried calling Tara to no avail. On the Friday afternoon that Tara's roommate went home to visit her parents, Tara overdosed on a full bottle of acetaminophen. Her body was discovered by her roommate in their apartment, who immediately called the emergency services, when she returned home Sunday night. Paramedics who arrived on the scene called the medical examiner's office when they found her body pulseless, lifeless, stiff, and cold. No suicide note was found.

Was there a missed *tell* in Tara's original assessment? Was she in fact not suicidal when her psychiatrist saw her, but then became so afterward? But Tara denied suicidal ideation, one might say. Was she lying? If she had no previous history of a suicide attempt, and if there was no (known) substance use in the picture, it could be argued that the decision to do no more than was initially done conformed to all the available data at the time, despite the unfortunate catastrophic outcome. A review of 22 studies found that 50% of people with suicidal thoughts deny having them, as do 50% of suicide completers and 30% of suicide attempters during the preceding month (Obegi, 2021).

There is no way to predict suicide attempts or completions, and if clinicians rounded up and detained everyone with depressed mood who expressed any form of suicidal thinking (or, as in Tara's case, denied suicidal thinking but presented with sufficient levels of interpersonal or other psychosocial stress that we are not *entirely* surprised by the catastrophic outcome of events), there would be almost no further decision-making to undertake, just custodial retention. Even if Tara had been hospitalized, there is a high likelihood her inpatient stay would have been short and not necessarily equipped her with better tools to manage her feelings or impulses after discharge.

L ALTERNATIVES TO HOSPITALIZATION

So-called "medical necessity," or grounds for inpatient hospitalization, nowadays tends to revolve around clinical situations involving either an imminent risk to a patient's own safety or the safety of others (note that if Tara denied suicidal thinking in an emergency room she quite likely would have been discharged and offered a less restrictive outpatient treatment, such as a crisis management appointment). Grounds for hospitalization also arise when patients are gravely impaired, as evidenced by marked inattention to self-care, eating, hygiene, toileting, getting out of bed, and essentially being able to perform basic normal everyday tasks. The decision to hospitalize someone has evolved from what was once a potential long-term (weeks to months) proposition to a much shorter undertaking that tends to be geared more toward crisis resolution and redirection to more intermediate levels of care such as partial hospital or day treatment programs. Hospitalization makes sense when someone's condition has not improved (or has deteriorated) despite less-structured or restrictive levels of care. In someone who presents emergently with a high level of acuity and severity, particularly with a significant level of risk, efforts to avert hospitalization may become heroic. Viable alternatives to hospitalization – such as crisis intervention services – may be more feasible when the patient is already receiving treatment in an established relationship with a mental health clinician. Hospitalization tends not to be so compelling an option when there is reason to think someone is unlikely to benefit from being hospitalized, or if the nature of their psychopathology is such that they may become more regressed in their behavior and level of self-care in a hospital setting. Nonhospitalization options also may be preferable when there may be an alternative specific modality for treatment that could be more easily procured outside of an inpatient treatment setting, which is not superseded by the need for closely supervised monitoring, as illustrated in Clinical Vignette 5.5.

Clinical Vignette 5.5

Maria was a 57-year-old divorced woman with chronic depression and borderline personality disorder, who experienced chronic suicidal thinking, with several lifetime instances of suicide gestures (most often overdoses on relatively small quantities of medications that led to no medical repercussions). When she felt overwhelmed with suicidal thoughts, she would at times call her psychiatrist and ask if she should present to a psychiatric emergency department, and had had several brief hospitalizations, which generally led to a reconstitution of her functioning without any changes in pharmacology, although her chronic depression generally persisted through such times. On one such occasion of intensified suicidal thinking her psychiatrist actively dissuaded her from presenting to an emergency room and instead made arrangements for her to receive intravenous ketamine from a colleague within 24 hours of her outreach. Subsequently, Maria noted a marked improvement in mood and rapid reduction in the frequency and intensity of suicidal thinking within 24 hours of a first dose of ketamine.

Maria's case differentiates the notion of a decision to hospitalize someone for purposes of safekeeping versus providing them access to a treatment specific for their ailment. ECT counts as a good example that straddles this decision-making fence, as when someone who is depressed and gravely impaired may warrant inpatient admission and ECT is one of several viable treatment options that happens to often be more accessible most expeditiously through an inpatient than outpatient point of entry to a healthcare system. To pursue newer high-potency treatments that are typically outpatient-based, such as intravenous ketamine or theta-burst TMS, hospitalization may currently represent an obstacle to care.

Which patients further decompensate, psychologically regress, or otherwise clinically worsen in an inpatient hospital setting (making it wiser to pursue alternative high levels of care)? Clinical lore has long been that this description pertains to individuals with borderline personality disorder, or potentially those with other (e.g., dependent) personality disorders on the assumption that prolonged hospitalization is at cross purposes with fostering someone's sense of autonomy and competence to negotiate life stresses in a less-protected environment. Hospital settings that provide highly structured psychotherapeutic programs (such as intensive DBT) may lessen that dichotomy. They can help to refocus treatment-plan decisions more toward the delivery of high-intensity therapeutic interventions rather than simply the idea of 24/7 monitoring and potential nominal changes to a pharmacology regimen that may take weeks to gauge pharmacodynamic effects.

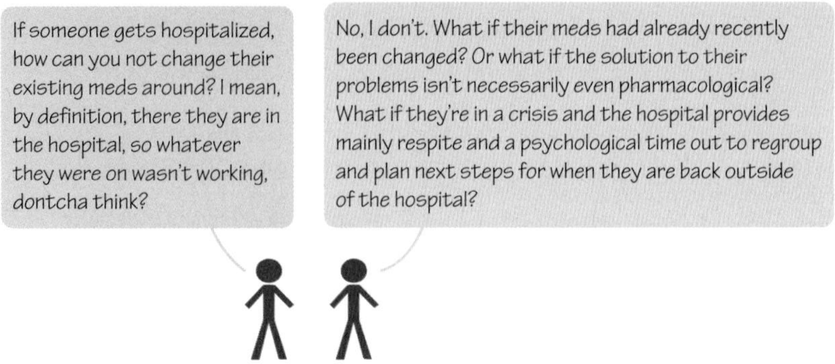

M IT TAKES A VILLAGE

How does a clinician decide when a treatment team is more appropriate than treatment via an individual clinician? The degree of intensity, and extent of personnel, best involved in treating a mental health condition largely depends on the level of symptom severity and functional disability caused by the problem itself. Much the way an intensive care unit with round-the-clock professional staffing is vital for life-threatening medical conditions, so too does matching the proper level of care with the magnitude and severity of a mental health problem. Box 5.7 summarizes levels of mental healthcare by increasing levels of intensity

Box 5.7

Increasing levels of care based on symptom severity and functional impairment

- Self-help books or online courses or information sites
- Self-help support groups
- Digital apps
- Peer support coaching
- Counseling services
- Individual and/or group psychotherapy
- Medication management (with or without psychotherapy)
- Crisis outreach programs (mobile crisis units)
- Intensive outpatient programs
- Day treatment programs
- Partial hospital programs
- Intensive community-based support services (e.g., assertive community treatment programs)
- Hospitalization
- Residentially based long-term care facilities

(and degrees of restrictiveness) as well as the extent to which individuals continue to live independently in the community versus within a supportive living setting such as a hospital or residential facility.

Some serious forms of mental illness require long-term residentially based treatment because no known pharmacological or other behavioral intervention has been shown to afford a sufficient level of symptom manageability to allow for safe independent living in the community. Consider the example in Clinical Vignette 5.6.

Clinical Vignette 5.6

Valerie was a 22-year-old unemployed woman who had dropped out of college, stating she had no idea what she wanted to do with her life. She reported a history of longstanding emotional abuse from her parents while growing up and as an adult tended to have tumultuous and unsustained relationships with friends or potential romantic partners. When upset, she would make suicide gestures by tying an electric cord around her neck or cutting her arms longitudinally with a razor, occasioning multiple trips to the emergency department for suturing of lacerations and emergent psychiatric assessments, and sometimes leading to short inpatient stays mainly for observation. As an outpatient, Valerie was referred to a succession of psychotherapists and psychopharmacologists, who alternately identified her as having dysthymic disorder, an unspecified anxiety disorder, PTSD, borderline personality disorder, and bulimia nervosa. There was no known history of substance use disorders. She was treated with a litany of antidepressants, antipsychotics, lithium, and anticonvulsants all with no significant impact on her mood or impulsive self-destructive behavior. She would purge up to several times daily and once developed a Mallory-Weiss tear. Her mother brought her for a "psychopharmacology evaluation" and was dismayed when told that it was unlikely there existed a medication that would fundamentally yield substantial improvement in any of Valerie's many target symptoms but, instead, long-term residential placement seemed to be the most viable management strategy.

N TREATMENT ENDPOINTS AND THE ART OF DEPRESCRIBING

Clinicians seldom have specific endpoints in mind when starting a psychotropic drug – unlike nonpsychiatric physicians who may prescribe a specified course of an antibiotic, steroid, or proton pump inhibitor, it is far less often the case that mental health prescribers focus on the termination of a course of treatment – whether pharmacological or psychotherapeutic. Underlying the indefinite use of a psychotropic medication is the premise that the ailment under treatment is itself a long-term if not lifelong condition for which treatment is suppressive rather than disease-modifying, and cessation would expectably lead to clinical worsening. Such may be the case with schizophrenia, highly recurrent depression, bipolar disorder, and at least some anxiety disorders. On the other hand, some practice guidelines advise that in patients with schizophrenia, antipsychotic medications might cautiously be discontinued in those who have been symptom free for at least one year (Lehman et al., 2004). The Expert Consensus Guideline Series for the Treatment of Patients with Bipolar Disorder also proposes that after a single manic episode, prophylactic pharmacotherapy could be cautiously discontinued after 1 year of full stability (Sachs et al., 2000).

However, controversy abounds as to whether and when such planned discontinuations could lead to inevitable relapse. Some studies that argue there are definable subpopulations of individuals with serious forms of mental illness such as schizophrenia for whom long-term pharmacotherapy may be unnecessary are limited by their observational, nonrandomized study designs (Harrow and Jobe, 2013) – that is, patients who remain well off medications for extended periods of time may simply be self-selected good-prognosis patients, precluding causal relationships about pharmacotherapy and long-term outcome. Similarly, in patients with bipolar disorder, one observational study followed 213 patients who had been stable for at least 2 years in which 54 were slowly tapered off lithium; mean time until relapse was 1.33 years among those who stopped lithium versus 7.33 years among those who remained in treatment (Biel et al., 2007). Sometimes, parameters such as gradual versus abrupt treatment cessation may influence the rate or magnitude of relapse (see Box 5.8) but, by and large, stopping long-term pharmacotherapy in stable bipolar disorder appears to inevitably lead to relapse in the majority of patients without clearly identified protective patient characteristics.

Box 5.8

Does abrupt lithium cessation hasten relapse?

The oft-cited admonition that abrupt lithium discontinuation (i.e., cessation over less than 2 weeks rather than over 2-4 weeks) increases relapse risk in bipolar disorder comes from one nonrandomized (observational) study of patients who were deemed stable for at least 18 months and wished to stop treatment altogether (rather than switch to an alternative regimen); over the next 5 years, "abrupt" discontinuers were 2.8 times more likely to have an episode than those whose treatment cessation occurred over a 2-4-week period (Faedda et al., 1993). It is unknown whether this increased relapse risk might be less if abrupt lithium cessation precedes an alternative therapy as opposed to no pharmacotherapy at all.

Because there exist few long-term pharmacotherapy trials involving randomized discontinuation, it is hard to know empirically if there are in fact "optimal" durations of treatment, beyond which time further therapy to prevent relapse may be unnecessary. Medication de-prescriptions often result by happenstance, as when a patient misses several doses and then chooses to stop their own treatment (i.e., nonadherence), if a drug becomes unavailable due to a change in insurance reimbursement coverage, a shortage in the marketplace, or if a toxicity occurs (e.g., with lithium) that prompts an abrupt cessation of the drug. Patients who overdose on a particular medication are sometimes perceived to no longer be an appropriate candidate to continue the drug for its previously intended therapeutic purposes, although there is little research on the rationale or outcome for such decisions.

Medications typically are purposefully discontinued when it becomes apparent that their risk–benefit ratio becomes significant and there is not a viable mitigation strategy to continue. Gray zones often exist, as might be the case for a patient with lithium-responsive bipolar disorder who experiences a declining estimated glomerular filtration rate, or if significant iatrogenic weight gain occurs alongside metabolic dysregulation with a second-generation antipsychotic medication despite heroic mitigation strategies. Table 5.3 describes several representative examples.

Table 5.3 Adverse drug effects: to mitigate or not to mitigate?

Adverse effects without viable risk-mitigation strategies	Adverse effects with viable risk-mitigation strategies
Clozapine-induced myocarditis	Use of vesicular monoamine transporter type 2 inhibitors to allow continued use of antipsychotic medications in the setting of tardive dyskinesia
Severe cutaneous reactions	Use of beta-blockers to overcome nontoxic tremors
Neuroleptic malignant syndrome	Cevimeline or pilocarpine to manage dry mouth
	Lithium to boost white blood cell production in patients with near-leukopenia taking clozapine
	Weight gain from second-generation antipsychotic medications managed with an array of potential pharmacological antidotes, including metformin, phentermine, topiramate, amantadine, zonisamide, and/or glucagon-like peptide-1 agonists

Optimal durations of treatment are unfortunately subject more to clinical impressions than a robust evidence base composed of randomized discontinuation trials – which may be the only way to know with some statistical confidence the risk for relapse and recurrence after a treatment is withdrawn. Nevertheless, at least for mood disorders, there are a number of useful concepts that bear on long-term clinical decision-making about therapeutic endpoints, as summarized in Box 5.9.

Box 5.9

Considerations for optimal duration of pharmacotherapy in mood disorders

- After the resolution of a single episode of major depression, practice guidelines tend to favor continued treatment for a period of 4–9 months before contemplating cessation of therapy in order to minimize recurrence. A Danish population-based cohort study of 89,442 adults treated with antidepressants for major depression found that the likelihood for requiring reinitiation of antidepressant medication after cessation was highest in those who had stopped their initial treatment less than 10–12 months after recovery (Liu et al., 2021).
- The risk for relapse across psychiatric disorders (that is, a return of the symptoms associated with an index episode) is generally considered to pertain to the first 6 months following remission; recurrence (that is, the occurrence of a new episode) pertains to symptoms or full episodes that occur after this time window. As a rule of thumb, patients who can traverse a 6-month time window without residual or relapsing symptoms following an index episode of nearly any psychiatric disorder are at lower risk for recurrence than are patients who fail to maintain that approximate 6-month time frame without residual or relapsing symptoms.
- Optimal duration of an adjunctive second-generation antipsychotic medication (added to an antidepressant) in major depression is unstudied, but likely impacted by metabolic, neurological, and cognitive tolerability concerns that require long-term monitoring.
- After resolution of an acute manic episode with an antimanic mood stabilizer plus a second-generation antipsychotic medication, retention of the adjunctive antipsychotic significantly reduces the risk of recurrence for up to 24 weeks but beyond that time the potential for metabolic changes may offset more modest additional prophylactic efficacy beyond a mood stabilizer alone (Yatham et al., 2016).

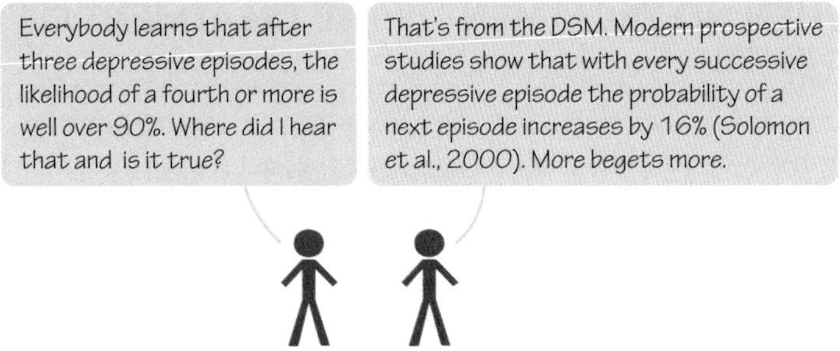

O DEPRESCRIBING AFTER LACK OF EFFICACY

It is hard to justify the indefinite retention of a medication that is clearly ineffective while psychiatric symptoms persist without improvement. After the elapse of an adequate trial, however one chooses to define the concept for a given population (one that may be unusually chronic, treatment-resistant, or comorbidly afflicted), it makes for good pharmacological hygiene to assess in a binary fashion whether a treatment is or is not conferring a benefit (and then, separately, the magnitude of that benefit). Such appraisals pertain equally to psychosocial as well as pharmacological interventions. The slowly growing literature on the concept of formal "deprescribing" of psychotropic medications also points out the need to recognize:

- when the evolving balance of treatment risks versus benefits may become unfavorable
- when an unwieldy pharmacology regimen may simply invite nonadherence
- when polypharmacy regimens may have outlived their usefulness (as when an initial sedative–hypnotic medication that may have been intended to alleviate transient insomnia or anxiety becomes retained on a long-term basis for no explicit reason)
- when polypharmacy regimens involve mechanistic redundancies or drug interactions (including with nonpsychiatric medications) that may pose unnecessary risks or foreseeable hazards over time.

Gupta and Cahill (2016) point out that, when deprescribing, clinicians should avoid obvious times of crisis or life transitions, pay attention to potential disruptions that may already exist in the therapeutic alliance, tread carefully if there is alcohol or illicit substance use in the clinical picture, survey a patient's knowledge and perception of specific medication effects to frame risk–benefit discussions, and engage patients' own thoughts and concerns about medications being targeted for discontinuation, with contingency plans outlined in the event that a discontinued drug might subsequently warrant reintroduction.

P WHEN NO TREATMENT IS THE TREATMENT OF CHOICE

Contrarian as the notion might seem, there are instances in which psychiatric treatment may be inappropriate or contraindicated, at least at a given point in time for a given set of circumstances. Apart from situations in which a psychiatric disorder is obviously absent, there are times when a mental health clinician may deem it wisest to refrain from recommending any specific treatment at a given time. Such situations might occur when a full assessment has not been completed and there may be no clear diagnostic impression; when complaints may be in evolution and an extended evaluation may itself be the only recommendation; in the setting of adjustment disorders with only mild symptoms for which even formal psychotherapy recommendations may be a matter of judgment; for instances in which malingering appears to be a salient concern (see Chapter 3, Box 3.1); or when facing a complex family or other systems issue and it may be unclear who constitutes the identified patient (see Chapter 3, Section B), and further assessment may be necessary to determine what exactly is the object and recipient of any psychiatric intervention.

Francis and Clarkin (1981), focusing mainly on psychotherapy as the primary intervention, identify patients whom they consider to be at risk for a negative therapeutic response and those at high risk for nonresponse, or who may be unable to make productive use of therapeutic resources. We might update their perspective to include instances in which neither pharmacotherapy nor psychosocial interventions are likely to offer an expectable benefit, in which case there may be value in taking a break from the pursuit of psychiatric treatment and allow for the emergence of a clearer picture of whatever problems may persist, with the option for future reassessment if appropriate.

TAKE-HOME POINTS

- Differential therapeutic options involving pharmacotherapy or psychosocial interventions should be tailored to individual patient needs. Decisions about treatment modalities should depend on patients' preferences as well as symptom severity, functional impairment, past treatment outcomes, and recognizing symptom targets that may require skill-building
- Medications can target specific symptoms within the broader constellation of a psychiatric syndrome; recognize instances in which medications are or are not likely to be beneficial to thereby choose treatment recommendations judiciously
- Choose levels of care and individual versus team-based treatment plans based on a patient's level of severity, distress, and anticipated frequency of needed engagement
- Recognize endpoints for both pharmacotherapy and psychosocial interventions in relation to fulfilling the objectives of an intended treatment plan
- Periodically review the risks and benefits of any intervention in order to flexibly modify a treatment plan as clinical conditions evolve over time

References

American Psychiatric Association. Diagnostic and Statistical Manual of Mental Disorders, 5th edition, text revision. Washington, DC: American Psychiatric Association, 2022

Bibring E. Psychoanalysis and the dynamic therapies. J Amer Psychoanalytic Assoc 1954; 2: 745–770

Biel MG, Peselow E, Mulcare L, et al. Continuation versus discontinuation of lithium in recurrent bipolar illness: A naturalistic study. Bipolar Disord 2007; 9: 435–442

Black D. Efficacy of combined pharmacotherapy and psychotherapy versus monotherapy in the treatment of anxiety disorders. CNS Spectr 2006; 10: 29–33

Choy Y, Fyer AJ, Lipsitz JD. Treatment of specific phobias in adults. Clin Psychol Rev 2007; 27: 266–286

Cleare A, Pariante CM, Young AH, et al. Evidence-based guidelines for treating depressive disorders with antidepressants: A revision of the 2008 British Association for Psychopharmacology guidelines. J Psychopharmacol 2015; 29: 459–525

Corbisiero S, Bitto H, Newark P, et al. A comparison of cognitive-behavioral therapy and pharmacotherapy vs. pharmacotherapy alone in adults with attention-deficit/hyperactivity disorder (ADHD) – a randomized controlled trial. Front Psychiatry 2018; 9: 571

Crow SJ. Pharmacotherapy of eating disorders. Psych Clin N Amer 2019; 42: 253–262

Cuijpers P, Sijbrandij M, Koole SL, et al. The efficacy of psychotherapy and pharmacotherapy in treating depressive and anxiety disorders: A meta-analysis of direct comparisons. World Psychiatry 2013; 12: 137–148

Cuijpers P, Sijbrandij M, Koole SL, et al. Adding psychotherapy to antidepressant medication in depression and anxiety disorders: A meta-analysis. World Psychiatry 2014; 13: 56–67

Cuijpers P, Oud M, Karyotaki E, et al. Psychological treatment of depression compared with pharmacotherapy and combined treatment in primary care: A network meta-analysis. Ann Fam Med 2021; 19: 262–270

De Leo D, Cerin E, Spathonis K, et al. Lifetime risk of suicide ideation and attempts in an Australian community: Prevalence, suicidal process, and help-seeking behavior. J Affect Disord 2005; 86: 215–224

Faedda GL, Tondo L, Baldessarini RJ, et al. Outcome after rapid vs. gradual discontinuation of lithium treatment in bipolar disorder. Arch Gen Psychiatry 1993; 50: 448–455

Forbes D, Creamer M, Bisson JI, et al. A guide to guidelines for the treatment of PTSD and related conditions. J Traumatic Stress 2010; 23: 537–552

Francis A, Clarkin JF. No treatment as the prescription of choice. Arch Gen Psychiatry 1981; 38: 542–545

Garakani A, Buono FD, Larkin K, et al. Development and validation of a new scale to measure chronic suicidal ideation: The Chronic Suicidal Ideation Inventory-5 (CSI-5). J Affect Disord 2022; 140: 160–164

Gelenberg AJ, Kane JM, Keller MB, et al. Comparison of standard and low levels of lithium for maintenance treatment of bipolar disorder. N Engl J Med 1989; 321: 1489–1493

Gelenberg AJ, Freeman MP, Markowitz JC, et al. Practice Guideline for the Treatment of Patients with Major Depressive Disorder, 3rd edition. Washington, DC: American Psychiatric Association, 2010

González-Rodriguez A, Guàrdia A, Palao JD, et al. Moderators and mediators of antipsychotic response in delusional disorder: Further steps are needed. World J Psychiatry 2020; 10: 34–45

Gupta S, Cahill DJ. A prescription for "deprescribing" in psychiatry. Psychiatr Serv 2016; 67: 904–907

Harrow M, Jobe TH. Does long-term treatment of schizophrenia with antipsychotic medications facilitate recovery? Schizophr Bull 2013; 39: 962–965

Huang X, Fox KR, Ribeiro JD, et al. Psychosis as a risk factor for suicidal thoughts and behaviors: A meta-analysis of longitudinal studies. Psychol Med 2018; 48: 765–776

Huhn M, Nikolakopoulou A, Schneider-Thoma J, et al. Comparative efficacy and tolerability of 32 oral antipsychotics for the acute treatment of adults with multi-episode schizophrenia: A systematic review and network meta-analysis. Lancet 2019; 394: 939–951

Ingehoven T, Lafay P, Rinne T, et al. Effectiveness of pharmacotherapy for severe personality disorders: Meta-analyses of randomized controlled trials. J Clin Psychiatry 2010; 71: 14–25

Jakobsen JC, Hansen JL, Simonsen S, et al. Effects of cognitive therapy versus interpersonal psychotherapy in patients with major depressive disorder: A systematic review of randomized clinical trials with meta-analyses and trial sequential analyses. Psychol Med 2012; 42: 1343–1357

Laska KM, Gurman AS, Wampold BE. Expanding the lens of evidence-based practice in psychotherapy: a common factors perspective. Psychotherapy (Chic) 2014; 51: 467–481

Laws KR, Darlington N, Kondel TK, et al. Cognitive behavioural therapy for schizophrenia – outcomes for functioning, distress and quality of life: A meta-analysis. BMC Psychol 2018; 6: 32

Lehman AF, Lieberman JA, Dixon LB, et al. Practice Guideline for the Treatment of Patients with Schizophrenia, 2nd edition. Washington, DC: American Psychiatric Association, 2004

Leucht S. Measurements of response, remission, and recovery in schizophrenia and examples for their clinical application. J Clin Psychiatry 2014; 75 (suppl 1): 8–14

Liu X, Momen NC, Molenaar N, et al. Discontinuation of antidepressants: Is there a minimum time on treatment that will reduce relapse risk? J Affect Disord 2021; 290: 254–260

Mataix-Cols D, de la Cruz LF, Nordsletten AE, et al. Towards an international expert consensus for defining treatment response, remission, recovery and relapse in obsessive-compulsive disorder. World Psychiatry 2016; 15: 80–81

Morrison AP, Law H, Carter L, et al. Antipsychotic drugs versus cognitive behavioural therapy versus a combination of both in people with psychosis: A randomised controlled pilot and feasibility study. Lancet Psychiatry 2018; 5: 411–423

Obegi JH. How common is recent denial of suicidal ideation among suicidal ideators, attempters, and suicide decedents? A literature review. Gen Hosp Psychiatry 2021; 72: 92–95

Oldham JM, Gabbard GO, Goin MK, et al. Practice Guideline for the Treatment of Borderline Personality Disorder. Washington, DC: American Psychiatric Association, 2001.

Roshanaei-Moghaddam B, Pauly MC, Atkins DC, et al. Relative effects of CBT and pharmacotherapy in depression versus anxiety: Is medication somewhat better for depression, and CBT somewhat better for anxiety? Depress Anxiety 2011; 28: 560–567

Rothschild AJ, Wilner J, Flint AJ, et al. Missed diagnosis of psychotic depression at 4 academic medical centers. J Clin Psychiatry 2008; 69: 1293–1296

Sachs GS, Printz DJ, Kahn DA, et al. The Expert Consensus Guideline Series for the Treatment of Bipolar Disorder. Memphis, TN: Physicians Postgraduate Press, 2000

Solomon DA, Keller MB, Leon AC, et al. Multiple recurrences of major depressive disorder. Am J Psychiatry 2000; 157: 229–233

Stein MB, Goin MK, Pollack MH, et al. Practice Guideline for the Treatment of Patients with Panic Disorder, 2nd edition. Washington, DC: American Psychiatric Association, 2010

Varker T, Kartal D, Watson L, et al. Defining response and nonresponse to posttraumatic stress disorder treatments: A systematic review. Clin Psychol: Science and Practice 2020; 27: e12355

Weisaeth N. Vulnerability and protective factors for posttraumatic stress disorder. Psychiatry Clin Neurosci 1998; 52: S39–S44

Yatham LN, Beaulieu S, Schaffer A, et al. Optimal duration of risperidone or olanzapine adjunctive therapy to mood stabilizer following remission of a manic episode. Mol Psychiatry 2016; 21: 1050–1056

6 Measurement-Based Care and Applying Statistical Concepts to the Individual Patient

LEARNING OBJECTIVES

- ☐ Define and describe the key elements of measurement-based care
- ☐ Describe commonly used diagnostic screening tools and symptom rating scales used in psychiatry, and their basic interpretation
- ☐ Understand clinical versus statistical significance and effect sizes
- ☐ Be able to tabulate whether symptom rating scales for a given patient have or have not changed significantly over the course of a treatment period
- ☐ Understand the concept of individualized treatment rules (ITRs) and how previous illness features or treatment results can inform outcomes during iterative pharmacotherapy trials
- ☐ Understand the role of machine learning algorithms and "training samples" to inform possible outcomes for future patients based on their clinical profiles

"Measurement-based care" (MBC) refers to the systematic assessment of patients' symptoms over the course of some observation period in order to glean information about likely treatment effects. The concept grew mainly from the world of clinical trials and US Food and Drug Administration registration studies, where efforts to judge the efficacy of an intervention depended on reliable quantifiable measures to track changes in symptoms or clinical status over time. In this chapter, our interest in MBC pertains mainly to describing the ways in which it can impact hypothesis-testing, decision-making, and outcome-tracking in clinical practice rather than in research settings.

Fewer than 20% of mental health clinicians report that they integrate MBC into routine clinical practice (Zimmerman and McGlinchey, 2008; Lewis et al., 2019). Reasons they cite for this include skepticism that MBC tools would be helpful or more useful than simple clinical judgment, perceptions that MBC tools are too time-consuming, and a lack of training (or perhaps lack of interest in training?) in their proper use. Psychometric rating scales (even self-report forms) typically require at least some degree of training in their proper administration and interpretation, but seldom is the task onerous. The pay-off for clinical care comes from confidence in being able to know if an intervention truly produced a meaningful effect, having a common language for communicating with colleagues, being able to compare the magnitude of effect of one treatment relative to another, and eliminating nebulous conclusions about whether or not the perceived benefits of a medication or other therapy outweigh its risks.

A DO RATING SCALES IMPROVE CLINICAL OUTCOMES?

It makes intuitive sense to think that objective assessment of clinical phenomena leads to a more precise awareness of target symptoms and related features (e.g., their functional impact), which, in turn, one would think can only facilitate shared decision-making by making therapeutic accomplishment or failures more explicit. Elsewhere in medicine it is impossible to perform treatment without objectifying and quantifying the clinical problems of interest. In an extensive and comprehensive literature review of the impact of MBC on mental health outcomes, studies by Peterson et al. (2018) yield a number of pertinent observations, as summarized in Box 6.1.

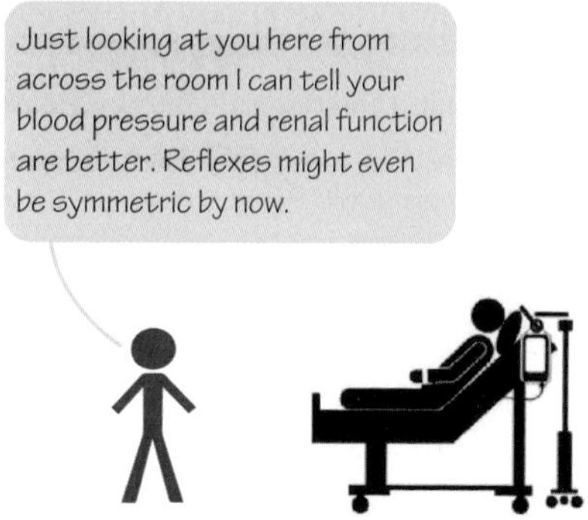

Box 6.1

Outcome findings from studies of measurement-based care in psychiatry

- At least some degree of improvement in patients' sense of overall distress was observed in most studies
- In three randomized trials examining quality of life, improvement was observed in one
- Three randomized trials studying patient satisfaction with care found improvement among patients with schizophrenia but declines in patients with mood or anxiety disorders
- No data are available regarding the impact of MBC on suicidal behavior, patient missed appointments or treatment dropout, or medication adherence
- In patients in severe crisis, MBC has been associated with poorer outcomes based on one randomized trial

Not mentioned in the above-noted Department of Veterans Affairs review by Peterson et al. (2018) was a 24-week randomized comparison of MBC versus standard treatment in 120 outpatients with moderate-to-severe depression, which found significantly higher rates of response (86.9% for MBC versus 62.7% with standard treatment) or remission (73.8% versus 28.8%, respectively) (Guo et al., 2015). Interestingly, patients randomized to MBC had significantly more treatment adjustments and ultimately higher antidepressant medication doses as compared to those receiving standard treatment. In other words, quantitative monitoring of depression (especially in the first few weeks of treatment) may drive more aggressive pharmacotherapy adjustments, which in turn minimize the risk of subtherapeutic dosing.

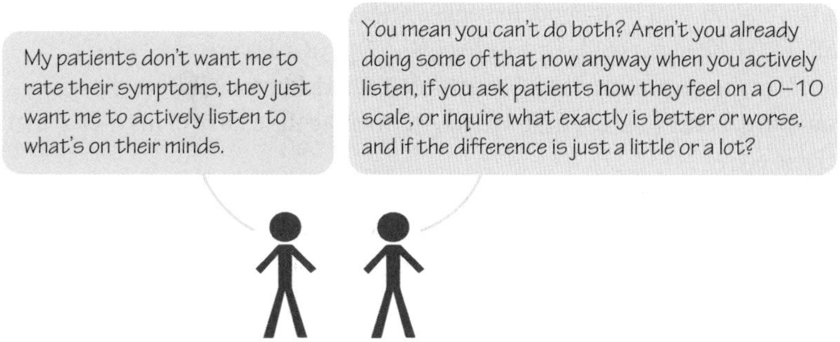

B WHAT TO MEASURE?

A range of clinical parameters can be codified, quantified, operationalized, or otherwise converted into measurable ratings that can describe overall or detailed aspects of a psychiatric condition being treated. When it comes to describing both the overall severity of a clinical condition as well as the degree to which global improvement is or is not evident, let us start with, arguably, the simplest and perhaps most versatile of all standardized measures, the Clinical Global Impressions (CGI) scale (Guy, 1976a). This 0–7 rating scale, described in Box 6.2, has valid psychometric properties, meaning that biostatisticians have shown that it accurately does measure the characteristics it intends to measure (at least, when it is rated by a clinician). It can be applied to any ailment to describe current degree of symptom prominence or severity (CGI-S) as well as the degree to which improvement has or has not occurred over time (CGI-I).

Box 6.2

The Clinical Global Impressions Scale

Severity	Scoring	Improvement
Normal, not at all ill	1	Very much improved
Borderline mentally ill	2	Much improved
Mildly ill	3	Minimally improved
Moderately ill	4	No change
Markedly ill	5	Minimally worse
Severely ill	6	Much worse
Among the most severely ill	7	Very much worse

With its seven-point spread, the CGI-S and CGI-I scales provide a nice degree of variance for which numerical trends over time can be mapped for a given patient. So, for example, suppose that Keenan has obsessive–compulsive disorder (OCD) and struggles with checking compulsions and intrusive thoughts about contamination, and he is about to begin a selective serotonin reuptake inhibitor (SSRI) trial. Keenan could self-rate his CGI-S and CGI-I score, say, twice a week over the course of 6 weeks, to provide a metric for tracking his change in symptom severity over the trial. We can summarize the course of his *n*-of-1 trial in Table 6.1.

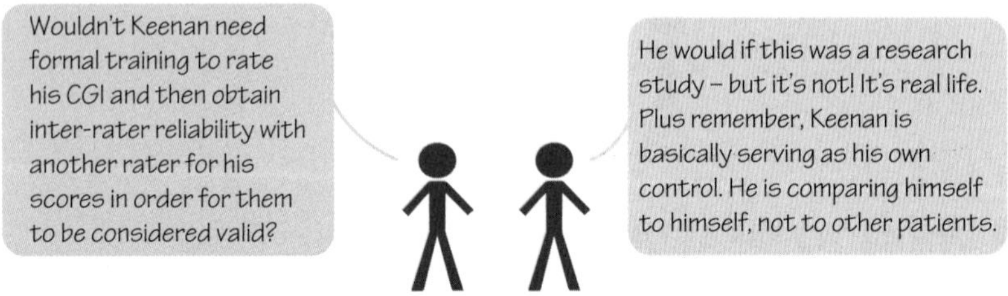

Table 6.1 Is Keenan's OCD improving with fluoxetine?

	Week 1	Week 2	Week 3	Week 4	Week 5	Week 6	Week 7	Week 8
Fluoxetine dose	10 mg	20 mg	20 mg	30 mg	40 mg	60 mg	60 mg	60 mg
CGI-S	Mon: 6	Mon: 6	Mon: 5	Mon: 4	Mon: 4	Mon: 6	Mon: 5	Mon: 4
	Thurs: 6	Thurs: 5	Thurs: 6	Thurs: 5	Thurs: 4	Thurs: 4	Thurs: 5	Thurs: 5
Weekly mean score	6.0	5.5	5.5	4.5	4.0	5.0	5.0	4.5

Now it is time for some back-of-the-envelope statistics. We would like to know if the trajectory of changes in Keenan's CGI-S semi-weekly scores (going from a mean of 6.0 to 4.5 over 8 weeks) was significantly different from baseline. We can calculate this for Keenan using a one-sample *t*-test, which compares the changes in his mean scores over time against the baseline starting value. For anyone who especially likes math, the *t*-test statistic can be calculated by hand using the equation in Formula 6.1:

$$t = \frac{\bar{x} - \mu_0}{s} \cdot \sqrt{n} \qquad (6.1)$$

where $\bar{x}$ is the sample mean ($[6 + 6 + 6 + 5 + 5 + 6 + 4 + 5 + 4 + 4 + 6 + 4 + 5 + 5 + 4 + 5] \div 16 = 5$), μ_0 is the hypothesized population mean (we will take this as

6, Keenan's baseline score), s is the sample standard deviation (0.625), and n is the sample size ($n = 16$ data points), which gives us:

$$\frac{5-6}{0.625} \times (4) = 6.40$$

For all the rest of us, go find a handy online calculator for one-sample t-tests (e.g., www.statology.org/one-sample-t-test-calculator/), enter in Keenan's CGI-S scores, and use a hypothesized population mean of "6" (his baseline score) and we find a t-value of 6.40 with 15 degrees of freedom (n minus 1) and two-tailed p-value of 0.0001. What do we conclude? Keenan's OCD symptoms (based on his self-reported CGI severity) improved significantly over 8 weeks. The p-value means that if we gave Keenan this treatment over 1,000 different times, the probability of seeing different results is about zero, so this was no random fluke. However, before we begin any victory laps, bear in mind that Keenan went from feeling "severely ill" to feeling midway between "moderately" and "markedly" ill. Better, but not fixed.

Tip

"Degrees of freedom" means the maximum number of independent values that can vary in a data set.

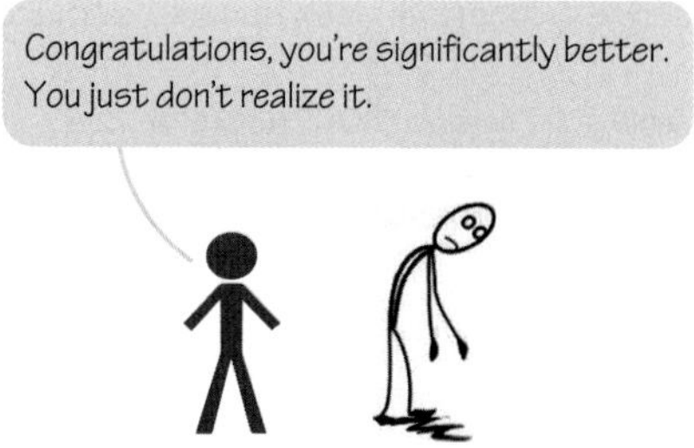

How clinically meaningful was this change? We can calculate a within-group effect size for a one-sample t-test, based on Keenan's CGI-S scores, according to the formula in Formula 6.2:

$$\text{Cohen's } d = \frac{\text{Keenan's mean score} - \text{Baseline score}}{\text{Pooled SD}} \quad (6.2)$$

That is,

$$\frac{5-6}{0.625} = 1.6$$

A Cohen's d of 1.6 is a very large effect size, which is clinically meaningful.

So, decision-wise, is fluoxetine a keeper? Technically, yes, it produced a significant improvement and clinically large effect over 8 weeks. It would therefore not make sense to abandon it. Should the dose be raised further? Should it be augmented with a second agent? Should we just give it more time to see if time alone will further increase its efficacy? All good ideas – none is wrong. The only wrong idea would be to abandon fluoxetine altogether or to conclude it was utterly ineffective.

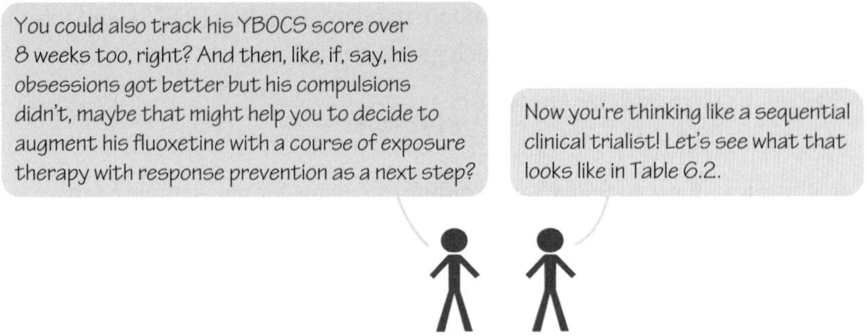

We can separately rate the five Yale–Brown Obsessive–Compulsive Scale (YBOCS) items that measure obsessions and the five YBOCS items that measure compulsive behaviors, with individual items rated from 0 (none) to 1 (mild) to 2 (moderate) to 3 (severe) to 4 (extreme). Mean weekly scores for each subscale across Keenan's 8-week fluoxetine trial are listed in Table 6.2.

Table 6.2 Keenan's YBOCS subscores

	Week 1	Week 2	Week 3	Week 4	Week 5	Week 6	Week 7	Week 8
YBOCS - obsessions	14	14	12	13	11	9	9	8
YBOCS - compulsions	9	10	8	9	9	8	8	8

Visual inspection of Table 6.2 shows that most of Keenan's CGI-S changes likely reflect improvement in obsessive thoughts rather than compulsive behaviors ("Keenan, your obsessions improved by 43% but your compulsions were reduced only 11%")

Math

$[(14-8) \div 14] \times 100 = 43\%$

$[(9-8) \div 9] \times 100 = 11\%$

Another back-of-the-envelope t-test shows significant reductions in Keenan's YBOCS obsession subscale scores ($t = 3.27$, $p = 0.007$), but the change in YBOCS compulsion subscale scores is nonsignificant ($t = 1.43$, $p = 0.099$). From a decisional standpoint, a quick MedLine check finds evidence that sequential cognitive–behavioral therapy added after a partial response to pharmacotherapy yields significantly greater improvement in both obsessions and compulsions of OCD than continued pharmacotherapy alone (Tenneij et al., 2005), and that the combination of behavior therapy with an SSRI for OCD was more effective in reducing obsessions specifically than was the case for behavior therapy alone (Hohagen et al., 1998).

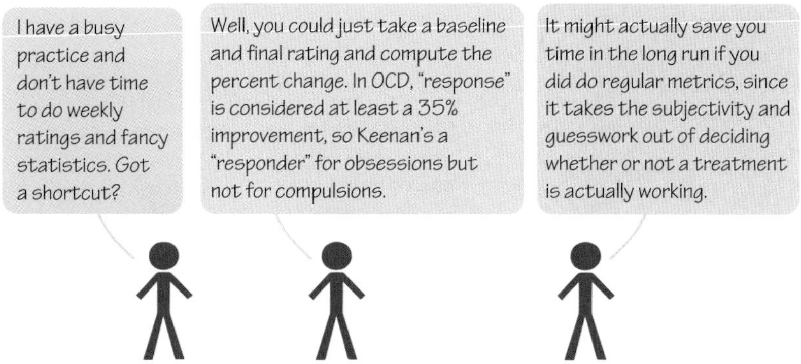

C PSYCHOMETRIC VALIDATION OF RATING SCALES

In real-world clinical practice, and outside of the realm of formal clinical research trials, there are a number of ways one can track patient progress short of eyeballing things and just asking, "So, are you better or not?". "Crude" measures are better than no measures, and there is nothing wrong with asking patients to make a 0–10 visual analog severity scale (as is commonly done in pain medicine) and track their symptom severity over time, as occurred for Diana's anxiety in Clinical Vignette 6.1.

Clinical Vignette 6.1

Diana was a 64-year-old woman with longstanding generalized anxiety disorder (GAD), who had experienced various side effects from serotonergic antidepressant medications over the years, which she felt outweighed any benefit, and instead found herself relying on lorazepam 0.5 mg twice a day as the mainstay of her GAD treatment. Along came Dr. Gallahad, who proposed trying pregabalin as a non-serotonergic pharmacology strategy for GAD. He also suggested that Diana track her anxiety symptoms twice a day (mid-day and evening) on a scale from 0 to 10 with "0" reflecting no anxiety at all and "10" being the worst anxiety she has ever experienced. They would use this scale to track progress with pregabalin as her dose went up. He then asked Diana if she would agree that "9" was unacceptable and not tolerable and that "1" was acceptable and tolerable, which she did. He suggested that somewhere between 2 and 8 was a border threshold for intolerability and asked her to think about what that threshold number likely was. He offered "5" or "6" for consideration and she agreed. He then further suggested that she convert her lorazepam use to only as needed, based on 0–10 scores of "5" or higher and use it as a "rescue" for intolerable symptoms, and said that they would tally up her need for lorazepam rescues as a "secondary outcome measure" of pregabalin's success (or lack thereof) over the coming weeks of the trial.

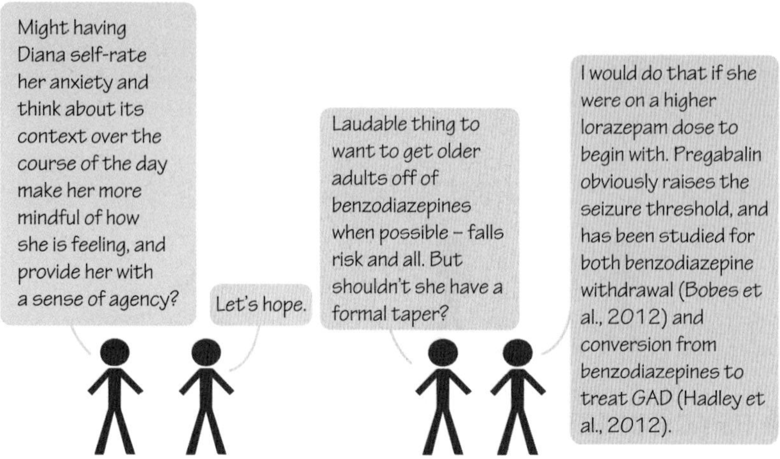

There are a plethora of published scales to quantify and rate threshold criteria for a plethora of psychiatric symptoms and conditions. Is there a reason we cannot just home-grow our own scale to measure something we think is important and then use that? One certainly could devise an original measure, but the problem is in knowing with statistical confidence that a home-grown rating instrument actually measures the relevant features of the phenomenon we are interested in tracking. Suppose you wanted to devise a new scale to track depression and, in your opinion, excessive daydreaming, social isolation, and time spent playing video games were salient elements of depression. You could put together a measure that certainly captures these features but it would be hard to know if they were truly integral components of depression – as opposed to, say, social anxiety, cannabis use, or schizoid personality traits. What if you left out critically important features of the phenomenon of interest, or gave unequal weight to some features more than others? How do we know that the items in the scale are all inter-related as a coherent entity? How do we know if the elements in the scale are stable constructs or sensitive to change over time (height would be a bad item

Tip

Patients tend to be more inclined to undertake ongoing self-rating scales when they are symptomatic and may be less likely to maintain formal metrics when they are well.

Tip

Remember from Chapter 1: *validity* means that the construct being measured actually and accurately measures what it claims to measure. Valid means *accurate*. *Reliability* means that a *consistent* finding is observed over time – regardless of whether it is valid. (Ideally, both exist.)

to include, even if one hypothesized that stature influences depression). Until someone administers your scale to large and well-defined clinical groups over time, and then demonstrates that the items in the scale are meaningfully inter-related, and unrelated to concepts that are not relevant, the scale will not have established validity. Sometimes it is also important to know what the effects are of repeatedly administering the same scale to the same individual – for example, when performing cognitive tests, patients can develop greater ability to perform because of practice effects (either in a good way, showing that learning has occurred; or in a bad way, showing that the test is not so useful to administer on a regular basis because the results become a less meaningful measure of someone's cognitive skills if they are "contaminated" by learning effects).

The types of statistical validity that are relevant to scales that measure psychiatric symptoms are summarized in Table 6.3.

Table 6.3 Types of validity

Type of validity	What that means
Face	A test or rating scale measures, at a superficial or face-value level, what it claims to measure
Convergent	Two different rating scales are correlated and measure the same basic construct; helpful especially when a first scale is well established and a newly developed scale purports to measure something similar
Discriminant	Two different scales are unrelated and capture separate independent phenomena - even if they may have some superficial overlap (e.g., a sleep scale and a pain scale may both be relevant to someone with depression, but tap different core constructs)
Construct	How well does the measure detect information about the theoretical concept (the construct) of interest? Construct validity depends on establishing both convergent and discriminant validity.

Lastly, it is important to know how well inter-related and cohesive the individual items are within a given measurement scale. If a depression scale included items about food preferences, they might not necessarily align well with other questions about sleep, energy, and anhedonia. The inter-relatedness among individual items of a scale is a type of reliability that is typically measured by a statistic called Cronbach's alpha, which is basically a correlation among the individual items that comprise a scale. Scores range from 0 to 1. Those ≥ 0.90 are considered excellent, 0.9–0.8 are good, and 0.8–0.7 acceptable. Once again, for math afficionados, the equation by which to calculate Cronbach's alpha is shown in Formula 6.3:

$$\alpha = \frac{k}{k-1}\left(1 - \frac{\sum_{i=1}^{k}\sigma_y^2}{\sigma_x^2}\right) \tag{6.3}$$

where k is the number of items in the scale, σ^2_y represents the variance associated with each item, and σ^2_x represents the variance associated with the total scores of the scale. For the rest of us, we just need to know that if we choose to use a rating scale that has convergent and discriminant (i.e., construct) validity, and high internal consistency (with a Cronbach alpha preferably in the 0.90 neighborhood), we have a well-calibrated tool to track the phenomenon we want to measure.

Before we move on to consider some examples of specific measurement scales for major psychiatric disorders, and their practical utility for clinicians, let us first talk about using screening tools to detect the presence of psychiatric conditions. Many psychiatric diagnostic screeners are self-reported measures, which (for better or worse) rely on the patient's intact ability to recognize and self-report the presence of symptoms – which sometimes may be easy and obvious (e.g., depression) and at other times not so much (e.g., dementia).

D DIAGNOSTIC SCREENS

Screening tools are just that – screens, and not proxies for diagnoses. They are meant to cast a wide net in order to identify *possible* cases without missing too many, if any, real cases. Here, we need to consider the concept of **true positives** (**TP**s; i.e., real cases) and **true negatives** (**TN**s, i.e., real non-cases) and their discrimination from **false positives** (**FP**s; i.e., looks like a duck and walks like a duck but it is really a goose) and **false negatives** (**FN**s, i.e., you are trying to identify real cases of a disorder but erroneously miss one by the screen). Screens try to minimize false negatives (think, if this were malignancy screening, one would hate to miss true cases, hence casting the wide net) and are generally more tolerant of false positives (better to biopsy someone who actually did not need it than to skip a biopsy on someone who did).

Think back to epidemiology coursework you may have taken in a past life and you may well remember Table 6.4, sometimes referred to as a **confusion matrix**. How is this relevant to a mental health clinician? It is fundamental, because it gives us succinct information about whether the assay we are using is any good at ruling in versus ruling out cases. And, as we will see a little later, a confusion matrix is often a key element in machine learning and something called **predictive analysis**, when we want to gauge the likelihood of an event occurring based on probabilities gleaned from previous treatments or assessments in a given patient.

Table 6.4 Confusion matrix

		Predicted condition	
		Positive	Negative
Actual condition	Positive	TP	FN
	Negative	FP	TN

Recall four key parameters related to this table, known as test characteristics: sensitivity, specificity, positive predictive value (PPV), and negative predictive value (NPV), which are defined in Table 6.5.

Table 6.5 Key parameters derived from a confusion matrix

Parameter	Equation	What it means
Sensitivity	TP ÷ (TP + FN)	The test does not miss anybody; if there is any chance that somebody is a case, the test will identify them
Specificity	TN ÷ (TN + FP)	If the test identifies someone as a case, they really are a case and very unlikely something else
Positive predictive value (PPV)	TP ÷ (TP + FP)	If someone has a positive screen score, what is the probability that they *really do* have that condition based its prevalence?
Negative predictive value (NPV)	TN ÷ (TN + FN)	How well the test rules out false cases

Let us take a real-life example. The Mood Disorders Questionnaire (see Table 6.6) is a psychometrically standardized self-report screening tool for bipolar disorder. When it is given across multiple clinical populations, we obtain the test characteristics shown in Table 6.6.

Table 6.6 Test characteristics for the Mood Disorders Questionnaire

	Number of studies	Total sample size	Sensitivity	Specificity	PPV	NPV
General population	3	1,875	0.259	0.979	0.431	0.956
Psychiatric outpatients	3	943	0.647	0.823	0.388	0.931
Mood disorder patients	10	2,052	0.647	0.811	0.687	0.782

Based on data from Zimmerman and Galione (2011). Note, traditionally confusion matrix values are expressed as decimals, which are interchangeable with fractions.

What do we make of Table 6.6? First, for the busy practitioner with not enough time to evaluate everything worth evaluating, look at the NPVs across populations – they are quite high. That means that if a patient self-administers the MDQ and scores *below* the established threshold level of 7 or more on the 13 core items, there is roughly a 90% chance that they do not have bipolar disorder – so stop wasting time and move on to ask about other disorders. Second, the specificity of the MDQ is relatively high in the general population but more modest in mood disorder patients (with about a 20% rate of false positives, meaning around one in five MDQ+ mood disorder patients does not actually have bipolar disorder). Its PPV is rather weak, especially in the general population and in psychiatric outpatients. How can that be if the specificity is high in those groups? When the prevalence of a condition is low (bipolar disorder affects only about 2% of the population), the PPV of a screen is often low because more false positive cases tend to occur than when disease prevalence is high. In other words, a screen-positive rating requires a more extensive assessment to affirm casehood and rule out false positives, even when specificity and sensitivity are high.

Certain factors may confound both the discriminant and convergent validity of a screening tool. In psychiatric inpatients with mood symptoms and active substance use, for example, screening for bipolar disorder with the MDQ found relatively poor concordance with expert clinician semi-structured diagnostic interviews, largely because patients' affirmative MDQ item responses did not take into account the effects of intoxication and withdrawal states on self-identified mood symptoms (Goldberg et al., 2012). In that study group, the MDQ had only modest sensitivity (0.52) and low PPV (0.38), and there was poor concordance between clinicians' versus patients' ratings of items such as irritability, racing thoughts, or distractibility. However, when the MDQ was then used as a clinician- rather than patient-rated instrument, with clarifications of patients' intended responses when sober versus nonsober (e.g., "times when you were much more social" or "times when you did things that were unusual for you"), substantial improvement occurred in scale specificity (0.95), sensitivity (0.97), PPV (0.99), and NPV (0.99).

Let us next consider an instrument that is not explicitly a diagnostic screening tool so much as a compendium of clinical features that becomes corroborative of a clinical diagnostic impression, but not explicitly synonymous with its diagnostic criteria. As such, a scale like this generates more of a predictive model for a possible diagnosis, rather than a formal screen. As an example, the Bipolarity Index (Aiken et al., 2015) is a descriptive rating scale that largely captures the stigmata of bipolar disorder rather than its direct features – such as, being married more than three times, having repeated incarcerations or frequent job changes, and obtaining more than two advanced degrees, with differing weights accorded to each such item. While the scale reported very high sensitivity (0.90) and specificity (0.90) in a single-site study of outpatients (Aiken et al., 2015), the absence of its established discriminant validity from other conditions (such as antisocial personality disorder or borderline personality disorder) makes it more of a corroborative tool than a differential diagnostic probe.

Table 6.7 presents examples of a number of diagnostic screening tools commonly used for a representative (and by no means exhaustive) list of major psychiatric disorders.

Table 6.7 Examples of diagnostic screening tools

Disorder	Diagnostic screen	Description
Adult attention deficit-hyperactivity disorder (ADHD)	World Health Organization Adult ADHD Self-Report Scale (ASRS; Ustun et al., 2017)	18 self-report questions, each scored from 0 ("never") to 4 ("very often"). Scores of 17–23 are considered "likely" casehood and > 24 are considered "highly likely" casehood. However, it may overestimate true casehood by 7–10-fold (Chamberlain et al., 2021).
Alcohol use disorder	Alcohol Use Disorders Identification Test (AUDIT; Saunders et al., 1993)	10-item questionnaire, scoring range 0–40; scores ≥ 8 are associated with hazardous or harmful alcohol use
Bipolar disorder	Mood Disorder Questionnaire (MDQ; Hirschfeld et al., 2003)	13 self-report items keyed to historical symptoms of mania; scores ≥ 7 are screen (+)
	Rapid Mood Screener (RMS; McIntyre et al., 2021)	Six-item self-report screen for bipolar disorder; scores ≥ 4 are considered to be consistent with a bipolar disorder diagnosis
Generalized anxiety disorder	Generalized Anxiety Disorder-7 (GAD-7; Spitzer et al., 2006)	Seven-item self-report questionnaire (each scored from 0 to 3), originally developed in primary care to screen for GAD; scores > 10 are consistent with a diagnosis of GAD
Major depressive disorder	Patient Health Questionnaire-9 (PHQ-9; Kroenke et al., 2001)	Nine-item symptom rating scale used for both diagnostic screening and monitoring of symptom severity; see Table 6.8 for scoring details
Posttraumatic stress disorder (PTSD)	The Posttraumatic Stress Disorder Checklist for DSM-5 (PCL-5; Weathers et al., 2013)	20-item self-report measure keyed to DSM-5 (American Psychiatric Association, 2013) symptoms of PTSD with scoring from 0 to 80; scores > 31–33 are considered to indicate probable PTSD
Sleep disorders	Epworth Sleepiness Scale (ESS; Johns, 1991)	Eight-item self-report questionnaire with each item rated 0–3; scores > 16 are associated with severe sleep apnea or narcolepsy

E RATING SCALES RELATED TO DEPRESSION

Depression is perhaps the clinical condition for which most efforts toward MBC have been implemented worldwide. Symptom rating scales provide a useful method not only for tracking overall changes in severity but also for following the trajectory of individual items of interest (such as low motivation, or suicidal thinking). Psychometrically validated self-administered as well as clinician-rated scales are ubiquitous. Before reviewing several specific examples, consider the points raised in Box 6.3 about the mechanics of administering a rating scale.

Box 6.3

Issues when administering a symptom rating scale

- What is the time frame for making comparisons across rating periods? Are symptoms being assessed in comparison to the previous assessment point, or to the initial starting point of treatment? (For example, the Columbia-Suicide Severity Rating Scale assesses potential treatment-emergent suicidal ideation by drawing comparisons to the patient's own recent history)
- How does one "rate" potential symptoms that are most likely an artifact of some cause other than the psychiatric condition of interest (e.g., fatigue or insomnia in the setting of physical illness, or a suspected medication adverse effect)?
- Pay attention to whether the endorsement of a symptom is being rated as present or absent; this can be confusing – is insomnia present, or is normal sleep absent? Different rating scales may tier responses with different orientations
- Psychometric scales that capture psychiatric symptoms may not necessarily be sensitive to detecting changes over time. For example, while the Patient Health Questionnaire-9 is widely used as a screen for major depression, it has not formally been studied to assess longitudinal changes in individual symptoms. In the case of major depression, would one expect that all symptoms within the broad constellation of a depressive episode are equally likely to change over time? In other words, are some symptoms more prone to early response versus later response, or even no response? Do all deserve equal weighting? (Is poor concentration as central to judging severity when considering antidepressant response as is, say, suicidal ideation?)
- Consider whether a scale has been used and validated in a particular clinical population (such as children, or older adults) or whether cultural factors might impact how someone responds to standardized questions that may have been normed in a nondiverse study group

In clinical trials, treatment efficacy focuses on an a priori designated primary outcome – that is, the scale or measurement tool that has been designated (often supplemented by one or more secondary outcomes of interest), quantified by validated rating scales. A fundamental shift occurred in psychiatric practice when an earlier, longstanding interview model of open-ended questioning (where patients were encouraged to tell their own narrative, and complaints, in their own style) became replaced by a much more structured focus on eliciting key pieces of information linked to diagnostic criteria or specific target symptoms. Clinicians became more formal evaluators rather than facilitators of a patient's ability to self-report their internal experiences. Indeed, the mindset of the clinician mainly as an "evaluator" or symptom rater can make them feel in some ways more like an umpire than a healthcare provider, with the risk of losing sight of the patient as a whole.

Raters focus on determining whether a patient meets operational criteria for a category (such as a diagnosis, or a status of treatment "responder" or "remitter"). Engaging patients in clinical trials depends heavily on determining if they meet inclusion and exclusion criteria based on measurable characteristics. The process is somewhat akin to deciding whether or not someone with cardiac valve disease or degenerative joint disease is a surgical candidate. Homogenizing diagnoses and quantifying symptoms provide an easier means by which to generate reproducible results, from which generalizable or probabilistic effects can be forecast for future patients, perhaps aiding the field more than the individual. On the other hand, imposing a quantitative measure of symptom change over time for an individual patient provides an opportunity to provide evidence for the fruit of mutual labors, and make the idea of improvement from psychiatric symptoms all the more tangible.

Tip

When assessing symptoms in the nonresearch clinical world, it is often useful to invite patients to use their own "personal best" as their point of comparison - that is, "as compared to when you've felt well" or "as compared to the last time you felt like your usual self," how is now different? This is tantamount to using the patient as their own case-control. Patients may have trouble making such a comparison if they have chronic or non-episodic conditions.

Table 6.8 provides several representative examples of current depression symptom rating scales and their interpretation.

Table 6.8 Symptom severity scales for mood disorders

Disorder	Rating scale	Description
Major depression	Patient Health Questionnaire-9 (PHQ-9; Kroenke et al., 2001)	Self-administered nine-item questionnaire originally developed as a depression screen, often used to track response; scores of 5-9 reflect "mild" depression, 10-14 are "moderate," 15-19 are "moderately severe," and ≥ 20 reflect "severe" depression
	Beck Depression Inventory-II (BDI-II; Beck et al., 1996)	21 self-report questions each scored from 0-3 (maximum score of 63); scores of 0–13 reflect "minimal symptoms," 14-19 are "mild," 20-28 are "moderate," and > 29 are "major"; the scale captures attitudes and distortions related to the cognitive theory of depression
	Hamilton Depression Rating Scale (HAM-D; Hamilton, 1960)	Originally a 17-item scale, with variations up to a 31-item scale and down to a 1- or 6-item measure; those with HAM-D_{17} total scores of 0-7 are considered "not depressed," 8-13 are "mild," 14-18 are "moderate," 19-22 are "severe," and ≥ 23 are "very severe"
	Montgomery-Åsberg Depression Rating Scale (MADRS; Montgomery et al., 1979)	10-item scale, each rated 0-6; scores of 7-19 are considered "mild," 20-34 are "moderate," and > 34 are "severe"; developed as a scale that is sensitive to change in symptoms over time
	Quick Inventory of Depressive Symptomatology (QIDS; Rush et al., 2003)	16-item self- or clinician-rated measure. Scores of 0-5 are considered "not depressed," 6-10 reflect "mild depression," 11-15 are "moderate," 16-20 are "severe," and scores ≥ 20 are "very severe"
Anhedonia	Snaith-Hamilton Pleasure Scale (SHAPS; Snaith et al., 1995)	14-item scale with scores from 0 to 14; scores ≥ 3 reflect an impaired capacity to feel pleasure
Suicidal ideation	Columbia-Suicide Severity Rating Scale (C-SSRS; Posner et al., 2011)	Six yes/no self-report questions regarding suicidal thoughts or behaviors over the preceding month, 3 months, and lifetime; affirmative responses to questions about specific suicide thoughts with intent to act are considered particularly high risk
Bipolar mania symptoms	Young Mania Rating Scale (YMRS; Young et al., 1978)	11-item clinician-rated scale; scores ≤ 12 reflect "remission," 13–19 reflect "mild symptoms," 20–25 reflect "mild mania," 26–37 reflect "moderate mania," and 38–60 reflect "severe mania"

Let us pause for a moment while considering measures for depression symptom severity and ask what the likelihood is that objective measures of depression correlate with subjective measures. One study of 274 outpatients treated for major depression (the Rhode Island Methods to Improve Diagnostic and Assessment Services, or MIDAS) found that about half of those who were technically deemed to be in remission (according to a 17-item Hamilton Depression Rating Scale (HAM-D) total score < 7) considered themselves still to be meaningfully symptomatic with depression (Zimmerman et al., 2012a). The opposite could also occur, in which a patient might report some subjective sense of improved well-being yet technically, formally, the target symptoms for which they are being treated could remain relatively unchanged – as was the case in about one-quarter of MIDAS patients (Zimmerman et al., 2012b). "Concordant" remitters in that study (i.e., those whose objective HAM-D scores were congruent with subjective ratings of remission) reported better quality of life, higher satisfaction with their overall mental health, and better coping ability.

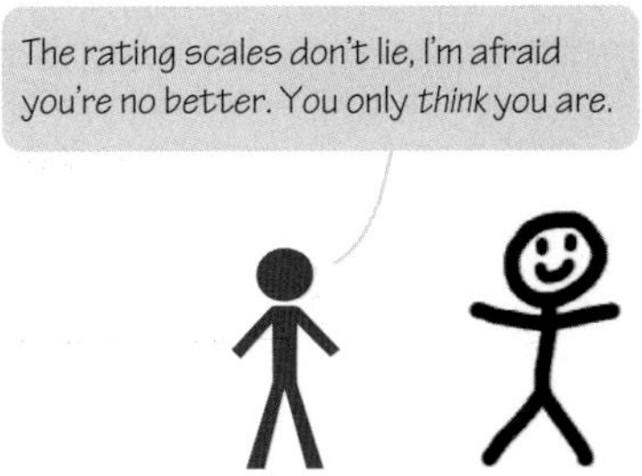

Disparities could also occur between self-rated versus clinician-rated measures of target symptoms. The Quick Inventory of Depressive Symptoms (QIDS) has both a self-report (SR) and clinician-rated (CR) version which have shown fairly robust inter-correlations from major depressive disorder patients seen in public sector settings (Bernstein et al., 2007). Studies using a 30-item forerunner of the QIDS, known as the Inventory of Depressive Symptoms (IDS), found that self-report versions tended to incur only slightly higher ratings than its clinician-rated version (Tondo et al., 1988). A self-administered version of the (traditionally clinician-rated) Montgomery–Åsberg Depression Rating Scale (MADRS) has been used with similar findings across both versions (Bondolfi et al., 2010).

In the case of cognitive complaints among mood-disordered patients, outpatients with bipolar disorder often overstated their own subjective cognitive complaints relative to objective performance-based assessments, or subjectively reported memory or attention problems without showing performance-based deficits when affective or anxiety symptoms were prominent (Burdick et al., 2005).

Yet another concern when rating depression is the question of whether a particular scale is tapping the *right* symptoms of depression. The HAM-D, for example, has undergone many iterations and, to varying degrees, is weighted rather heavily toward somatic symptoms, which could pose a confounding problem when used in medically ill populations; it may also under-identify elements of depression in patients for whom the cognitive rather than somatic symptoms of depression are paramount. The HAM-D and the MADRS also capture no symptoms of atypical depression (i.e., hypersomnia and hyperphagia), which has led some authors to question their relative usefulness for capturing features of, say, bipolar rather than unipolar depression.

Commonly used rating scales to measure symptom severity in anxiety disorders, OCD, and PTSD are presented in Table 6.9. Symptom measures commonly used in schizophrenia are summarized in Table 6.10, while common measures of objective cognitive function are summarized in Table 6.11.

Table 6.9 Symptom severity scales for anxiety disorders, OCD, and PTSD

Disorder	Rating scale	Description
Overall anxiety symptoms	Hamilton Anxiety Scale (HAM-A; Hamilton, 1959)	14-item clinician-rated scale capturing psychic and somatic anxiety subcomponents, with total scores from 0 to 54; scores ≤ 17 indicate mild anxiety; 18–24 indicate mild-moderate anxiety; scores ≥ 25 are considered moderate to severe
	State-Trait Anxiety Inventory (STAI; Spielberger et al., 1983)	40 self-report items, separately measuring state and trait anxiety features, with each subscale scored from 20 to 80
Social anxiety	Liebowitz Social Anxiety Scale (LSAS; Liebowitz, 1987)	24-item scale (either clinician- or self-administered) tapping performance anxiety and social situations; scores > 60 are associated with probable social anxiety disorder
OCD	Yale-Brown Obsessive-Compulsive Scale (YBOCS; Goodman et al., 1989)	Two subscales each of five items that rate obsessions and compulsions, each with scores ranging from 0 to 20 (summed up to 40 points); total scores < 7 are subclinical, 8-15 reflect mild OCD, 16-23 are moderate OCD, 24-31 are severe OCD, and ≥ 32 reflect extreme OCD
PTSD	Clinically Administered PTSD Scale (CAPS; Blake et al., 1990)	30-item semi-structured interview, scored by an algorithm according to DSM-5 criteria for PTSD

Table 6.10 Symptom severity scale for schizophrenia

	Measure	Description
Positive and negative symptoms, global psychopathology	Positive and Negative Symptoms Scale (PANSS; Kay et al., 1987)	Total scores < 58 reflect "mild," 59-75 are "moderate," 76-95 are "marked," and > 95 reflect "severe" illness (Leucht et al., 2005a)
Positive and negative symptoms	Scale for the Assessment of Positive Symptoms (SAPS; Andreasen, 1983) and Scale for the Assessment of Negative Symptoms (SANS; Andreasen, 1984)	The SAPS measures four domains (hallucinations, delusions, bizarre behavior, and formal thought disorder); the SANS captures five domains (affective flattening, alogia, avolition-apathy, anhedonia-asociality, and attention); SAPS and SANS items are each rated from 0 (absent) to 5 (severe)
General psychopathology	Brief Psychiatric Rating Scale (BPRS; Overall and Gorham, 1962)	18 clinician-rated items that tap a wide range of psychiatric symptoms (e.g., anxiety, emotional withdrawal, conceptual disorganization, mood); scores of about 31 correspond to "mildly ill," 41 corresponds to "moderately ill," and 53 equates to "markedly ill" (Leucht et al., 2005b)

Table 6.11 Examples of measures of cognitive function

Measure	Description
WAIS Digit Symbol Substitution Test	Subscale of the Wechsler Adult Intelligence Scale; measures processing speed, attention and working memory
Montreal Cognitive Assessment (MoCA; Nasreddine et al., 2005)	30-item test encompassing measures of attention, executive function, working memory, visuospatial processing, verbal memory, and fluency. Scores of 18–25 out of 30 suggest mild cognitive impairment; 10–17 indicate moderate cognitive impairment; scores < 10 reflect severe cognitive impairment.
Screen for Cognitive Impairment in Psychiatry (SCIP; Rojo et al., 2010)	Brief interview that captures list learning, attention, verbal fluency, delayed list learning, and visuomotor tracking. Total scores < 70 reflect cognitive impairment.

F PSYCHOSOCIAL FUNCTIONING

Practitioners tend to be less concerned than researchers might be in formally measuring psychosocial functioning and outcome. Perhaps that is because clinicians in practice, more than investigators in research studies, often spend considerable time qualitatively speaking with patients about their personal and professional lives and events therein, making work and social functioning nonamorphous and less in need of quantification. At the same time, when clinicians read and interpret clinical trials, it can be useful for them to know whether a treatment intervention merely (or only) improved targeted psychiatric symptoms or, moreover, led to benefits in work, social, or other areas of functioning. Recall also from Chapter 4, Section E, that patients themselves typically are more interested in the impact of psychiatric treatment on their daily lives, quality of life, and ability to fulfill role functions, rather than reducing symptoms alone. Table 6.12 describes several representative commonly used rating scales to measure aspects of psychosocial functioning.

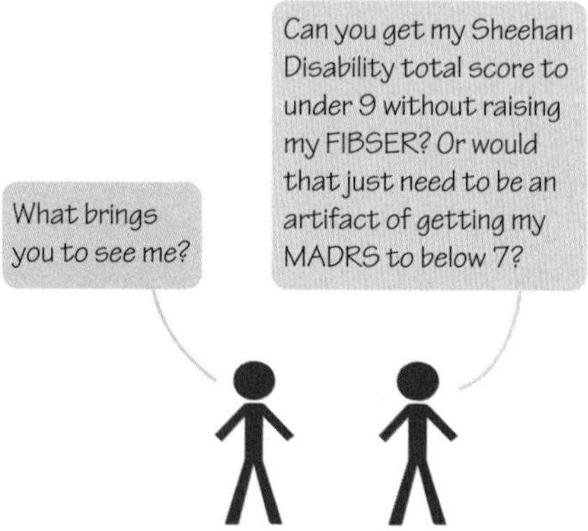

Table 6.12 Rating scales for psychosocial functioning

Domain	Measure	Description
Global functioning	Global Assessment of Functioning (GAF; American Psychiatric Association, 2000)	100-point scale with lower numbers reflecting greater impairment in symptoms, social, and work/school functioning
	World Health Organization Disability Assessment Scale (WHODAS; World Health Organization, 1988)	A detailed interview that replaced the GAF as a potentially more reliable component for the DSM-5
Quality of life	Quality of Life Enjoyment Satisfaction Scale (Q-LES-Q; Endicott et al., 1993)	14-item self-report scale with raw scores of 12–70

Table 6.12 (cont.)

Domain	Measure	Description
	Sheehan Disability Scale (SDS; Sheehan et al., 1996)	Three self-rated measures of work, social/leisure, and family/home activities, each scored from 0–10; for each subscale, 1-3 = "mild," 4-6 = "moderate," 7-9 = "severe," and 10 = "extreme" disability
Work and social functioning	Functional Assessment Short Test (FAST; Rosa et al., 2007)	24-item clinician-rated measure of six domains (autonomy, work functioning, cognition, financial issues, relationships, and leisure activity), each rated on a four-point scale from "no difficulty" (0) to "severe difficulty" (3)

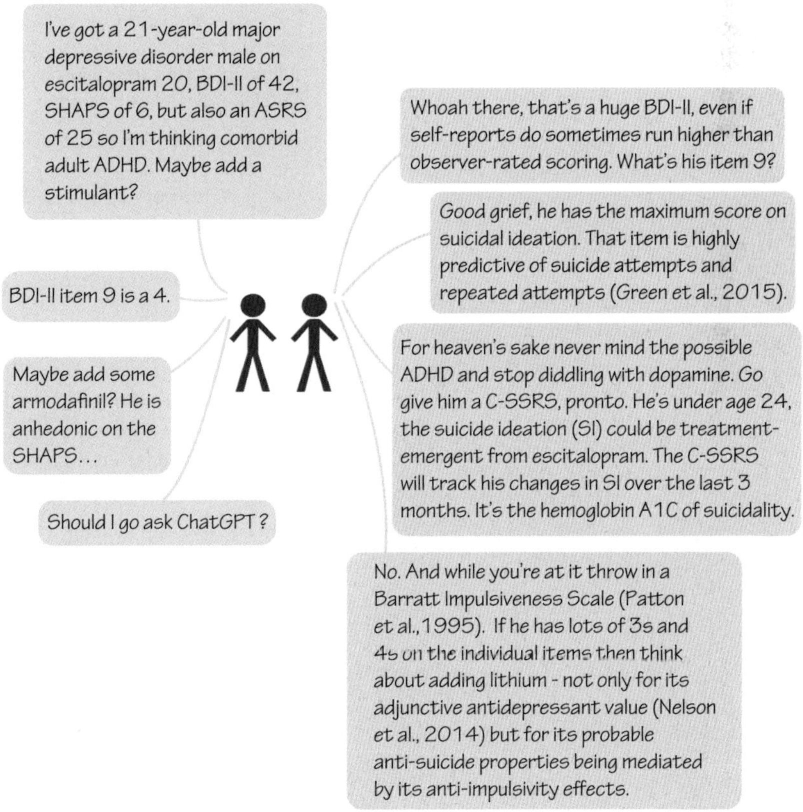

G MEASURING ADVERSE DRUG EFFECTS

A substantial problem when anticipating possible or probable medication side effects involves the extent to which a particular side effect of interest was formally and prospectively studied in published trials, or whether published reports of particular adverse drug effects rely solely on spontaneous patient reporting. Sexual dysfunction is notoriously one such common iatrogenic problem with many serotonergic and other medications, which is often under-identified in a manufacturer's product information due to a lack of prospective assessment (or, ratings of "WNL" – "we never looked"). Table 6.13 presents several examples of quantitative rating scales for medication side effects with their accompanying customary numerical interpretations.

Table 6.13 Rating scales to quantify medication side effects

Side effect	Rating scale	Description
Akathisia	Barnes Akathisia Rating Scale (BARS; Barnes, 1989)	Clinician-rated four-point scale assessing subjective and objective restlessness plus a five-point global assessment
	Simpson Angus Scale (SAS; Simpson and Angus, 1970)	Clinician-rated 10-item scale with total scores of 0–40; totals ≥ 6 prompt treatment reconsideration; > 12 "require attention," and ≥ 18 "almost certainly" require treatment modification
Overall side effects	Frequency, Intensity, and Burden of Side Effect Rating (FIBSER; Wisniewski et al., 2006)	Self-rated three-item scale rating interference with activities; scores of 0–2 = "mild," 3–4 = "moderate," and 5–6 = "severe" interference
Sexual dysfunction	Arizona Sexual Experience Scale (ASEX; McGahuey et al., 2000)	Self-rated five questions (total score = 3–30) addressing desire, arousal, erection or lubrication, orgasm, and satisfaction; "dysfunction" is reflected by a total score > 19 or ≥ 5 on one item or ≥ 4 on three items
Tardive dyskinesia	Abnormal Involuntary Movement Scale (AIMS; Guy, 1976b)	Seven core items each clinician-scored from 0 to 4; summed scores > 4 are considered strong evidence of tardive dyskinesia

H DISEASE STAGING

Other measurement-based tools for describing the nature and extent of psychiatric disorders are so-called staging models. Some staging models tend to focus on the number and types of failed medications for a given condition (as opposed to other types of indices of severity, such as hospitalizations, suicide attempts, degree of functional impairment). Others incorporate more varied dimensions of illness severity. A review of six staging models in depression (Ruhé et al., 2012) found variable predictive values of future treatment responses based on past treatment failures, but noted somewhat more robust values using the Maudsley Staging Model (Fekadu et al., 2009), which incorporates information on illness duration and symptom severity, as well as various augmentation and medication switching strategies. More detail regarding the Maudsley Staging Model for depression appears in Chapter 9, Table 9.2.

I TRANSLATING STATISTICAL CONCEPTS TO CLINICAL CARE DECISIONS

There are a number of key elements from the world of statistics and clinical trials that become relevant for making evidence-based treatment decisions in psychiatry: statistical significance and effect size are chief among these, along with replication and generalizability, and finally hypothesis-generating post hoc observations by the clinician-observer. Let us expand on these concepts in ways that can be useful to practitioners for decision-making purposes as well as patients for their part in shared decision-making – or at least recognizing the intended effects of a proposed intervention.

When we use formal measures to track target symptoms, as noted throughout this chapter, we have a way to tell if the changes we think we see over time are real or just a random occurrence. Engaging a patient to fill out a symptom rating form (or allowing the clinician to devote time to that) lets us then conclude with some degree of confidence that real change either has or has not occurred. This becomes critically useful when deciding between switching a treatment to an alternative versus augmenting it; it usually makes more sense to retain an initial therapy if we have some confidence that its contribution has been salient, meaning that it has made a significant and unambiguous difference. Whether or not we collect patient scores over an assessment period and formally run a statistical test on an app to measure whether change over time is real or random, or just compare the percentage of change from beginning to end, MBC can foster meaningful collaboration with patients.

The concept of statistical significance is relevant to direct patient care in at least two other aspects. First, let us consider the aphorism that we strive to change only one variable at a time. If multiple events occur simultaneously (such as stopping and starting multiple medications, adding a formal psychotherapy, or acknowledging major life events), causal relationships become harder to infer with confidence, and the presumptive "significance" of any one intervention can easily become lost. Statisticians refer to this problem as "multiplicity" or "simultaneous inference" – meaning that it is harder to judge with confidence the impact of a change in one variable when several are simultaneously in flux. Is it not always the case that multiple factors are in flux for people in real life? Of course! Which is why we strive to account for as many variables as possible when we ask why someone is better, or worse, or neither better nor worse. Confounders to treatment effects may be direct (such as nonadherence, or pharmacokinetic and pharmacodynamic interactions with other medications or psychoactive substances) or indirect (such as relationship stresses, physical illnesses, and the myriad of other life problems). Careful evaluators aim to determine which variables are a constant (are job or relationship stresses consistent or changing?) in order to allow an estimate of the impact of any one intervention on target symptoms, based on a guiding hypothesis.

A second relevant aspect to statistical significance comes from the basic premise of evidence-based medicine, in that the interventions which clinicians choose should, ideally, be supported by empirical precedent from clinical trials. Medications that have never been studied for a particular ailment, or have been studied and found to be no better than a placebo, become an iffy proposition when chosen blindly, and in favor of other options that may have a more supportive database. In the absence of empirical data, it is entirely consistent with evidence-based medicine to choose interventions mainly because they offer a compelling rationale and provide a way to test a hypothesis.

The expected or observed magnitude of change we see from an intervention captures the basic premise of an effect size – which is basically how much something has quantitatively changed from beginning to end after taking into account the variability seen in our measurements (as described in Formula 6.2). We can describe this to patients as how meaningful or impactful an intervention is on the target symptoms being treated. An effect size can be small, medium, or large. Patients may be surprised to learn that many pharmacotherapies have relatively small effect sizes (e.g., most monoaminergic antidepressant medications have small to medium effects, with a Cohen's *d* somewhere in the region of 0.30 (Goldberg, 2022)). In no small part, this is because placebo effects in depression are not trivial. They may be further surprised to learn that other treatment options can have much larger effect sizes (e.g., intravenous ketamine, or electroconvulsive therapy, with effect sizes of 0.80 or higher) when it comes time to weigh risks and benefits, or pros and cons. Recognizing treatment effect sizes removes another level of perceived arbitrariness from the decision-making dialogue and gives patients that much more insight and knowledge when they express a preference.

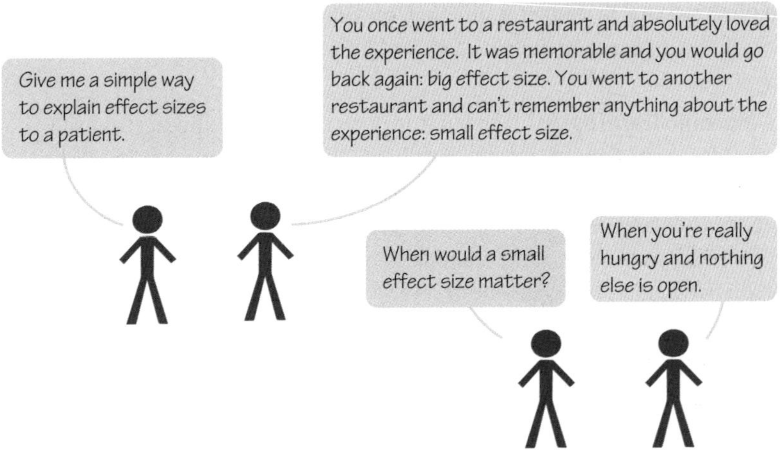

Ideally, we favor treatments that have been studied in large rather than small proof-of-concept studies, preferably in randomized trials so that likely cause-and-effect relationships are better supported. Case reports, open nonrandomized trials, or post hoc analyses and secondary data analyses from studies that were designed to measure a different question give us less confident information about treatment effects; such data are really more hypothesis-generating than hypothesis-testing.

Thus far we have been considering the use of metrics for individual patients to help facilitate clinical decision-making. Let us now consider the emerging role of big data and artificial intelligence as sources of information about clinical outcomes, and their applicability to definable patient subgroups.

J THE ROLE OF MACHINE LEARNING FOR MEASUREMENT-BASED CARE

Decisional analyses, which are discussed more explicitly in Chapters 7 and 8, provide a hierarchical summary of factors that collectively influence a decision point. In an area of statistics known as Bayesian analytics, when these factors involve likelihoods of an event occurring, they are called **prior probabilities**, or **posterior probabilities** when their values become updated with new information. The decision to discharge a suicidal patient from the emergency department may culminate from collective pieces of information that include as a prior probability the absence of a previous suicide attempt; once a suicide attempt has occurred, that information becomes a posterior probability relevant to the probability of future attempts. The decision to prescribe bupropion rather than an SSRI for depression may hinge on a clinical profile that includes obesity, smoking, seasonality, lethargy, inattention, minimal baseline anxiety, and the desire to minimize sexual dysfunction, although previous intolerance of a bupropion trial would be a posterior probability that could diminish enthusiasm for the decision to retry it.

Machine learning (**ML**), an outgrowth of artificial intelligence, aims to gather large amounts of information about a clinical subgroup (a "**training sample**") in order to then make quantitative predictions about a subsequent patient with respect to how their clinical profile conforms to the model generated by members of the training sample. It involves the generation of predictive models based on one of several approaches, such as decision trees or variations on regression analyses. Algorithms generate predictions with balanced accuracy that is sometimes expressed as an **F-1 score**, rated from 0 (worst) to 1 (best). Readers of this literature will encounter a variety of different ML algorithms, shown in Box 6.4.

Box 6.4

Subtypes of machine learning algorithms

- **Random forest**: an "ensemble" that combines the output of multiple decision trees that are built independently, then uses their averages (majority rules); often considered the most accurate learning algorithm
- **Support vector machine**: an ML algorithm in which a hyperplane (geometric subspace) divides different classes of subgroups based on characteristics of interest (say, suicide risk or likelihood of treatment nonadherence) from a training data set
- **Naïve Bayes classifiers**: a classification system that makes predictions on the basis of probabilities; it assumes the features of a measurement are independent ("naïve") of one another
- **Gradient-boosting decision tree**: similar to a random forest, where decision trees are combined, but building occurs at the beginning rather than the end of the analysis (trees are built one at a time rather than independently)
- **Extreme gradient-boosting**: a faster extension of gradient-boosting
- **Multilayer perceptron**: a so-called "feed forward" artificial neural network that iteratively adjusts weights in the network; it classifies data sets that are not linearly separable
- **Stochastic gradient descent**: a type of ML algorithm in which a single random sampling from a training data set (or a small batch taken from a larger training data set) is used to calculate a minimum value for the model being generated; it is a way to try to minimize the number of steps needed (and the potential for error) for an algorithm to "learn" from the training data set

The common thread among these various ML algorithms is that they each develop a way of making predictions about definable patient subgroups, based on collections of clinical or neurobiological characteristics. ML algorithms yield predictions with quantifiable accuracy, sensitivity, and specificity. One ML application focusing on a heterogeneous group of outpatients predicted psychotherapy outcomes with 67% balanced accuracy (using the 90-item psychiatric symptom checklist called the Symptom Checklist-90 (Derogatis et al., 2000) based on a combination of 16 predictor variables (Taubitz et al., 2022)). Another ML algorithm predicted the risk for emerging psychosis in an at-risk population with 85.5% balanced accuracy (Koutsouleris et al., 2021). A random-forest ML algorithm was developed to predict the emergence of "side effects" from psychotherapy (emergence of negative affect states, or worsening tension and anger), generating an F-1 score of 0.797 (Yao et al., 2020).

Regression is the overarching statistical approach that aims to form predictions about a dependent (outcome) variable while taking into account simultaneous previous information relevant to the immediate decision point. Factors might include demographic information, polygenic risk scores, and clinical information such as a history of trauma or suicide attempts. These relevant patient-specific parameters are called **individualized treatment rules** (ITRs). Optimal ITRs could, in principle, be inputted into a decision-tree regression model in order to yield quantitative output about the probability of response to a particular intervention. Such models in ML are known as decision trees for classification, and they depend on two key parameters: **entropy** (which refers to uncertainty in a group of observations) and **information gain** (a measure of how much information a feature provides about a class, which in turn helps to determine the order of attributes in the nodes of a decision tree).

Tip

Regression is a statistical approach for determining how much of the variability in a parameter of interest is explainable by a series of independent predictor variables, while accounting for each of their relative contributions and possible interactions with each other.

Tip

Polygenic risk scores are calculated weighted sums of gene variants (alleles) obtained from genome-wide association studies, which are used on an experimental basis to help explain complex heritable traits.

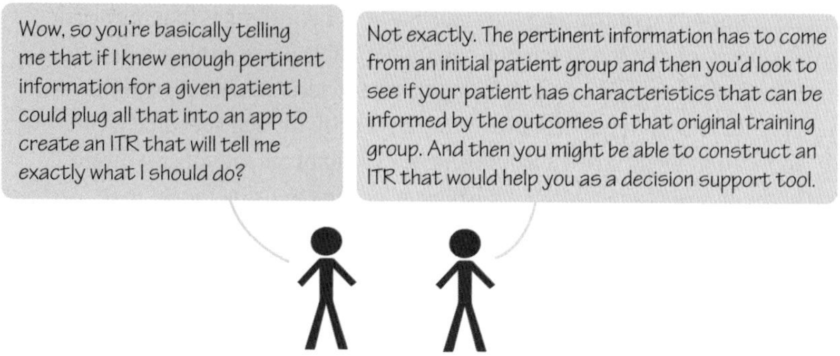

ML algorithms at present have been applied to *groups* of patients, rather than *individual* patients, based on learning from pre-existing data sets. Initial findings may help to shape the profile of optimal treatment responders to a given intervention by taking into account larger numbers of predictor variables than can be feasibly obtained from smaller data sets. Box 6.5 provides several representative examples from the literature on ML applications to fit predictive models of pharmacotherapy responses.

Box 6.5

Machine learning applications for predicting pharmacotherapy response

- Wu et al. (2020) undertook an ML approach to develop an ITR for choosing optimal pharmacotherapy for first-episode schizophrenia patients. Their training sample that provided clinical and demographic data was comprised of 32,272 patients from a national health insurance database. The resulting ITR yielded a significantly higher treatment success rate (51.7%) as compared to patients not within the ITR (44.5%) ($p < 0.001$).
- Del Fabro et al. (2023) reviewed the literature on ML as a decisional support tool for choosing antipsychotic medications for patients with schizophrenia. Among the variables they found that were entered successfully into predictive models were functional MRI, Positive and Negative Symptoms Scale (PANSS) baseline severity, and polygenic risk scores.
- In major depressive disorder, use of the Sequenced Treatment Alternatives to Relieve Depression (STAR*D) data set as a training sample allowed for the building of a tree-based random-forest model with approximately 25 predictor variables from STAR*D to characterize likelihood for remission (Salem et al., 2023); significant variables included baseline depression severity scores, age, education level, employment status, comorbidities, and a number of specific depression symptoms, side effects, and social supports. The resultant model achieved an 84.6% accuracy for predicting remission.

TAKE-HOME POINTS

- The use of psychometrically validated, quantitative measures of psychiatric symptoms can facilitate diagnostics, identification of target symptoms, and the tracking of progress over the course of a clinical trial
- Quantifiable changes in target symptoms using rating scales can facilitate decisions to continue, stop, switch, or augment a given treatment intervention
- Basic statistical concepts regarding effect sizes and the presence of statistically significant differences can be translated for patients to help their deliberations about pros and cons of relative treatment options
- Machine learning algorithms are being developed to help predict clinical outcomes for definable collections of subgroups according to collections of clinical, demographic, and neurobiological (neuroimaging, polygenic risk score) data

References

Aiken CB, Weisler RH, Sachs GS. The Bipolarity Index: A clinician-rated measure of diagnostic confidence. J Affect Disord 2015; 177: 59–64

American Psychiatric Association. Diagnostic and Statistical Manual of Mental Disorders, 4th edition, text revision (DSM-IV-TR). Washington, DC: American Psychiatric Association, 2000

American Psychiatric Association. Diagnostic and Statistical Manual of Mental Disorders, 5th edition. Washington, DC: American Psychiatric Association, 2013

Andreasen NC. The Scale for the Assessment of Negative Symptoms (SANS). Iowa City, Iowa: The University of Iowa, 1983

Andreasen NC. The Scale for the Assessment of Positive Symptoms (SAPS). Iowa City, Iowa: The University of Iowa, 1984

Barnes TR. A rating scale for drug-induced akathisia. Br J Psychiatry 1989; 154: 672–676

Beck AT, Steer RA, Ball R, et al. Comparison of Beck Depressive Inventories -IA and II in psychiatric outpatients. J Personality Assess 1996; 67: 588–597

Bernstein IH, Rush AJ, Carmody TJ, et al. Clinical versus self-report versions of the Quick Inventory of Depressive Symptoms in a public sector sample. J Psychiatr Res 2007; 41: 239–246

Blake DD, Weathers FW, Nagy LM, et al. A clinician rating scale for assessing current and lifetime PTSD: The CAPS-1. Behav Therap 1990; 13: 187–188

Bobes J, Rubio G, Téran A, et al. Pregabalin for the discontinuation of long-term benzodiazepines use: An assessment of its effectiveness in daily clinical practice. Eur Psychiatry 2012; 27: 301-307

Bondolfi G, Germann F, Weber Rouget B, et al. Self- and clinician-rated Montgomery–Åsberg Depression Rating Scale: Evaluation in clinical practice. J Affect Disord 2010; 121: 268-272

Burdick KE, Endick CJ, Goldberg JF. Assessing cognitive deficits in bipolar disorder: Are self-reports valid? Psychiatry Res 2005; 136: 43–50

Chamberlain SR, Cortese S, Grant JE. Screening for adult ADHD using brief rating tools: What can we conclude from a positive screen? Some caveats. Compr Psychiatry 2021; 106: 152224

Del Fabro L, Bondi E, Serio F, et al. Machine learning methods to predict outcomes of pharmacological treatment in psychosis. Transl Psychiatry 2023; 13(1): 75

Derogatis LR, Savitz KL. The SCL-90-R, Brief Symptom Inventory, and matching clinical rating scales. In Maruish ME (ed.), The Use of Psychological Testing for Treatment Planning and Outcomes Assessment. New York: Routledge, 2000, pp. 679–724

Endicott J, Nee J, Harrison W, et al. Quality of Life Enjoyment and Satisfaction Questionnaire: A new measure. Psychopharmacol Bull 1993; 29: 321–326

Fekadu A, Wooderson S, Donaldson C, et al. A multidimensional tool to quantify treatment resistance in depression: The Maudsley Staging Method. J Clin Psychiatry 2009; 70: 177–184

Goldberg JF. Perspectives on the success rate of current antidepressant pharmacotherapy. Expert Opin Pharmacother 2022; 23: 1781–1791

Goldberg JF, Garakani A, Ackerman SH. Clinician-rated versus self-rated screening for bipolar disorder among inpatients with mood symptoms and substance misuse. J Clin Psychiatry 2012; 73: 1525–1530

Goodman WK, Price LH, Rasmussen SA, et al. The Yale-Brown Obsessive-Compulsive Scale. I. Development, use, and reliability. Arch Gen Psychiatry 1989; 46: 1006–1011

Green KL, Brown GK, Jager-Hyman S, et al. The predictive validity of the Beck Depression Inventory suicide item. J Clin Psychiatry 2015; 76: 1683–1686

Guo T, Xiang Y-T, Xiao L, et al. Measurement-based care versus standard care for major depression: A randomized controlled trial with blind raters. Am J Psychiatry 2015; 172: 1004–1013

Guy W. Clinical Global Impressions. In ECDEU Assessment Manual for Psychopharmacology – Revised. Rockville, MD: US Department of Health, Education, and Welfare, 1976a, pp. 218–222

Guy W. Abnormal Involuntary Movement Scale (AIMS). In ECDEU Assessment Manual for Psychopharmacology – Revised. Rockville, MD: US Department of Health, Education, and Welfare, 1976b, pp. 534–537

Hadley SJ, Mandel FS, Schweizer E. Switching from long-term benzodiazepine therapy to pregabalin in patients with generalized anxiety disorder: A double-blind, placebo-controlled trial. J Psychopharmacol 2012; 26: 461–470

Hamilton M. The assessment of anxiety states by rating. Br J Med Psychol 1959; 32: 50–55

Hamilton M. A rating scale for depression. J Neurol Neursurg Psychiatry 1960; 23: 56–62

Hirschfeld RMA, Holzer C, Calabrese JR, et al. Validity of the Mood Disorder Questionnaire: A general population study. Am J Psychiatry 2003; 160: 178–180

Hohagen A, Münchau N, Hiss H, et al. Combination of behaviour therapy with fluvoxamine in comparison with behaviour therapy and placebo. Results of a multicentre study. Br J Psychiatry Suppl 1998; 35: 71–78

Johns MW. A new method for measuring daytime sleepiness: The Epworth Sleepiness Scale. Sleep 1991; 14: 540–545

Kay SR, Fiszbein A, Opler LA. The Positive and Negative Syndrome Scale (PANSS) for schizophrenia. Schiz Bull 1987; 13: 261–276

Koutsouleris N, Dwyer DB, Degenhardt F, et al. Multimodal machine learning workflows for prediction of psychosis in patients with clinical high-risk syndromes and recent-onset depression. JAMA Psychiatry 2021; 78: 195–209

Kroenke K, Spitzer RL, Williams JB. The PHQ-9: Validity of a brief depression severity measure. J Gen Int Med 2001; 16: 606–613

Leucht S, Kane JM, Kissling W, et al. What does the PANSS mean? Schizophr Res 2005a; 79: 231–238

Leucht S, Kane JM, Kissling W. Clinical implications of Brief Psychiatric Rating Scale scores. Br J Psychiatry 2005b; 187: 366–371

Lewis CC, Boyd M, Puspitasari A, et al. Implementing measurement-based care in behavioral health: A review. JAMA Psychiatry 2019; 76: 324–335

Liebowitz MR. Social phobia. Mod Probl Pharmacopsychiatry 1987; 22: 141–173

McGahuey CA, Gelenberg AJ, Laukes CA, et al. The Arizona Sexual Experience Scale (ASEX): Reliability and validity. J Sex Marital Ther 2000; 26: 25–40

McIntyre RS, Patel MD, Masand PS, et al. The Rapid Mood Screener (RMS): A novel and pragmatic screener for bipolar I disorder. Curr Med Res Opin 2021; 37: 135–144

Montgomery SA, Åsberg M. A new depression scale designed to be sensitive to change. Br J Psychiatry 1979; 134: 382–389

Nasreddine ZS, Phillips NA, Bédirian V, et al. The Montreal Cognitive Assessment, MoCA: A brief screening tool for mild cognitive impairment. J Am Geriatr Soc 2005; 53: 695–699

Nelson CJ, Baumann P, Delucchi K, et al. A systematic review and meta-analysis of lithium augmentation of tricyclic and second generation antidepressants in major depression. J Affect Disord 2014; 168: 269–275

Overall JE, Gorham DR. The Brief Psychiatric Rating Scale. Psychol Rep 1962; 10: 799–812

Patton JH, Stanford MS, Barratt ES. Factor structure of the Barratt Impulsiveness Scale. J Clin Psychol 1995; 51: 768–774

Peterson K, Anderson J, Bourne D. Evidence brief: Use of patient reported outcome measures for measurement based care in mental health shared decision making. Washington, DC: Department of Veterans Affairs (US), 2018

Posner K, Brown GK, Stanley B, et al. The Columbia-Suicide Severity Rating Scale: Initial validity and internal consistency findings from three multisite studies with adolescents and adults. Am J Psychiatry 2011; 168, 1266–1277

Rojo E, Pino O, Guilera G, et al. Neurocognitive diagnosis and cut-off scores of the Screen for Cognitive Impairment in Psychiatry (SCIP-S). Schizophr Res 2010; 116: 243–251

Rosa AR, Sánchez-Moreno J, Martínez-Aran A, et al. Validity and reliability of the Functioning Assessment Short Test (FAST) in bipolar disorder. Clin Pract Epidemiol Mental Health 2007; 3: 5

Ruhé HG, van Rooijen G, Spijker J, et al. Staging methods for treatment resistant depression. A systematic review. J Affect Disord 2012; 137: 35–45

Rush AJ, Trivedi MH, Ibrahim HM, et al. The 16-item Quick Inventory of Depressive Symptomatology (QIDS), clinician-rating (QIDS-C), and self-report (QIDS-SR): A psychometric evaluation in patients with chronic major depression. Biol Psychiatry 2003; 54: 573–583

Salem S, Huynh T, Topolski N, et al. Temporal multi-step predictive modeling of remission in major depressive disorder using early stage treatment data: STAR*D based machine learning approach. J Affect Disord 2023; 324: 286–293

Saunders JB, Aasland OG, Babor TF, et al. Development of the Alcohol Use Disorders Identification Test (AUDIT): WHO Collaborative Project on Early Detection of Persons with Harmful Alcohol Consumption – II. Addiction 1993; 88: 791–804

Sheehan DV, Harnett-Sheehan K, Raj BA. The measurement of disability. Int Clin Psychopharmacol 1996; 11 (Suppl 3): 89–95

Simpson GM, Angus JWS. A rating scale for extrapyramidal side effects. Acta Psychiatr Scand (Suppl) 1970; 212: 11–19

Snaith RP, Hamilton M, Morley S, et al. A scale for the assessment of hedonic tone the Snaith–Hamilton Pleasure Scale. Br J Psychiatry 1995; 167: 99–103

Spielberger CD, Gorsuch RL, Lushene RE, et al. Manual for the State–Trait Anxiety Inventory (Form Y). Palo Alto, CA: Consulting Psychologists Press, 1983

Spitzer RL, Kroenke K, Williams JB, et al. A brief measure for assessing generalized anxiety disorder: The GAD-7. Arch Int Med 2006; 166: 1092–1097

Taubitz FS, Büdenbender B, Alpers GW. What the future holds: Machine learning to predict success in psychotherapy. Behav Res Ther 2022; 156: 104116

Tenneij NH, van Megen HJGM, Denys DA, et al. Behavior therapy augments response of patients with obsessive–compulsive disorder responding to drug treatment. J Clin Psychiatry 2005; 66: 1169–1175

Tondo L, Burrai C, Scamonatti L, et al. Comparison between clinician-rated and self-reported depressive symptoms in Italian psychiatric patients. Neuropsychobiology 1988; 19: 1–5

Ustun B, Adler LA, Rudin C, et al. The World Health Organization Adult Attention-Deficit/Hyperactivity Disorder self-report screening scale for DSM-5. JAMA Psychiatry 2017; 74: 520–526

Weathers FW, Litz BT, Keane TM, et al. The PTSD Checklist for DSM-5 (PCL-5). Boston, MA: National Center for PTSD, 2013

Wisniewski SR, Rush AJ, Balasubramani GK, et al. Self-rated global measure of the frequency, intensity, and burden of side effects. J Psychiatr Pract 2006; 12: 71–79

World Health Organization. WHO Psychiatric Disability Assessment Schedule. Geneva: WHO; 1988

Wu C-S, Luedtke AR, Sadikova E, et al. Development and validation of a machine learning individualized treatment rule in first-episode schizophrenia. JAMA Netw Open 2020; 3(2): e1921660

Yao L, Zhao X, Xu Z, et al. Influencing factors and machine learning-based prediction of side effects in psychotherapy. Front Psychiatry 2020; 11: 537442

Young RC, Biggs JT, Ziegler VE, et al. A rating scale for mania: Reliability, validity and sensitivity. Br J Psychiatry 1978; 133: 429–435

Zimmerman M, Galione JN. Screening for bipolar disorder with the mood disorders questionnaire: A review. Harv Rev Psychiatry 2011; 19: 219–228

Zimmerman M, McGlinchey JB. Why don't psychiatrists use scales to measure outcome when treating depressed patients? J Clin Psychiatry 2008; 69: 1916–1919

Zimmerman M, Martinez J, Attiulah N, et al. Why do some depressed outpatients who are in remission according to the Hamilton Depression Rating Scale not consider themselves to be in remission? J Clin Psychiatry 2012a; 73: 790–795

Zimmerman M, Martinez J, Attiulah N, et al. Why do some depressed outpatients who are not in remission according to the Hamilton Depression Rating Scale nonetheless consider themselves to be in remission? Depress Anxiety 2012b; 29: 891–895

7 Hypothesis-Testing and Crafting Patient-Specific Decision Trees

LEARNING OBJECTIVES

- [ ] Understand the basic principles of hypothesis generation and testing as relevant to devising clinical diagnostic formulations, evaluating possible causal relationships between symptoms and treatments, and making generalizable versus provisional inferences about treatment effects
- [ ] Describe pattern recognition, template matching, prototype matching, and expectancy bias as influences on clinical reasoning and decision-making
- [ ] Describe the types of cognitive bias that can distort objective clinical inferences
- [ ] Define pseudospecificity
- [ ] Recognize the basic elements of crafting and using patient-specific decision trees

A EVERYTHING IS A TESTABLE HYPOTHESIS

Formulating and empirically testing hypotheses lies at the core of the scientific method, and is a cornerstone for practicing evidence-based medicine – especially if and when the evidence base for a given problem may not yet be so well developed in the literature. Whether we realize it or not, every clinical encounter is essentially the buildup to generating a hypothesis – a framework for explaining how and why a set of problems arose, and then figuring out whether the available information supports or refutes the proposed explanation. A hypothesis is a testable, falsifiable question posed about the association between two variables.

> **Tip**
> Approach every clinical problem with the mindset of generating a "differential diagnostic" list of plausible explanations.

For example, one might wonder if insomnia complaints reflect simple insomnia, restless legs, a medication side effect, a circadian rhythm disorder, sleep apnea, a sign of mania, or drug-seeking behavior for a controlled substance; or if increased motor activity represents mania versus substance misuse versus akathisia versus neurotoxicity from a pharmacokinetic interaction. One could hypothesize that poor interpersonal relatedness is more likely a sign of autism versus schizophrenia versus social anxiety, depending on the presence of other features, such as a formal thought disorder or disorganized speech. Or that poor medication adherence, rather than lack of drug efficacy, is a more likely explanation of relapse. Formulating viable and testable hypotheses pertains to both assessment and treatment, and becomes a prerequisite for both.

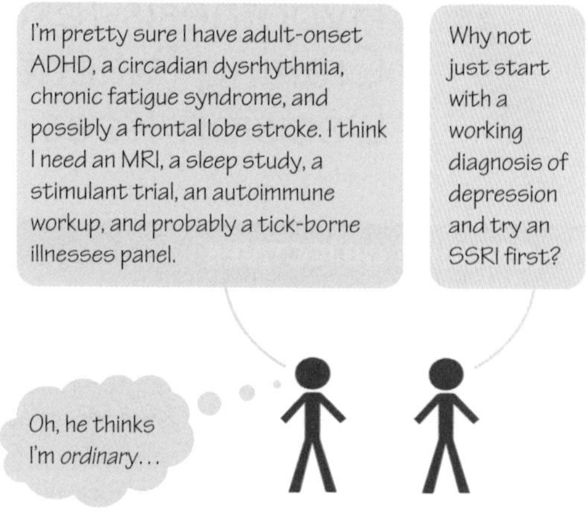

Clinicians make hypotheses when they surmise that a patient with a particular clinical profile might benefit from one treatment option more than another, or when they think that the presence of certain features must signal the presence of one disorder as more likely than another, or could be subsumed under another for explaining a clinical problem. Patients generate hypotheses all the time when they speculate about etiologies of a problem, or look for a way to try to explain one away (e.g., "I think the escitalopram, rather than my cocaine use, is causing my mood swings"). Our key interest in this chapter, for both patients and practitioners, involves first reviewing how to formulate cogent, plausible hypotheses (and teaching patients how to do this themselves), and then articulating a strategy to examine the evidence that supports or refutes a suspected hypothesis (something we usually must continually remind and re-teach ourselves as clinicians who want to follow a scientific methodology).

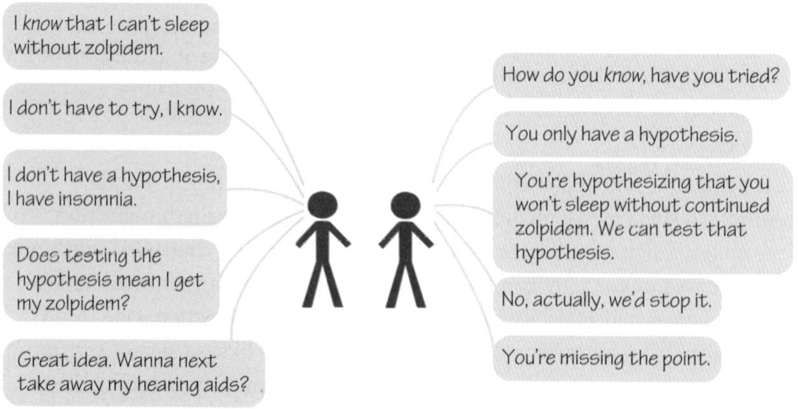

At the core of hypothesis-testing lies the distinction between the **null hypothesis**, designated $\mathbf{H_0}$ (i.e., the idea that a suspected observation is simply due to random chance, or a fluke event), versus an **alternative hypothesis**, designated $\mathbf{H_A}$ (i.e., that the suspected observation is real, and not due to random events or another more plausible explanation). One can also have multiple competing hypotheses, with a mental numerical designation (H_1, H_2, H_3, ...). Take as an example the hypothesis that an antidepressant medication has induced mania in a patient with bipolar disorder. Accepting the null hypothesis would mean that an observed case of mania following antidepressant exposure likely *did not result from* the antidepressant exposure, but instead occurred due to *random chance* (that is, simply the natural course of illness). Before one can decide whether to accept or reject the null hypothesis, we must establish a few core tenets:

- Affirm that the observed phenomenon is, indeed, the phenomenon of interest and not something else entirely. In this case, declaring the occurrence of mania means that one is fairly sure that mania is present, and not simply a remission from depression, the occurrence of akathisia, anxious distress, simple insomnia caused by a medication, or subthreshold irritability or agitation that is not necessarily a marker of mania as a full syndrome
- Determine a temporal association between the observed event (mania) and the suspected cause (antidepressant exposure); such an association contrasts with mania that may have been present before antidepressant medication exposure, became neither better nor worse afterward, but was only noticed after the exposure
- Consider whether there may be likely confounding factors that impact a suspected causal link. For instance, are we certain that the patient actually *took* the suspected offending antidepressant? Was there contemporaneous illicit substance use that might better account for the observed phenomenon? Was the patient unambiguously depressed prior to antidepressant exposure, or could their "newly emergent" mania have been misidentified as a continuation of an existing state that was unrecognized before starting an antidepressant medication? Are there other unaccounted-for factors that could trigger mania, such as steroid use or changes to a sleep schedule? What is thc patient's baseline frequency of episodes? Someone with true rapid cycling (four or more distinct episodes per year) is statistically predisposed to having more spontaneous mood episodes over time, independent of the treatments they receive, than someone whose last mania occurred in the remote past

Unaccounted-for confounding factors such as these could quickly torpedo the H_A of interest. In fact, the above process essentially means formulating a differential diagnosis (or, differential explanations) for an observed phenomenon, resisting the temptation to jump to a premature conclusion.

Before delving further into the mechanics of hypothesis generation and testing as it applies to individualized patient care, let us first consider how a clinician's prior experience shapes the way they perceive and process the clinical data they take in. That requires us to take a brief excursion into the cognitive process of pattern recognition.

B PATTERN RECOGNITION

We often make sense of new information and form impressions by recognizing familiar patterns in an unfolding narrative. For example, a clinician might instinctively think of obsessive–compulsive disorder (OCD) when they hear about a patient who is preoccupied with repetitive thoughts that seem senseless to him, or they might think of psychosis if the repetitive thoughts hold a strong belief-conviction. (One then might further hypothesize a role for serotonergic antidepressant medications in the first scenario but antipsychotic medications in the second.) "Anxiety" complaints fit a pattern of social phobia when they involve self-consciousness and feelings of being ridiculed or embarrassed, or they may instead fit a pattern of ideas of reference related to schizophrenia when they involve attributions about persecutory intent from other people.

Pattern recognition involves the ability to interpret incoming information into a coherent signal; it involves synthesizing parts into a comprehensible whole, based largely on past experience. Imagine conducting a diagnostic interview with Peggy, a 24-year-old unemployed woman, that elicits a hodgepodge of seemingly unrelated elements – mood dysregulation, impaired attention, poor impulse control, formal thought disorder, internal preoccupation, panic attacks, binge-eating/purging, sleep–wake cycle reversal, amotivation/apathy, body dysmorphic features, somatic preoccupations, autonomic hyperarousal in the context of past trauma .... We could go on, but it would be nearly impossible to leach out from such a litany of complaints a coherent and overarching organizing pattern, leaving most clinicians rightly confused about what could be going on with Peggy. Some might bypass that confusion or lack of a coherent signal and yield to the temptation to force-fit Peggy into a conceptual diagnostic framework that may not neatly capture the actual elements of her problems. In fact, who knows what could be wrong with Peggy unless we can render some sense of recognizable order from her variety of complaints. Relying on single overarching symptoms as being specifically diagnostic for one disorder over another remains a nosologically risky proposition (see Box 7.1).

Box 7.1

Are there pathognomonic signs of specific disorders?

At one time, there was considerable interest in trying to identify possible diagnostically unique features that would in themselves be considered high-probability indicators of a particular psychiatric condition. Historical examples in schizophrenia have included neologisms, verbigeration (i.e., the repetition of random words), and so-called first-rank symptoms (FRS) as originally described by the German psychiatrist Kurt Schneider (a collation of 11 symptoms that largely involve delusions or hallucinations notable for an external locus of control - such as thought insertion, thought withdrawal, thought broadcasting, "made" feelings or emotions, and "made" behaviors). A Cochrane review found that FRS had only a rather-*myeh* 58% sensitivity and 75% specificity in discriminating schizophrenia from other psychotic disorders (Soares-Weiser et al., 2015).

It is a tricky thing to think of "pathognomonic" signs for *any* psychiatric disorder because most symptoms have at least some potential overlap with other conditions. (Arguably, cataplexy is pathognomonic of narcolepsy because its occurrence in other disorders is exceedingly rare.)

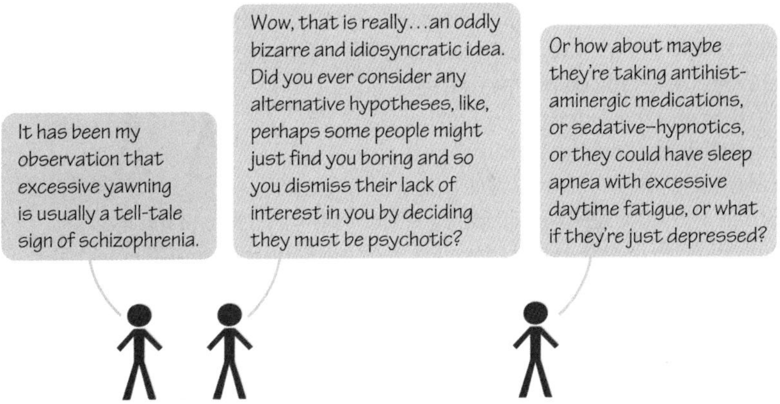

Psychologists refer to two processes involved in pattern recognition: **template matching** and **prototype matching**. **Template matching** involves comparing new information against an existing template of a known recognizable pattern. For instance, consider that a clinician's pre-existing template for assessing depression involves the pattern of observable decreased spontaneous movements, speech with diminished prosody, terse responses to questions, and apathy. Patients who report feeling depressed but fail to display the expected template pose an anomaly. Or imagine that the "template" for judging schizophrenia involves detecting poor interpersonal relatedness, concrete thinking, and bizarre speech content. One might have a vaguely similar but slightly different pattern in mind for detecting autism – perhaps sensing preoccupations with parts versus wholes, or sensing more curiosity than avoidance about the unknown. In short, when we take in new data we are primed to make it fit into a patterned context that makes sense based on our past experience.

> **Tip**
> Beware of the temptation to assume or imagine that missing elements of a diagnosis "must" be present because the known pattern calls for it. Don't assume obsessions necessarily involve compulsions, or that posttraumatic stress disorder (PTSD) expectably includes nightmares.

Powers of observation are integral to noticing pieces of a template, and can account for what might otherwise be called clinical intuition. Slowed gait with bradykinesia and masked facies connotes parkinsonism. Noticing bulging eyes and an apparent neck mass in a depressed middle-aged patient sets the wheels in motion for a line of inquiry that shapes the hypothesis of clinical hypothyroidism. Recognizing conjunctivitis in an amotivational young adult should prompt thinking about cannabis use. Predictable time courses also bear on expected patterns. A patient hospitalized for "psychotic mania" on a Friday night whose mental status clears entirely within 48 hours probably more closely fits a pattern of intoxication or delirium than true mania (the quick recovery time is inconsistent with the hypothesis that mania explains Friday night's mental status). Or a purported first lifetime episode of mania after age 60 does not fit the epidemiological template of prototypical bipolar disorder and that incongruence would drive the search for other hypotheses to explain a secondary mania – such as a more likely underlying endocrine, toxic–metabolic, or other medical/neurological cause.

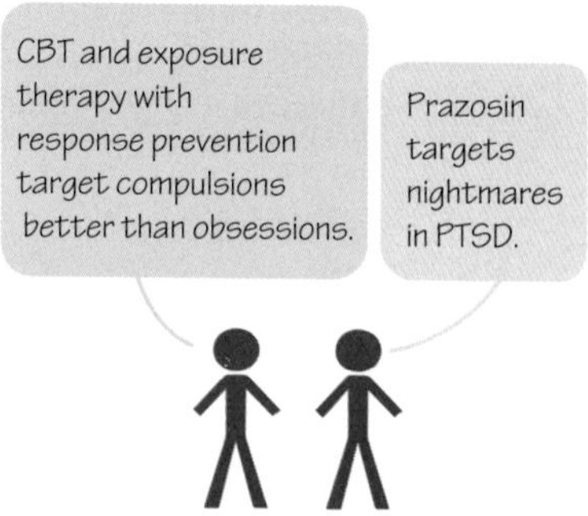

Box 7.1 summarizes a number of useful concepts worth considering that bear on pattern recognition for deducing likely hypotheses.

Prototype matching is a kind of variant of template matching; it involves drawing a more imperfect kind of association between new incoming information and an "average" or general kind of template – rather like fuzzy logic in the world of artificial intelligence. As an example, one might broadly lump all descriptions of anxiety under the overarching heading of "anxiety" – including somatic anxiety, panic attacks, free-floating generalized anxiety, phobias, and autonomic hyperarousal states. Once the prototype becomes matched, the

Box 7.1

Points to consider when formulating and evaluating a diagnostic hypothesis

- Do the chronology and time frame of events make sense?
- Does the presentation follow a known epidemiological pattern?
- How is the current clinical presentation similar to or different from previously known examples?
- What other factors could account for the observed phenomenon?
- Could medication effects (including side effects, drug interactions, or nonadherence) explain the symptoms of interest?
- In what psychosocial context do symptoms arise?

clinician may then impose corollaries about treatment that may sometimes run the risk of overgeneralizing from more specific past experiences. (If, for instance, alprazolam was known to stop a panic attack, the clinician might wrongly overgeneralize that benzodiazepines are the universal first-line approach to any and all forms of anxiety.) Or if a clinician subsumes all forms of depression under a single prototype (regardless of subtypes – anxious, agitated, melancholic, psychotic, atypical, bipolar, or mixed features), they may in turn assume that all forms of depression reflexively equate to the role for a selective serotonin reuptake inhibitor (SSRI) as a first-line intervention. Prototype matching can aid the diagnostic process when some but not all elements of a known clinical entity are present. The designation of "unspecified" subtypes of depression or bipolar disorder is useful when an insufficient number or duration of symptoms is present to match to an exact template. On the other hand, disparate symptoms that fail to map to any semblance of a known template pose a conundrum.

In Peggy's case, we could try to force-fit or even imagine a unifying, overarching pattern to explain her condition when no such rubric really exists. Maybe Peggy has bipolar disorder. Maybe borderline personality disorder. Maybe PTSD. Maybe major depression. Seeing or declaring a falsely imagined pattern, when no true pattern exists, is called *apophenia* – that is, perceiving meaningful connections among disparate elements when there is no unifying clinical, conceptual thread.

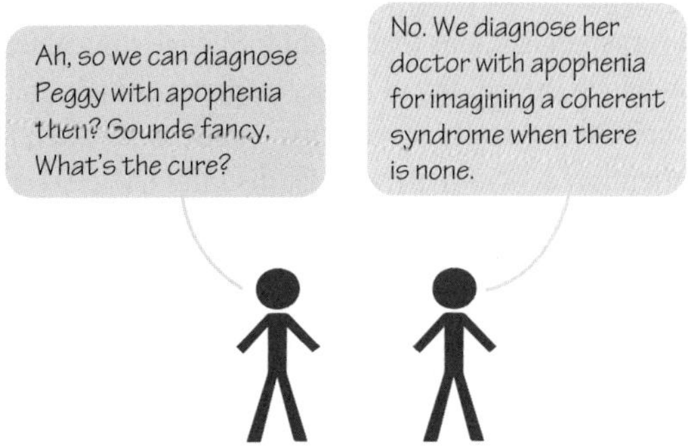

C APOPHENIC PSYCHOPHARMACOLOGY

Now, consider the potential for a clinician to develop wrongly biased templates about the pharmacodynamic effects of specific medications, and the resulting potential to form distorted hypotheses. Imagine that Dr. Bob perceives methylphenidate to be more potent than amphetamine (when in fact the opposite is true), believes that hydroxyzine reduces suicidal thinking (there are no reports of this in the literature), or that topiramate is a reliable and effective antimanic drug (even though there are multiple published negative placebo-controlled trials and no positive randomized adult trials; Kushner et al., 2006). Or suppose hypothetically that, in Dr. Sally's experience, she has come to form the impression that gabapentin is an excellent antimanic drug. Pretend the year is 1999, a time when there was a prevailing impression that anticonvulsant medications as a class likely possessed mood-stabilizing properties, and she even just read an enthusiastic recently published open trial showing that hypomanic bipolar patients had a favorable response to gabapentin (based on the symptomatically nonspecific Clinical Global Impressions (CGI) scale) with minimal side effects (Altshuler et al., 1999; never mind that the study only involved 18 patients). Cheerfully predisposed to what she has decided are solid, reliable, and generalizable pharmacodynamic benefits, she establishes a mental template for gabapentin-responsive bipolar disorder. She then imparts a positive outcome expectancy to patients and colleagues, perhaps unaware of the approximate 30% placebo response seen in studies of bipolar mania (Sysko and Walsh, 2007), and now embraces as a default conclusion that gabapentin has established efficacy in mania and may even represent the "easiest and safest" first-line treatment, especially for "soft" cases. She may even scoff at later randomized trials showing that it is in fact *inferior to placebo* in mania (Pande et al., 2000) because her template has become engrained. First impressions die hard. Can evidence-based data overcome entrenched distorted templates that are drawn from initial experiences? To paraphrase Samuel Clemens, never let the truth get in the way of good clinical apophenia.

Think of the many potentially distorted biases and apophenic overgeneralizations that might influence clinical templates, and the ways in which the validity of those templates either remains sacrosanct or can be subjected to scrutiny over time – such as: all attentional complaints equate to attention deficit–hyperactivity disorder (ADHD) and warrant a stimulant trial; irritability must be shorthand for bipolar disorder; inflammatory biomarkers should be measured in every depressed patient; or all hypersomnia must reflect sleep apnea until proven otherwise. Imagining patterns when there are none, or forming wrong conclusions about suspected patterns, closes off thinking to the generation of new hypotheses and discourages their testing.

With the above in mind, let us now turn to the process of hypothesis formulation and testing when working with patients.

D HYPOTHESIS GENERATION AND TESTING

We make predictions about associations between two variables – say, a symptom and its likely cause(s), or an interpersonal or other life stressor and the thoughts and feelings it stirs up – sometimes more as a passive than active process. Our goal here is to recognize when a relationship is clinically important and then make the process active. A first step in clinical hypothesis generation involves gathering pertinent data, checking these against previous experience, and then proposing a reasonable and testable explanation. Fundamentally, one is testing whether a suspected relationship between variables is true and not a red herring (meaning, an occurrence due only to random chance). A red herring in this case represents the null hypothesis – a random event.

> **Tip**
>
> **Falsifiability** refers to the ability to find empirical evidence that will refute a hypothesis. A hypothesis could be untestable or nonfalsifiable because of subjective factors (e.g., "escitalopram is a better drug than citalopram") or because empirical testing would be technically impossible (e.g., "stress causes depression").

> **Tip**
>
> Delusions, as fixed convictions, tend to resist being subjected to hypothesis-testing.

Suppose Alvin is a patient with hypertension and bipolar disorder who takes lithium and we measure his serum lithium level twice, one week apart: the first time, his level is 0.8 mEq/L and the second time it is 0.5 mEq/L. Is this an explainable result caused by some specific influence? Among various possible (and falsifiable) explanations, we could hypothesize that Alvin may have missed one or more doses of medication; may have gotten his second level drawn later in time after he last took lithium than occurred for his first level; or perhaps Alvin was taking a co-prescribed drug that could raise lithium levels (such as a nonsteroidal anti-inflammatory drug or a thiazide diuretic) prior to the first but not the second laboratory test, and we did not think to ask. Or was the drop in lithium levels just a random fluctuation (i.e., the null hypothesis) that has no clinical meaning behind it? What if the difference reflected a laboratory error – when should we simply re-order the test and not necessarily ascribe likely importance to the initial result? Added to this, how much does the numerical difference between the two laboratory values even matter clinically? A drop from 0.8 mEq/L to an undetectable level is stark, as is a rise from 0.8 mEq/L to 1.5 mEq/L, but how does the clinician know where to draw the line of what is clinically meaningful and worth investigating, before venturing into the realm of finding explanations for a phenomenon that may or may not even be nonrandom? Every plausible explanation constitutes a testable hypothesis, and hypothesis-testing is the only empirical way to deduce an evidence-based conclusion.

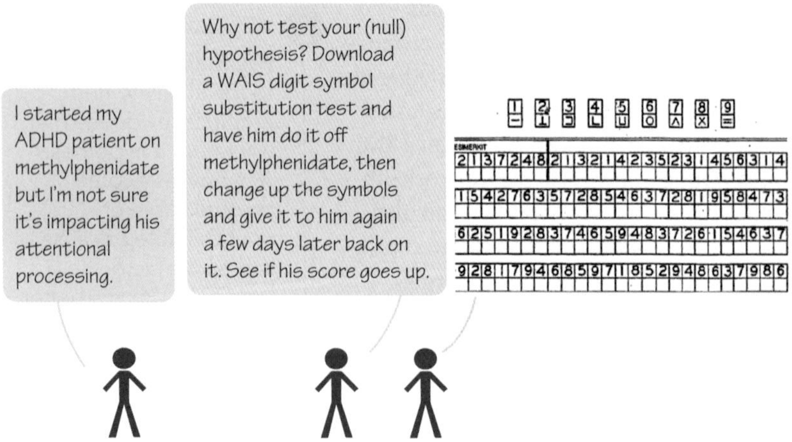

E HYPOTHESIS GENERATION VERSUS TESTING

We *generate* a hypothesis from observations that prompt us to consider explanations we had not previously thought of; we *test* a hypothesis when we have an explanation in mind at the outset and are able to account reasonably enough for all the possible red herrings that could otherwise intrude into a cause-and-effect explanation for our observations. As an example, consider a patient who switches from a brand name to a generic formulation of a drug that has a wide therapeutic window, and she feels that the generic is less effective. It is certainly possible, and plausible, that a generic drug could have lesser efficacy – the area under the curve for a generic drug must be anywhere between 80% and 120% of the equivalent level for the brand name, and demonstrated efficacy is typically not required for manufacturing approval of a generic drug. What stops us from declaring as a conclusion that generic drugs are inferior to branded formulations? Many things. For one, unless the patient is somehow blinded to knowing whether they are taking a branded or generic formulation, the hypothesis is contaminated by expectancy bias. (It helps support the hypothesis if the patient truly did not realize that a switch from branded to generic occurred.) A second consideration involves the magnitude of difference they perceive in efficacy between the branded and generic formulations; if the patient's symptoms were only partially improved with the branded formulation, and they experienced a subjective worsening of symptoms, it would be hard to know if the worsening resulted *from* the formulation switch or *despite* the formulation switch, inasmuch as the residual symptoms that were present before the switch may have simply worsened due to the natural course of illness. The process of clinical evaluation and decision-making is not immune to the impact of expectancy bias.

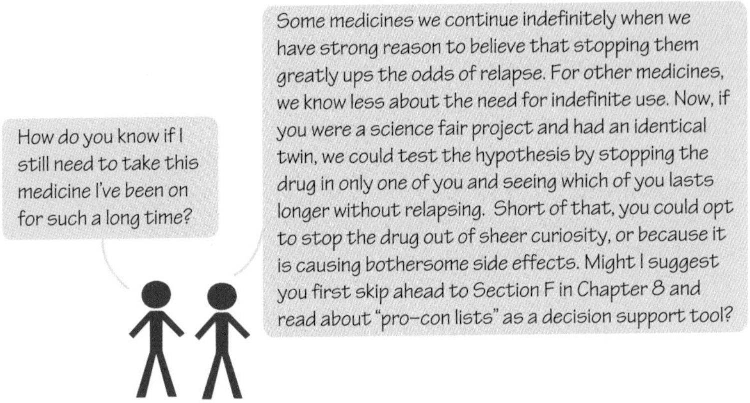

F WHAT IS EXPECTANCY BIAS AND HOW DOES IT INFLUENCE ASSESSMENT AND DECISION-MAKING?

Expectancy bias is a thorn in the side of practically all things remotely therapeutic. It is a form of cognitive bias in which one's belief in a hypothesis may lead to ignoring or outright discarding information that could contradict an embraced hypothesis. Expectancy bias can prompt clinicians (or patients) to cling to an ongoing useless treatment after it has failed to show efficacy ("it should start to work any day now … because it is *supposed* to work"); to eschew treatments that they perceive with disfavor (e.g., "monoamine oxidase inhibitors are dangerous" or "lamotrigine makes your skin fall off") or to discard alternative hypotheses without their proper vetting (for instance, expecting that depression will eventually improve once the "right" antidepressant medication is found could bias someone against forming and exploring other hypotheses to explain treatment resistance, such as poor adherence, undetected hypothyroidism, psychosis, or psychoactive substance use). For better or worse, expectancy bias can also inflate placebo responsivity – as when a new medication enters clinical practice amid a flurry of enthusiasm about its novelty and anticipated superiority over its predecessors.

Doherty and Carroll (2020) note four types of cognitive bias that could distort clinical decision-making, as summarized in Box 7.2.

Box 7.2

Types of cognitive bias in clinical decision-making

- **Confirmation bias** involves selectively gathering information that conforms to a held hypothesis (e.g., a conviction that a tick-borne illness must explain chronic fatigue, despite negative serology or known exposures)
- **Anchoring bias** refers to prioritizing data in ways that best support an embraced hypothesis (such as focusing on depressive symptoms over autonomic signs of alcohol withdrawal; or relentlessly searching for evidence of previous trauma if one staunchly holds the hypothesis that depression "must" almost always have such developmental roots)
- **Affect heuristic** is a type of bias that describes a clinician's emotional reaction to a patient or their symptoms as influencing their assessment or treatment decisions (e.g., refusing to consider the use of psychostimulants for ADHD in patients with a substance use disorder history, based on assumptions that prescribed stimulants would expectably become abused, and despite evidence to the contrary regarding their safety and efficacy in that setting (Faraone and Wilens, 2007))
- **Outcome bias** refers to assumptions that prior experiences will *predictably and necessarily* inform future experiences – as could happen if, say, a patient suicides while taking a particular antidepressant, prompting the clinician to never again prescribe that specific antidepressant medication; or, when a patient develops a skin rash with a particular drug, biasing the clinician against using that medication in other patients because of an overgeneralized expectation about the drug's assumed proclivity to cause cutaneous reactions

G WHEN ANECDOTAL OBSERVATIONS INSPIRE HYPOTHESIS FORMULATION

Hypothesis generation becomes a scientifically elegant process when anecdotal observations lead to formulating a hypothesis that then stands up to empirical assessment. Suppose that while treating a number of depressed patients with ketamine or esketamine, researchers notice that not only do depressive symptoms in general improve but that suicidal thoughts in particular seem to dramatically lessen. They could generate a hypothesis that ketamine might have specific anti-suicide properties. At what point can they convert this hypothesis to a fact, or generalizable conclusion? The observation would need to be replicated (preferably more than just once or twice, in different settings) – preferably, in a planned study that was prospectively designed specifically to test this as an a priori hypothesis, with a large enough group of patients to allow for generalizability. One would also need to consider accounting for other pertinent factors that could intrude on my suspected hypothesis between ketamine-taking and suicide reduction – such as: When is suicide reduction merely an artifact of an overall antidepressant effect? Or did the duration of suicidal ideation before ketamine influence its apparent "success"? What if ketamine "reduced" suicidal ideation only in people who had never before made a suicide attempt? Or in those for whom anxious ruminations about suicide were present – and then we would formulate a new hypothesis that ketamine reduces suicidal ideation by virtue of an anti-ruminative effect.

If a single symptom improves mainly by virtue of the effect of a treatment on a broader syndrome (think antibiotics improving cough in someone with bacterial pneumonia), we ask if the effect on the particular symptom is *pseudospecific*, as described further in Box 7.3.

Box 7.3

What is pseudospecificity?

The term "pseudospecificity" is sometimes used in the world of clinical trials to describe apparent treatment effects on a particular symptom that are actually just an artifact of some broader effect on an overall syndrome. For example, if a drug has a soporific effect in the context of treating depression, we cannot (necessarily) surmise that it would make a good sleep aid for any and all forms of insomnia. Or if a drug improves cognitive functioning in the context of treating depression, one could *hypothesize* that it might possess a distinct pro-cognitive effect (in turn raising further hypotheses about its possible utility for other types of cognitive disorders, such as ADHD). But how do we know whether the supposed pro-effect is not merely a byproduct of treating depression (that is, a *pseudospecific* improvement in just the domain of cognition)?

This is exactly the scenario that occurred in the case of vortioxetine in major depression: the active drug showed greater improvement than a placebo on performance-based measures of attentional processing. To account for possible pseudospecificity, the authors performed a type of regression analysis called path analysis, which statistically controlled for improvement in mood symptoms while assessing changes in cognitive performance, and found a significant independent effect on cognition (McIntyre et al., 2014). That finding, in turn, generated additional (and as-yet untested) hypotheses about whether vortioxetine can treat other forms of cognitive dysfunction, such as ADHD, or the cognitive symptoms of schizophrenia.

H PROBABLE VERSUS IMPROBABLE CONSEQUENCES

Some pharmacological outcomes have higher or lower (or, purely theoretical) likelihoods of an adverse outcome. Some may also have outcomes that are either mechanistically implausible or otherwise fail to account for confounding factors that might provide an alternative or more compelling hypothesis that explains the observed phenomena. Several examples are described in Table 7.1.

Table 7.1 Just how probable are some reported adverse outcomes?

Scenario	Likely? Clinically meaningful?
Hypertension from a serotonin-norepinephrine reuptake inhibitor (SNRI)	Certainly possible, and reported, but rare. For example, in US Food and Drug Administration (FDA) registration trials of *venlafaxine XR* across all indications, 1.4% of patients experienced a diastolic blood pressure rise of $\geq$15 mmHg, and a value of >105 mmHg, on at least three occasions; for *desvenlafaxine*, mean changes in diastolic blood pressure across dosages in major depressive disorder ranged from 0.7 mmHg to 2.3 mmHg, with sustained hypertension occurring in less than 1.3% of patients taking up to 200 mg/day; for *duloxetine*, across all indications, blood pressure changed a mean of 2.1 mmHg systolic and 2.3 mmHg diastolic; and short-term trials of *levomilnacipran* in major depressive disorder yielded a mean change from baseline of 3 mmHg systolic and 3.2 mmHg diastolic blood pressure
Serotonin syndrome from combining a selective serotonin reuptake inhibitor (SSRI) with trazodone or buspirone or lithium	It is theoretically possible that the putative serotonergic properties of all these agents could, in combination, cause serotonin syndrome; but if one scours the literature, there are only a small handful of individual case reports of alleged serotonin syndrome when combining buspirone with an SSRI, and no published reports when combining an SSRI with trazodone or with lithium
Lithium-induced mania (Yuvarajan and Yousufzai, 1988) 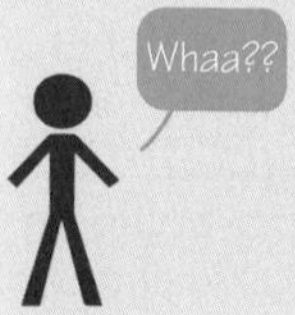	In an anomalous single case report, the authors hypothesize that lithium might somehow "over-potentiate" antidepressant properties to cause mania. An alternative hypothesis may be that lithium augmentation simply failed to avert an impending mania
Failure of brexpiprazole to treat mania better than placebo (Vieta et al., 2021)	Two negative randomized trials failed to prove the hypothesis that brexpiprazole has antimanic properties. That conclusion is entirely possible, although it is hard to account for why a dopamine D_2 antagonist would not treat mania - unless the placebo effect was unusually high, causing a failed rather than a negative trial

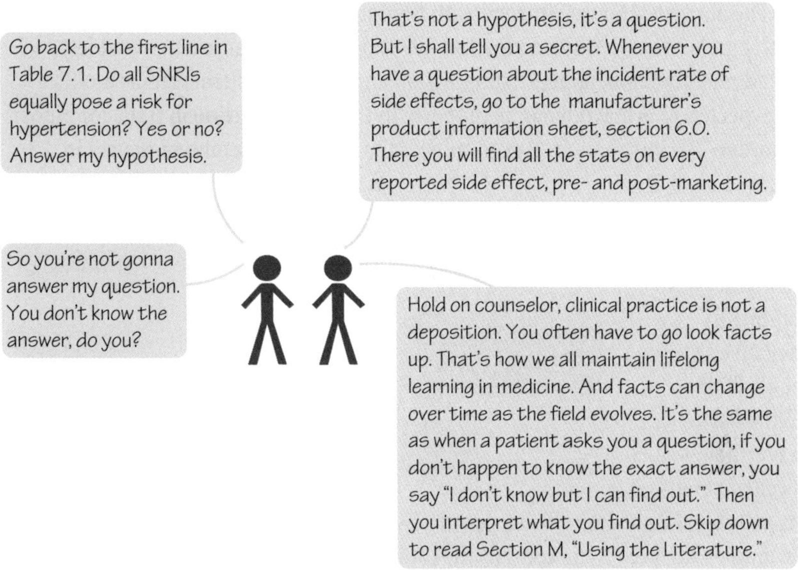

I HYPOTHESIS FRAMING: ASK TANGIBLY ANSWERABLE YES/NO QUESTIONS

Yes/no questions have their appeal. Multiple factors often influence treatment outcomes, and outcomes are often conditional (e.g., low bioavailability means that drug X works less well if not taken on an empty stomach; drug Y may be less effective if the patient is a cytochrome P450 2D6 ultra-rapid metabolizer; drug Z produces improvement in some but not all symptoms of a syndrome). But, consider the intellectual value of framing a hypothesis for which there is indisputably a binary yes/no conclusion. Such as: a dual orexin receptor antagonist either will or will not improve sleep; either moving from an SSRI to an SNRI will yield a better antidepressant effect or it will not; either amphetamine will help reduce distraction and bring thoughts into clearer focus or it will not. Avoid being misled by tangential issues or pharmacodynamic effects that are extraneous to the hypothesis of interest, which may arise in the course of starting a treatment.

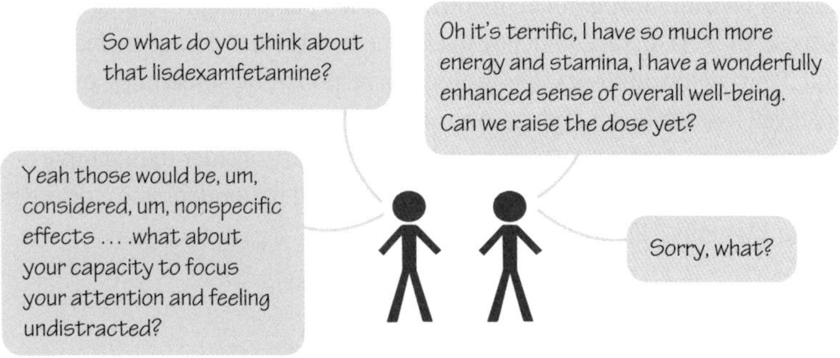

The above lesson was learned with topiramate in the course of clinical trials with bipolar disorder during the late 1990s. Before it became a more widely noted phenomenon, appetite suppression and weight loss emerged as a rather unexpected pharmacodynamic property in the course of clinical trials for bipolar disorder – to the point that, even though the primary outcome measures in those clinical trials, focusing on reductions in mania, were uniformly negative (Kushner et al., 2006) enthusiasm nevertheless swelled about its possible weight-loss effects, practically overshadowing any attention paid to leveraging affective symptoms as the intended hypothesis being studied.

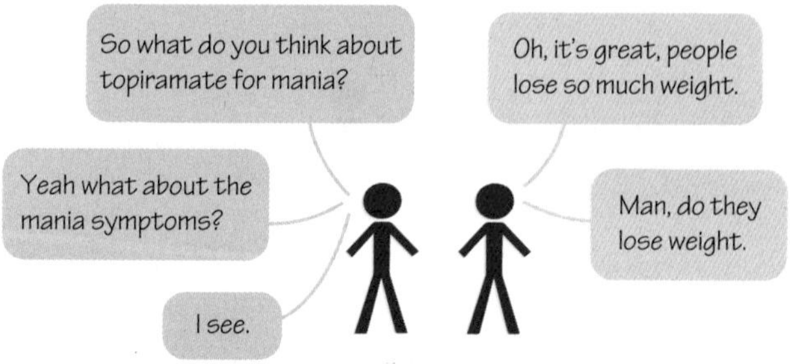

Of course, the history of psychopharmacology is filled with serendipitous observations that have led to hypotheses being generated about previously unrecognized pharmacodynamic effects. Recall that the antidepressant properties of monoamine oxidase inhibitors arose from studies of iproniazid for tuberculosis; or that imipramine was developed initially as a modification of chlorpromazine in an effort to develop a new antipsychotic medication. A cautious approach is essential when anecdotal observations prompt the generation of a hypothesis (some might call this "prescribing-based evidence" as opposed to "evidence-based prescribing"), particularly in light of the risk for affect heuristic bias and other types of cognitive biases that can reinforce tendencies for a clinician to see what they want to see, as described earlier in Box 7.2.

J BIASES ABOUT MEDICATION DOSE–RESPONSE RELATIONSHIPS

Clinicians and patients alike often presume the existence of linear dose–response relationships with most if not all medications. If a partial improvement is perceived, there is often a tendency to assume that further dosage increases would likely yield additional fine-tuning of a response; or, sometimes, one might even assume that a high or even supratherapeutic dose of a medication may expectably convert a nonresponse to a response. Consider the example of the dose–response relationship for desvenlafaxine in major depressive disorder (Clinical Vignette 7.1).

Clinical Vignette 7.1

Dr. Timido was a third-year psychiatry resident treating Ben, a 26-year-old man having a first lifetime major depressive episode that was initially unresponsive to escitalopram 20 mg/day. After being switched to desvenlafaxine 50 mg/day for a month, Ben's Patient Health Questionnaire-9 (PHQ-9) score was reduced from 19 to 16. Hoping to amplify this initial improvement, Dr. Timido's supervisor, Dr. Altezzoso, encouraged Dr. Timido to increase Ben's desvenlafaxine dose to 100 mg/day, which he did. After no further improvement occurred in the ensuing month, Dr. Altezzoso suggested further increasing the dose to 150 mg/day. Dr. Timido asked if it was likely that a response that apparently plateaued at 50 mg/day with no further improvement at 100 mg/day would further improve at higher doses. He asked if it would be wiser to switch Ben to a different medication altogether. Dr. Altezzoso assured Dr. Timido that he has seen such things happen many times, and also encouraged Dr. Timido to order pharmacogenetic testing for Ben to determine if he might be an ultra-rapid metabolizer, for whom higher-than-usual doses may be more beneficial. From the standpoint of evidence-based medicine, what is wrong with this picture?

What is wrong with this picture is, basically, everything. First, Ben's measly 16% improvement on a standardized rating scale for depression falls flat. While the decision to augment versus switch agents after an initial partial response is not dogmatic, and depends in part on patient preference, two important tenets must hold: first, deciding what constitutes a partial response upon which to build; and second, recognizing when dosing optimization has or has not yet occurred. **"Partial response" in major depressive disorder is conventionally taken to mean an improvement of >25% but <50% from baseline with a clinical global impression rating of "minimally improved"** (Nierenberg and DeCecco, 2001), making Ben's 16% quite the shortfall. Would higher doses likely yield further improvement, as Dr. Altezzoso hypothesizes? Let us consult the clinical trials literature for guidance. In FDA registration trials of desvenlafaxine for major depressive disorder, no clear further improvement in depressive symptoms was observed for patients dosed above 50 mg/day, as shown in Table 7.2.

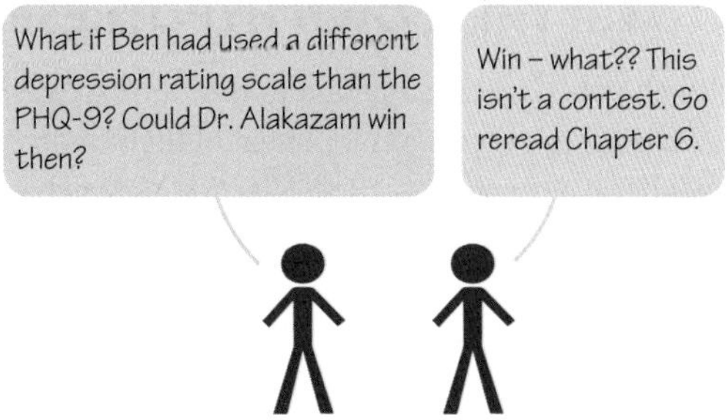

Table 7.2 Depressive symptom improvement with desvenlafaxine or placebo across escalating doses*

	50 mg/day	100 mg/day	200 mg/day	300 mg/day
Mean final difference in Hamilton Depression Rating Scale (HAM-D) scores versus placebo	−2.5	−3.0	−2.0	−3.1

* Based on manufacturer's product information.

While it is certainly possible that in some patients a dose greater than 50 mg/day could, maybe, perhaps, now and then, sometimes, potentially yield greater efficacy, there is no evidence base to support this as a generalizable hypothesis. A literature search for supportive data reveals only noncontrolled, open trials in which dosing was begun at 200 mg/day and rapidly titrated to 400 mg/day – rather than assessing high dosing in patients after an inadequate response to usual dosing (Ferguson et al., 2012).

As a general principle, there is merit to Dr. Altezzoso's general proposition that if Ben were an ultra-rapid metabolizer he might require a higher-than-usual dose of medication to achieve a response. However, in this case, desvenlafaxine does not undergo hepatic metabolism before being excreted, making pharmacogenetic testing to assess that hypothesis not relevant. This is a good example of when pharmacogenetics would *not* be helpful to answer the specific question of what to do with the medicine the patient is now taking, based on the known pharmacokinetics of the drug in question.

An evidence-based approach would favor Dr. Timedo sticking to his guns and trying some alternative to desvenlafaxine rather than either raising its dose or augmenting it, given Ben's meager initial benefit seen with standard dosing.

K TEACHING PATIENTS HOW TO FORMULATE AND TEST THEIR OWN HYPOTHESES

When patients ask if a symptom they are experiencing is the likely result of a medication, versus a component of their underlying ailment, or when they wonder if a particular course of action they may be curious about (such as taking a nutritional supplement) could be useful for them, it can be helpful to reframe their query as a hypothesis and encourage their inner scientist to help formulate a way of testing their theory. Not only does an approach such as this help to foster a collaborative, shared decision-making process, as discussed in Chapter 4, but moreover it provides patients with a sense of agency and affords them a more proactive role in understanding and managing their symptoms and psychological reactions to the phenomena they experience. Table 7.3 provides some examples, while Table 7.4 presents examples of more complex hypotheses and testable strategies that might be co-formulated with a treating clinician.

Table 7.3 A methodology to help patients self-formulate clinical hypotheses

What problems are you noticing?	Proximity and context: what events if any preceded their onset?	Plausible hypotheses	Ways to collaboratively hypothesis-test
Insomnia	Nothing unusual	Am I taking my Adderall XR 20 mg in the morning too late?	Does taking it earlier mitigate insomnia?
		Arthritic pain could be keeping me awake	Does a non-steroidal anti-inflammatory drug trial improve sleep?
		Caffeine in afternoon might be the culprit	Does abstinence from caffeine after noon for a week improve insomnia?
		Am I depressed and don't realize it?	Take a depression screener
Feeling more depressed	Stopped oral contraceptive 3 months ago	Could absence of estrogen supplementation cause depression relapse?	Able to resume the contraceptive?
		Was contraceptive affecting metabolism of any other medicines?	Discuss with prescriber or pharmacist the possibility of drug interactions
Feeling flat and dull	Began an SSRI a few months ago	Flat and dull feelings could signal depression even if I'm not really feeling sad or down	Discuss with therapist any life issues that might be contributing to feeling less engaged
		Could the SSRI be causing an apathy syndrome?	Discuss with prescriber the possibility of medication-induced apathy … recognizing she may counter-hypothesize I am smoking too much weed 😉
Skin rash	Pills look different	New generic formulation of an existing drug may have excipients (inactive ingredients) that are responsible	Track down and switch back to previous manufacturer's formulation
Do I need to take all these pills?	Just tired of taking so many medicines	Will I relapse if any of my medicines are reduced or stopped?	Could cautiously, systematically reduce one drug at a time and watch closely

Table 7.4 Reframing complaints as testable hypotheses

Complaint	Proximity and context	Plausible hypotheses	Ways to collaboratively hypothesis-test
Recently began to notice cheek muscles twitching	Restarted amphetamine salts after a 2-month hiatus, also have been taking lurasidone for about 2 years	H_1: Amphetamine could be causing tics H_2: Muscle twitches could be signs of emerging tardive dyskinesia (TD)	Stop amphetamine to determine if twitches abate Abnormal Involuntary Movement Scale (AIMS) exam to evaluate TD
Patient with bipolar II disorder reports feeling drowsy	Taking divalproex 500 mg plus lamotrigine 300 mg/day; stopped divalproex and drowsiness abated; mood is euthymic	H_1: Was divalproex the culprit? H_2: Was lamotrigine the culprit, by virtue of its having been effectively doubled in dose (tantamount to 600 mg/day) when co-prescribed with divalproex?	Watch and wait. If mood symptoms worsen, might then increase lamotrigine while watching for any worsening of sedation to test H_2. If mania symptoms recur, might restart divalproex but then halve lamotrigine to test H_2

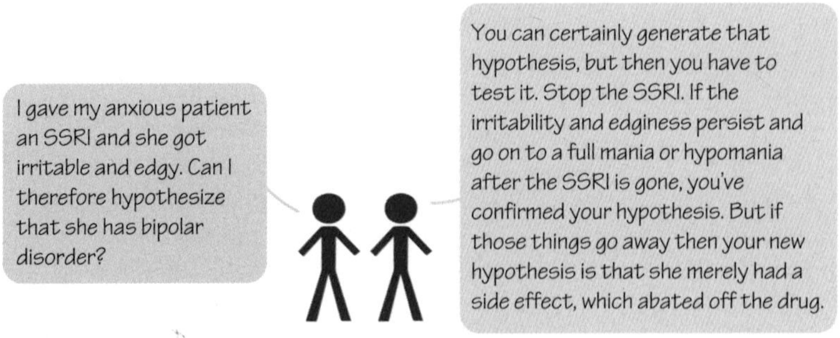

L CRAFTING PATIENT-SPECIFIC DECISION TREES

Decision trees, unlike generic treatment algorithms, are basically visually mapped-out contingency plans. They are conceptually different from treatment algorithms, which merely present a summary of available options and the extent to which a panel of experts feels their use is supported by varying levels of evidence. Decision trees present options in a hierarchical format based on successive levels of information that are pertinent to making an ultimate decision. Traditional guideline-based algorithms tend not to take into account the particular characteristics of a given patient that might influence drug response or tolerability, nor do they particularly account for what to do in the setting of previous treatment failures or complications such as adverse drug events or patient-specific contraindications to a particular treatment option. By contrast, the idea of a decision tree essentially means creating a blueprint for successive steps that can or should be taken after an inadequate treatment response or undesired result. Forecasting such an iterative process assures both the patient and the clinician that there is a sense of order driving the care plan, removes the arbitrariness with which one treatment might be favored over another, and provides a long-range perspective about problems that may not necessarily have simple short-term solutions.

L.1 Patient-Tailored Decision Trees

Sketching out the fundamental components of a decision tree as a joint undertaking with a given patient underscores the collaborative nature of medical decision-making, fosters an appreciation for the inherent risks of any treatment (or nontreatment) among all parties, and helps minimize concerns about what to do if the first intervention fails. The process is somewhat akin to writing a computer program, building in language that captures contingencies ("if" statements) and next steps depending on the outcome of previous steps.

It is useful to begin with a summary statement that succinctly captures the nature of the clinical problem coupled with the acceptability parameters around possible treatment options, followed by a list of the viable options, accounting for known information about increasing levels of breadth of spectrum and efficacy in the setting of a nonresponse or intolerance. Let us start with the example of major depression with prominent baseline anxiety. Why that? Because we know from studies like the Sequenced Treatment Alternatives to Relieve Depression (STAR*D) that anxiety symptoms occur in over half of patients with major depression and represent a common cause for poor treatment response; additionally, treatment trials for anxious depression tend to take longer, given that most anxious-depressed patients in STAR*D who responded to an intervention did so only *after* 6 weeks (Fava et al., 2008). Let us use Katie as a case example in Clinical Vignette 7.2.

As shown in the decision tree example in Figure 7.1, we begin with vilazodone as a first pharmacotherapy option. This starting point was chosen because, in clinical trials, vilazodone was one of the few medications for which baseline anxiety scores were shown not to diminish responsivity of depression symptoms (Thase et al., 2014). Additionally, vilazodone has shown superiority to placebo in clinical trials focused on the treatment of GAD (Durgam et al., 2016).

Clinical Vignette 7.2

Katie is a 42-year-old woman with persistent depressive disorder (formerly known as chronic major depression) and comorbid generalized anxiety disorder (GAD). She has been in and out of treatment with both pharmacotherapy and psychotherapy since her 20s, and previously was given paroxetine 10 mg/day and escitalopram 10 mg/day (each stopped after several months due to sedation and weight gain). She has been out of treatment for about 2 years but is now seeking a consultation. Her PHQ-9 score is 16 (reflecting a moderate level of depression symptom severity) and her GAD-7 score of 11 also indicates a moderate level of anxiety symptoms. She currently takes no medications and has no unstable medical conditions. She is especially worried about any medications that might cause sedation or weight gain, although her body mass index is 25 and she has no cardiometabolic risk factors.

How might we best craft a personalized treatment decision tree for Katie?

Figure 7.1 A decision tree for Katie's anxious depression.

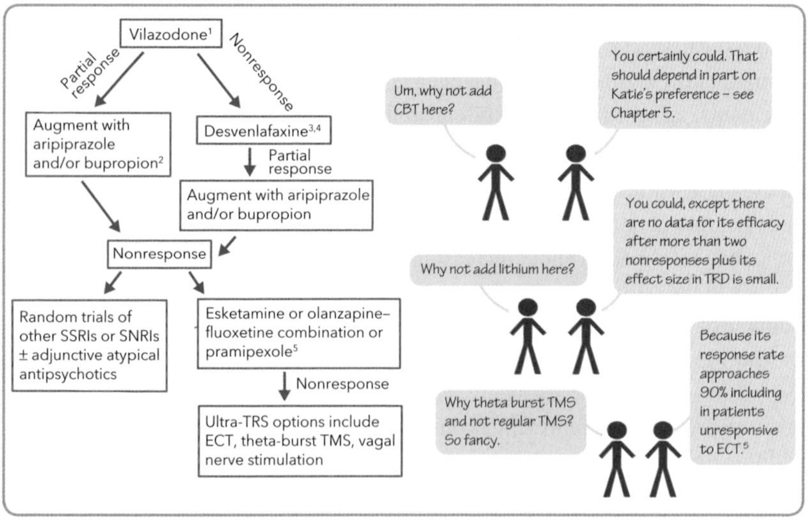

Rationales:

[1] Evidence base in anxious depression (Thase et al., 2014);

[2] Adjunctive aripiprazole better than bupropion in the Veterans Affairs Augmentation and Switching Treatments for Improving Depression Outcomes (VAST-D) trial (Mohamed et al., 2017);

[3] Switching from a purely serotonergic to an SNRI has ~6% greater chance for response (Papakostas et al., 2007);

[4] Desvenlafaxine is excreted without being metabolized (cf. venlafaxine);

[5] All are evidence-based options after nonresponse to more than two monoaminergic antidepressants. Abbreviations: ECT, electroconvulsive therapy; TMS, transcranial magnetic stimulation; TRD, treatment-resistant depression; TRS, treatment-resistant schizophrenia.

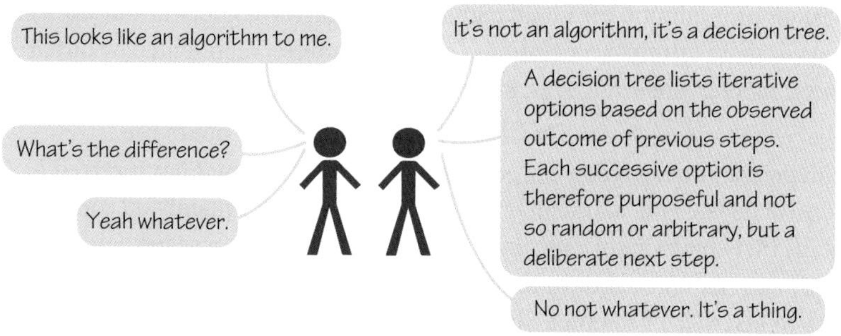

Decision trees are commonly used in large-scale machine learning, in which a model becomes developed or trained based on the inclusion of thousands (or more) of studied patients. Patient-specific information can then be inputted and an estimate of a particular outcome can then be made based on an algorithm using the characteristics of the originally studied group. An example would be calculating a Framingham risk score to estimate an individual's risk for having a heart attack or stroke over the next 10 years. Derived from risk scores inputted from an original cohort of over 5,000 patients enrolled in the Framingham Heart Study beginning in 1948 (with many hundreds of subsequent waves of enrollees) an algorithm was developed such that a *new* patient's risk for an event (heart attack or stroke) could be estimated based on a series of parameters around their age, sex, blood lipid values, blood pressure, diabetes, and smoking status. Adapting this approach to personalized medicine, imagine using such an algorithm of clinical characteristics to try to predict the response to a particular psychotropic medication, risk for making a suicide attempt, or even predicting treatment nonadherence, based on a composite summary of clinical features known to be pertinent for the outcome of interest.

The field of data analytics has not, as yet, developed clinician-friendly "Framingham-like" apps or other computer programs of wide practical utility to quantify probabilities of an outcome of interest in psychiatry, based on machine learning paradigms derived from "training samples" of thousands of patients. We provide some further discussion on the topic of machine learning and automated decision support in Chapter 6. But clinicians can in the meantime recognize clinical parameters that collectively increase (or decrease) the likelihood of a desired clinical outcome for a broad patient group, and collate that information through a series of steps that comprise a descriptive decision tree.

Decision trees can be formally mapped out as a pathway involving a central starting point (say, a clinical group of interest), known as a **root node**, which then undergoes a series of decision points (called subnodes, also known as **parent** and **offspring** or **child nodes**, designated by ovals) that are "split" (meaning, typically, decisions are made about how to proceed down the tree based on yes/no decisions or minimum threshold parameters). A series of nodes ultimately leads to one or more terminal conclusions (called **leaf nodes**, represented by boxed terms), all interconnected by branches of the tree.

Let us take an example. The decision about whether or not to use antidepressant medications for patients with bipolar disorder has received extensive debate and commentary in the literature, based mainly on concerns that (a) they might induce mania or accelerate cycling patterns in some predisposed patients, and (b) they have not robustly shown efficacy as compared either to placebos or to mood-stabilizing drugs such as lithium or divalproex alone. Let us not here and now resurrect the particulars of this ongoing scholarly–clinical debate but, rather, synthesize a decision-analytic tree, shown in Figure 7.2, which reflects findings from the literature on clinical factors that bear on the probable outcome of the use of antidepressant medication in bipolar disorder.

Figure 7.2 Decision tree for using antidepressant medications in bipolar depression

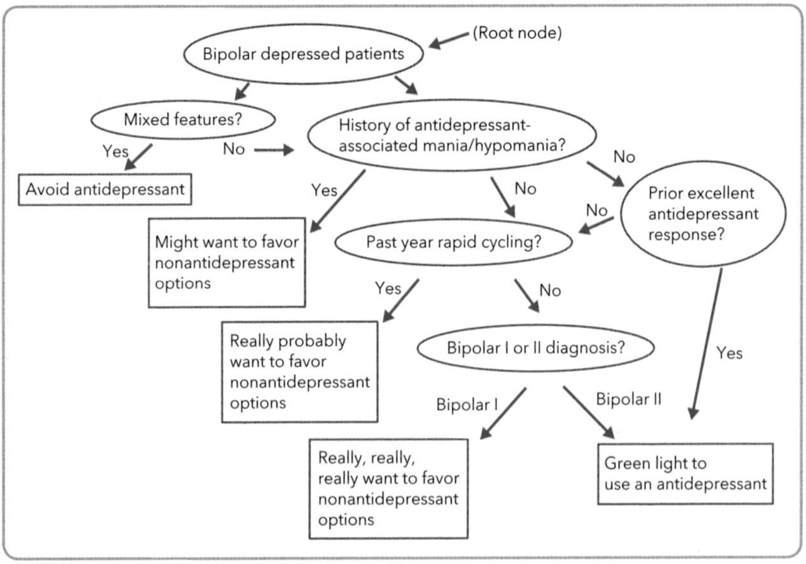

Figure 7.2 enumerates a series of such factors relevant to the final decision point, although we have no reason to think one factor holds more weight than another, and the *hierarchy* for considering the relative importance of one factor relative to another is subject to our whims (meaning that subsequent decisions are not *necessarily* predicated on the response to questions or issues posed in earlier parent nodes). We made this particular hierarchical decision tree based on our understanding and interpretation of the literature – we invoke literary license, authorship privileges, and the like – but suppose you, the

reader, disagreed with our sequencing and decided that a specific patient's past responder status to an antidepressant should carry more weight in Figure 7.2 than it now does relative to the nodes that we have placed before it. You can readily modify your own decision tree to the specifications of your own patient. For instance, what if your patient had a particularly severe manic episode in response to an antidepressant medication, or suppose another patient had a more virulent form of illness, or a rapid cycling course; you could readily transpose nodes to fit the hierarchical importance of a decision as you (and your patient) see fit.

Let us take as another example: the decision of whether to continue or discontinue an adjunctive long-term second-generation antipsychotic medication for a particular patient after successful treatment for a nonpsychotic mood disorder, as described in Clinical Vignette 7.3. This one is harder because it has more contingencies.

Clinical Vignette 7.3

Lou was a 52-year-old man with a history of hypertension and prediabetes, who was treated successfully by his psychiatrist, Dr. Mountainjar, for recurrent major depression with the combination of vortioxetine 20 mg/day and aripiprazole 5 mg/day. Previous trials of sertraline or escitalopram augmented with quetiapine yielded incomplete responses and led to up to a 20-pound weight gain. Though Lou was never psychotic and had no history of a lifetime mania or hypomania, aripiprazole augmentation converted a partial response to a marked improvement over vortioxetine alone. Lou has been well for over a year. Recent routine labs found a low-density lipoprotein cholesterol of 167 mg/dL and a fasting glucose of 104 mg/dL despite co-therapy with metformin 1,000 mg/day, and with a body mass index (BMI) of 32, his primary care doctor advised him to "try to get off the psych medicines that are making it hard for you to lose weight."

Before making a decision tree, let us list the salient issues for consideration, as summarized in Box 7.4.

There is no established calculus á la Framingham risk score to quantify Lou's specific risk for a serious adverse consequence if he were to continue taking aripiprazole, just as there is no clear statistic from randomized discontinuation trials to predict the likelihood that his depression would recur after stopping it, or that Lou's metabolic dysregulation will inevitably worsen. It would indeed be a helpful thing for the field if some altruistic research enterprise were to some day conduct an adequately powered randomized discontinuation trial of an antidepressant medication plus atypical antipsychotic medication versus adjunctive placebo after remission from nonpsychotic major depression, in

Box 7.4

Considerations for decision-making about Lou

- Lou is now psychiatrically well on his current regimen, and has a history of treatment-resistant depression that is now stable
- If aripiprazole were stopped and Lou's depression relapsed, would the plan then be simply to resume it?
- Should aripiprazole be switched to a different and more metabolically neutral augmentation to the vortioxetine? If that happened but was ineffective, what would be the back-up plan if his depression recurred?
- Lou's metformin dose could be further increased to better counteract insulin resistance; and, with a BMI > 27 coupled with two obesity-related medical problems (prediabetes and hyperlipidemia), he is also a candidate to take a glucagon-like peptide-1 (GLP-1) agonist such as semaglutide, which can cause *dramatic* weight loss
- Is Lou not a candidate for a statin?
- While we are considering potential long-term risks, Lou has several risk factors for tardive dyskinesia with continued use of a dopamine blocker (or partial agonist), namely, age > 50, presence of a mood disorder, and, potentially, diabetes

order to provide empirical information on these parameters. Until then, the risk–benefit decision for Lou remains not so measurable, and hence poses a more qualitative than quantitative predicament.

We *can* cheat slightly – since concern for Lou's actual risk for a myocardial infarction (MI) is highly relevant – and speaking of Framingham, we actually can calculate a more modernized version of a Framingham risk score for an MI, known as a pooled cohort risk equation, to help us forecast an important piece of information about Lou's cardiometabolic risk (clincalc.com/Cardiology/ASCVD/PooledCohort.aspx). This is shown in Figure 7.3.

The risk calculator places Lou's risk of having an MI in the next 10 years as 7.4%, which is only just a tad shy of the threshold for clinical significance of 7.5%, alongside a calculated lifetime risk of 46%. While these numbers do technically fall just a hair below the risk threshold, they are not far from it. His risk is far from nil, and so caution is in order.

Working with the above imperfections, let us then construct the decision tree analysis, framed along conditional parameters, shown in Figure 7.4.

Obviously, much will depend on Lou's own preference about how to proceed. Figure 7.4 could provide a useful framework for shared decision-making with Dr. Mountainjar, as discussed in Chapter 4. It articulates the salient decision-

Figure 7.3 Lou's risk for atherosclerotic cardiovascular disease (ASCVD)

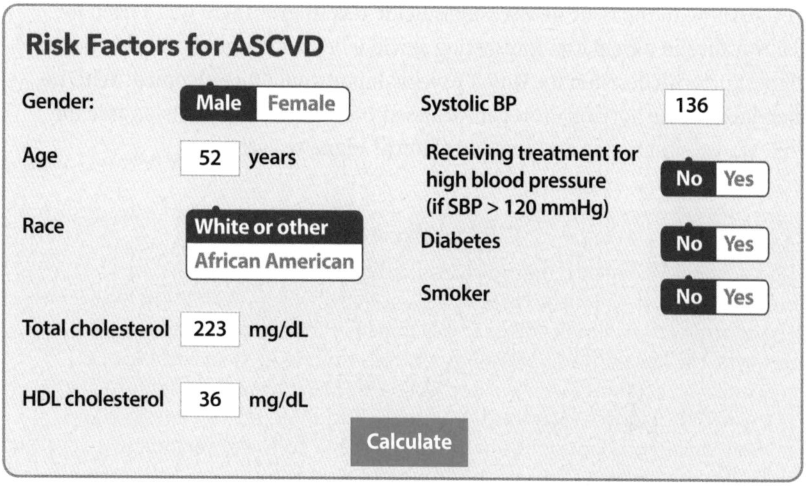

Figure 7.4 To continue or not to continue an atypical antipsychotic medication?

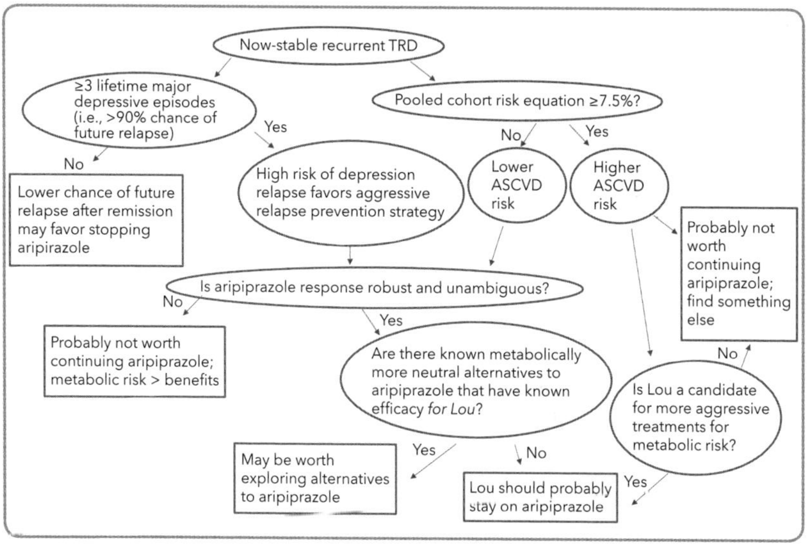

making points for both parties to discuss. For his part, Lou may prioritize metabolic concerns more highly than concerns about a potential relapse of depression; or he may be more optimistic than Dr. Mountainjar about finding a suitable alternative to adjunctive aripiprazole, should depression recur. The decision tree, once again, provides more of a blueprint for discussion than a dogmatic algorithm for what to do next in any and all circumstances.

Let us consider one last example of constructing a patient-specific decision tree, turning to the issue of assessing suicide risk. If ever there was a need for clairvoyance in psychiatry, forecasting suicidal behavior would probably be the highest priority decision for which psychic input would be welcomed. With no such luck on the horizon, how can we assemble a reasonable decision tree for Phil, whose situation is described in Clinical Vignette 7.4?

Clinical Vignette 7.4

Phil was a 44-year-old unemployed bisexual man living alone and supported by psychiatric disability benefits who spent much of his time "hanging out" and socializing at psychiatric club houses and drop-in centers. He has carried various diagnoses that have included bipolar disorder, schizoaffective disorder, dysthymic disorder, borderline personality disorder, posttraumatic stress disorder, and an unspecified anxiety disorder. He would often bring himself to the emergency department "complaining of thoughts of harming [him]self" because of "too much stress in [his] life." Sometimes he would be admitted for several days and then discharged; seldom had he had any lengthy hospital stays and rarely had changes been made to his longstanding psychotropic regimen of lithium carbonate 900 mg/day, risperidone 1 mg at night, clonazepam 0.5 mg at night, hydroxyzine 25 mg at night, and quetiapine 25 mg at night. Phil has made three serious and violent lifetime suicide attempts (hanging, stabbing, and overdosing on pills). He recreationally uses 3,4-methylenedioxymethamphetamine (MDMA) and snorts street ketamine to get high. On a cold and rainy Friday night he comes to the emergency department around midnight where he says he is having thoughts of harming himself, and "this time [he] means it."

Most psychiatrists, at some point in their careers, have met a Phil, and when recounting tales of patient care to colleagues or junior staff, the Phils of the world tend to stand out as examples of making clinicians feel "damned if you do" and "damned if you don't" with respect to decision-making. If only Phil had never

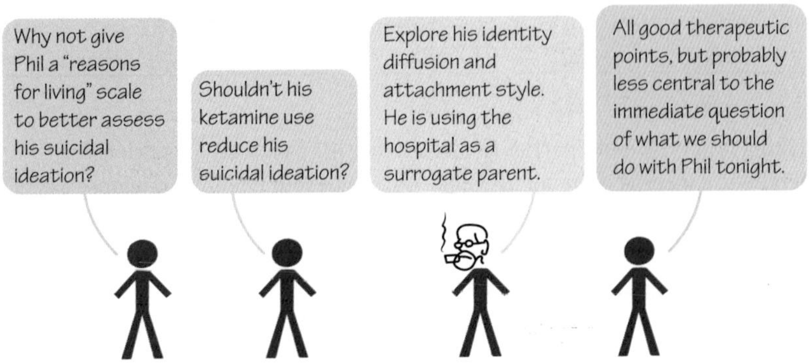

made a serious suicide attempt, or had only made obvious gestures as leverage for some outcome other than death, then we could focus on malingering and secondary gain, or manipulation based on his personality structure and efforts to procure some desired end result. If only Phil had no substance use disorder, then we could discuss premeditation versus chemically assisted loss of impulse control. If only Phil had a more stable social support system and a work identity, we could speak more about the anti-suicide protectants in his life in the community outside of institutions. If only there was some clear mental health benefit that hospitalization provided to Phil. If only Phil were stably in a meaningful psychotherapy. If only Phil did not make clinicians feel like if they called his bluff about suicide he would show them how wrong they were. If only there were a decision tree to solve Phil's situation – if not once and for all, then at least for tonight. Phils' decision tree appears in Figure 7.5.

Figure 7.5 Should Phil get hospitalized tonight?

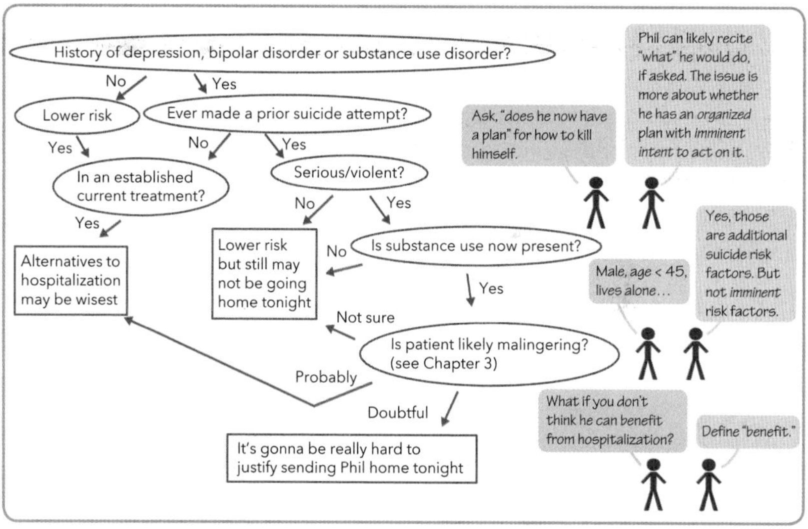

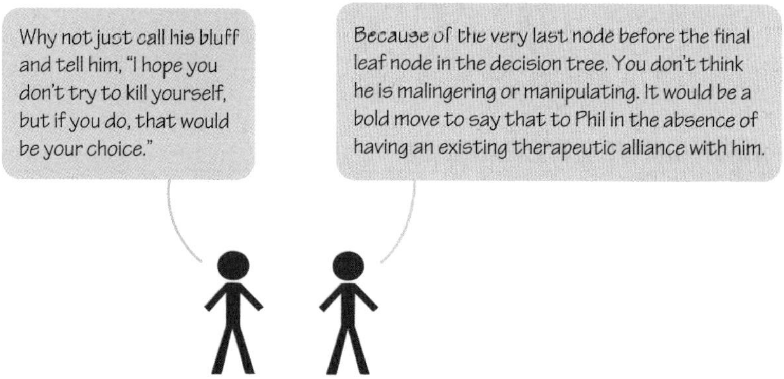

Well, the way out of this dilemma may very much hinge on the difference between what to do on this cold and rainy Friday night versus what to do longer term. Some patients with serious mental illnesses, who have certain personality structures along with institutional transferences, may actually benefit from being hospitalized, even if it is just for a few hours. Why? Not for psychopharmacological or meaningful psychotherapeutic purposes, and not even necessarily to devise new outpatient long-term treatment plans. It may be more like touching home base when playing freeze tag – it confers a sense of safety and reassurance before going back out into the world. Is that kind of respite a wise use of medical resources? That might very well depend on the individual patient. Phil has shown the clinical world that he can mean business when he wants to, and even an accidental death from a "botched" suicide attempt counts as a medical disaster that becomes practically indefensible after the fact if no solid alternative to hospitalization is spelled out with all its contingencies. Could, and should, Phil develop better coping strategies so that "stress" does not inevitably lead him down the path of suicidal thinking? Well, certainly – but that is not something likely to happen this Friday night and, if anything, Phil's presence in the emergency department is a signal that whatever outpatient efforts are now being deployed on his behalf to better engrain those skills seem not to be working well. There will be many things to consider come Monday morning, but the decision tree in Figure 7.5 is specific to the immediate circumstances – like a time-limited contract that contains specified clauses, it is a here-and-now roadmap with no indefinite expiration date.

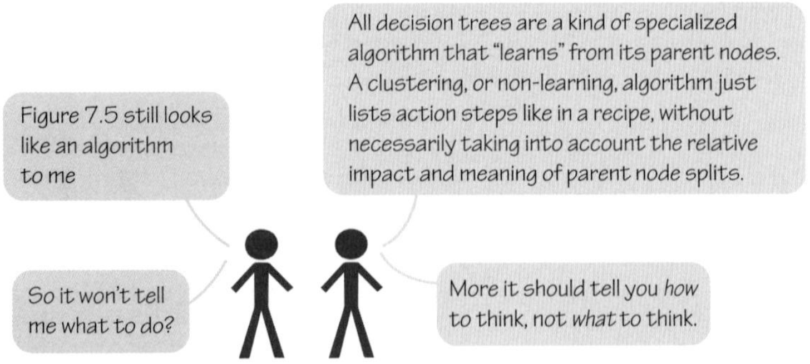

Ⓜ USING THE LITERATURE

Before closing out this chapter and moving on to a more in-depth discussion of decision points in Chapter 8, we are taking the opportunity here to remind readers that the world of evidence-based medicine is literally at your fingertips and the current empirically based answer to almost every clinical question is merely a few clicks away in the land of PubMed®, courtesy of the National

Library of Medicine. Hypothesis-testing goes nowhere if we do not have some database or frame of reference for providing empirically based answers to questions. Sometimes, direct clinical experience provides that database, as when we tell patients, "In my experience, it is quite uncommon for amphetamine to cause sedation, so I would not advise taking a higher dose to see if that was more activating." Other times, the answers to clinical questions warrant more empirical investigation. Facts change as the field evolves. Hypotheses that may apply to one population may not translate so easily to another. Extrapolation and interpretation are the clinical tools we apply to raw empirical information.

TAKE-HOME POINTS

- Translate clinical questions into testable hypotheses whenever possible, as a means of organizing pertinent clinical information. Hypotheses should provide a falsifiable statement that allows one to tell if a potential correlation or explanation exists for observed phenomena. It should help clarify whether the phenomena are genuinely connected to a plausible explanation, or are instead merely random events due to chance
- Think of clever ways to engage patients in testing hypotheses about their condition and their treatment, rather than just agreeing or disagreeing with a possible plan of action
- Delineate the most pertinent information that applies to decisions about a specific clinical problem. Make a patient-specific decision tree if a visual depiction would help provide a focal organizing point for decision-making

References

Altshuler LL, Keck PE Jr., McElroy SL, et al. Gabapentin in the acute treatment of refractory bipolar disorder. Bipolar Disord 1999; 1: 61–65

Cole EJ, Stimpson KH, Bentzley GS, et al. Stanford Accelerated Intelligent Neuromodulation Therapy for treatment-resistant depression. Am J Psychiatry 2020; 177: 716–726

Doherty TS, Carroll AE. Believing in overcoming cognitive biases. AMA J Ethics 2020; 22(9):E773–E778

Durgam S, Gommoll C, Forero G, et al. Efficacy and safety of vilazodone in patients with generalized anxiety disorder: A randomized, double-blind, placebo-controlled, flexible-dose trial. J Clin Psychiatry 2016; 77: 1687–1694

Faraone SV, Wilens TE. Effect of stimulant medications for attention-deficit/hyperactivity disorder on later substance use and the potential for stimulant misuse, abuse, and diversion. J Clin Psychiatry 2007; 68 (suppl 11): 15–22

Fava M, Rush AJ, Alpert JE, et al. Difference in treatment outcome in outpatients with anxious versus nonanxious depression: A STAR*D report. Am J Psychiatry 2008; 165: 342–351

Ferguson JM, Tourian KA, Rosas GR. High-dose desvenlafaxine in outpatients with major depressive disorder. CNS Spectrums 2012; 17: 121–130

Kushner SF, Khan A, Lane R, et al. Topiramate monotherapy in the management of acute mania: Results of four double-blind placebo-controlled trials. Bipolar Disord 2006; 8: 15–27

McIntyre RS, Lophaven S, Olsen CK. A randomized, double-blind, placebo-controlled study of vortioxetine on cognitive function in depressed adults. Int J Neuropsychopharmacol 2014; 17: 1557–1567

Mohamed S, Johnson GR, Chen P, et al. Effect of antidepressant switching vs. augmentation on remission among patients with major depressive disorder unresponsive to antidepressant treatment: The VAST-D randomized clinical trial. JAMA 2017; 318: 132–145

Nierenberg AA, DeCecco LM. Definitions of antidepressant treatment response, remission, nonresponse, partial response, and other relevant outcomes: A focus on treatment-resistant depression. J Clin Psychiatry 2001; 62 (suppl 16): 5–9

Pande AC, Crockatt JG, Janney CA, et al. Gabapentin in bipolar disorder: A placebo-controlled trial of adjunctive therapy. Gabapentin Bipolar Disorder Study Group. Bipolar Disord 2000; 2: 249–255

Papakostas GI, Thase ME, Fava M, et al. Are antidepressant drugs that combine serotonergic and noradrenergic mechanisms of action more effective than the selective serotonin reuptake inhibitors in treating major depressive disorder? A meta-analysis of studies of newer agents. Biol Psychiatry 2007; 62: 1217–1227

Soares-Weiser K, Maayan N, Bergman H, et al. First rank symptoms for schizophrenia. Cochrane Database Syst Rev 2015; 1: CD010653

Sysko R, Walsh BT. A systematic review of placebo response in studies of bipolar mania. J Clin Psychiatry 2007; 68: 1213–1217

Thase ME, Chen D, Edwards J, et al. Efficacy of vilazodone on anxiety symptoms in patients with major depressive disorder. Int Clin Psychopharmacol 2014; 29: 351–356

Vieta E, Sachs G, Chang D, et al. Two randomized, double-blind, placebo-controlled trials and one open-label, long-term trial of brexpiprazole for the acute treatment of bipolar mania. J Psychopharmacol 2021; 35: 971–982

Yuvarajan R, Yousufzai NM. Mania induced by lithium augmentation. A case report. Br J Psychiatry 1988; 153: 828–830

8 Decision Points in Iterative Pharmacotherapy

LEARNING OBJECTIVES

- ☐ Understand the ways in which iterative psychopharmacology means thinking about the implications of one treatment decision relative to the next
- ☐ Recognize, and delineate, the pros and cons from a summary of viable treatment options
- ☐ Understand how to construct a decision-analytic matrix and use it to map out patients' and clinicians' individual priorities as a strategy to find convergence for joint decision-making about the basis for preferred treatment options
- ☐ Devise back-up plans and present to patients a comprehensive strategy with contingency plans spelled out in the event that initial recommendations fail to achieve their objectives

More often than not, an initial intervention in psychiatry requires modification. Sometimes sooner than later, the clinician must judge whether a medication dose needs adjustment, an augmentation is warranted, or an outright change should occur when something has been tried and deemed to be unsuccessful. Perhaps a new additional diagnosis comes to light (such as alcohol or substance use disorder) requiring its own treatment. Or an insurmountable medication intolerance develops. Or the originally identified target symptoms worsen, metamorphose, or persist long enough after a previous medication change to warrant a further alteration. Other times, changes to a regimen happen not necessarily because sufficient time has elapsed to deem a change necessary, but because a patient's (or significant other's) capacity to tolerate negative affect or other elements of distress become saturated, prompting entreaties or outright demands to "do" something that seems more proactive. In all such instances, there is seldom if ever only one correct approach to iterative pharmacotherapy.

One useful guiding principle might be that, ideally, no decision should be random or arbitrary (unless indeed only relatively arbitrary decisions can be made – such as choosing one selective serotonin reuptake inhibitor (SSRI) versus another after a first one has failed; or when the probable efficacy or side effects of one drug are about the same as another). Our goal in this chapter is not so much to help the reader find the needle-in-the-haystack *definitive* or *ideal* medication but rather to assure that they have clarified all the salient issues necessary to articulate viable treatment options for a given clinical situation. That means spelling out the relative pros and cons of each approach, contextualizing those pros and cons relative to the patient's (and prescriber's) prioritized treatment objectives, and identifying back-up plans for what to do next in case a first or second or subsequent attempt fails. We would note that the shared decision-making process, formally discussed later in this chapter, is inherently more difficult, but not altogether impossible, with patients who have diminished capacity to comprehend and participate in this kind of joint operation; such important conundrums are discussed more specifically in Chapter 4, Section G.

A CHOOSING FROM AMONG APPROPRIATE AGENTS

What defines an *appropriate* treatment? Finding the right tool for the right job depends first on making a carefully rigorous assessment, as discussed in earlier chapters. That could mean "clinching" a discrete categorical diagnosis (e.g., the syndrome of major depression, panic disorder, or dementia) or honing in on a core feature (e.g., recognizing poor impulse control or affective lability in the setting of exquisite mood reactivity; realizing when wrong, rigid thinking indicates psychosis; when self-proclaimed "anxiety" really means "paranoia"; or "social phobia" really means "impaired social reciprocity" as in autism). For any definable clinical presentation, clinicians should have a firm sense of what treatments are appropriate, evidence-based, and nonarbitrary. Chain saws are wonderful power tools for cutting wood but not quite right for sanding. Wrenches are better for tightening nuts around bolts than for smashing nails into walls. So too should the right pharmacological tool(s) be identified for a clearly definable given clinical job. For illustrative purposes here, consider several examples of less-than-appropriate decisions with rather flimsy (if any) rationales:

- Prescribing lamotrigine for acute mania, or for the sheer diagnosis of bipolar disorder, without considering as an intended purpose the targeting of depressive rather than manic symptoms
- Treating the syndrome of depression solely with sedative–hypnotic anxiolytic medications
- Deciding to prescribe antipsychotic medications as interchangeable within-class entities, for purposes other than treating psychosis (e.g., favoring risperidone to target depressive symptoms in bipolar disorder in the absence of any supportive controlled trials; using perphenazine for anergic nonpsychotic depression when no data support such use; using quetiapine to target inattention in a nonpsychotic, nonanxious, non-mood-disordered patient with attention deficit–hyperactivity disorder (ADHD))

- Making egregious choices that are devoid of even a plausible rationale (e.g., stimulants to treat psychosis; anticholinergic drugs to treat delirium; opting *not* to use an antidepressant to treat severe, melancholic depression in a euthyroid, medically healthy patient with no history of mania or hypomania)

Pharmacology decision points also entail understanding the context for choosing among appropriate options, as exemplified in Clinical Vignette 8.1.

Clinical Vignette 8.1

Jenny was a 22-year-old college student with generalized anxiety disorder, a history of alcohol use disorder (abstinent by self-report for the past 8 months), and body dysmorphic concerns about being overweight. She stopped taking sertraline 100 mg/day because she felt it was preventing her from losing weight but was happy to continue taking topiramate 100 mg/day (presented to her as having possible "off-label" value for weight loss, though data about its utility to reduce alcohol craving or binge drinking was not shared). After about a month she called to request a prescription for alprazolam because she was now having "panic attacks."

A rudimentary level of assessment is necessary before making a decision about, and framing a cogent response to, Jenny's request. The immediate considerations are:

- What does Jenny mean by a "panic attack"? Is she identifying a phenomenon other than true panic attacks – such as discontinuation effects from sertraline? Or alcohol withdrawal? Or an interpersonal conflict that has left her upset?
- Has there been a resurgence of anxiety, more broadly, in the absence of sertraline – for which a discussion is in order about the pros, cons, and alternatives to resuming sertraline?
- If Jenny is truly having panic attacks, or other manifestations of anxiety, but does not wish to resume sertraline, are there not better and safer options than a benzodiazepine for someone with recent and perhaps shaky abstinence (short of being in a more meaningful program of recovery) from alcohol use disorder?

"What to do" with Jenny's request really depends on the outcome of exploring the above concerns – in ways that no algorithm for treating anxiety or panic attacks per se can take into account. Jenny has bought herself an assessment of her current condition as the proper response to her inquiry.

B ADOPTING AN ITERATIVE CLINICAL MINDSET: BECOMING A PHARMACOLOGICAL CHESSMASTER

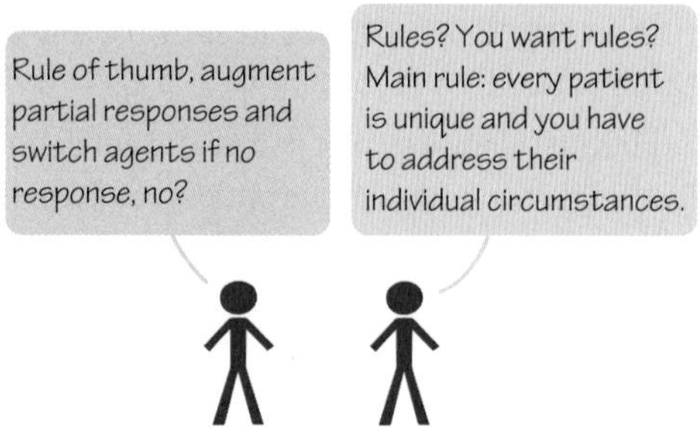

One of the most vexing aspects of psychopharmacology research has been the relative failure to establish evidence-based guidance about "what to do next" when a first intervention fails. "Failure" in itself becomes a relative concept when defining iterative decision points. Absence of meaningful improvement after an adequate trial generally invites a change to a regimen, although many qualifying factors often impinge, including:

- The decision to retain (and then augment) a drug that has produced a partial response (as opposed to discontinuing and replacing it altogether) is often a matter of preference; while outright replacement is often more parsimonious, it may be more practical to retain a partially efficacious drug that can be augmented when pharmacodynamically viable options exist, alternatives may be few or arbitrary, and past treatment failures have been extensive
- Drug intolerances signal the decision point to (a) encourage acclimation with further time and/or dosage reductions – particularly if alternative options are few or (b) abandon an intolerable treatment if the intolerance is deemed insurmountable, assuming that viable alternative therapeutic options exist
- The period needed to define an adequate trial is often longer in chronically ill populations (e.g., 12 weeks rather than 6 weeks in the case of persistent depressive disorders)
- Clinical worsening may not necessarily signal a therapeutic failure; the natural course of illness may sometimes follow a deteriorating trajectory but the intended intervention may not yet have produced its fullest effect, requiring the clinician to stand fast and resist the temptation to prematurely abandon an appropriate intervention before an adequate trial (dose + duration) has elapsed
- Time and episode number may exert significant influence over decision points to a treatment regimen insofar as chronicity, duration of untreated illness, and increasing episode number often hold negative prognostic implications. In other words, after the passage of several episodes (at least in the case of mood disorders), an eventual favorable response may become increasingly elusive. That suggests value in an especially rigorous approach *early* rather than later in the course of illness. Hence, ensuring optimized dosing and adequacy

of trial durations (without hasty or premature switches from one drug to another) may be most crucial at a time when a fledgling psychiatric illness may be most malleable

C LIMITATIONS OF TREATMENT ALGORITHMS AND PRACTICE GUIDELINES

Treatment algorithms essentially delineate sequential options for plausible interventions but a frequent shortcoming is their failure to account for the conditional probability that a next intervention will work in the setting of nonresponse to a previous agent (for more discussion see Box 8.1). In fact, this becomes one of the greatest conundrums for practicing psychopharmacologists: how to answer the question of "what should I do next?" based on an evidence base, or at least a rationale, rather than from a sheer litany of otherwise arbitrary options. In highly refractory patients, we would note that this sometimes becomes a vexation in the setting of a consultation: a consultant can always scrape the bottom of the pharmacological barrel to find *some* ostensibly "appropriate" agent that has not yet been tried, but without offering a probability that the untried option has a greater or lesser likelihood of being efficacious in the context of multiple previous nonresponses. As has been noted elsewhere (Goldberg, 2018), the pursuit of numerous iterative pharmacotherapy trials with consistently poor outcomes runs the risk of engendering demoralization for both the prescriber and the patient, and indeed may inadvertently create an operant conditioning paradigm in which each repeated sense of failure serves only to further galvanize a sense of futility. Such dilemmas regarding pharmacological futility are further discussed at the end of this chapter (Section M) as well as in Chapter 10, Section L.

Box 8.1

The limitations of treatment algorithms

Treatment algorithms and guidelines generally delineate a consensus-based hierarchy of viable therapeutic options drawn mainly from the copiousness of an existing database for each option relative to the others. Copiousness is largely driven by the resources of pharmaceutical industry sponsorship for drugs while they remain proprietary entities. Seldom if ever does a depression guideline, for example, rank order antidepressant choices based on their relative effect sizes, or stratify effect sizes based on the extent of previous treatment resistance. Concerns about tolerability or adherence are usually addressed by opinion in accompanying text, such as expressing lower enthusiasm for a drug with high metabolic liability or significant cardiovascular risk. Algorithms tend not to address differential therapeutics in the presence versus absence of specific psychiatric comorbidities. Specific recommendations often rapidly become outdated

Box 8.1 (cont.)

and require regular and frequent touch-ups. Guidelines generally do not help clinicians decide which antidepressant medication is best in an obese stroke patient, or which antipsychotic drug to use for chronic psychosis in someone with poorly controlled diabetes. Simply opting for the least "offensive" agent offers little help for the practitioner who must weigh the risks and benefits of using (or avoiding), say, clozapine in a deteriorated patient with multi-drug-resistant schizophrenia and poorly controlled diabetes. Guidelines also provide no calculus for anticipating the chances that a high-metabolic-liability drug such as clozapine or olanzapine, if successful, might prompt lifestyle changes that in turn lower other health risks. What if olanzapine helps reduce cigarette smoking (Rohsenow et al., 2008), or clozapine fosters better insight and adherence to following a diabetes treatment regimen? Treatment algorithms can provide a concise summary of the magnitude of an overall evidence base at the time of their writing to achieve response or remission for a single psychiatric condition. As such they serve more as a possible component of decision-making, rather than a substitute for that process itself.

With the foregoing in mind, let us for now step back from the unique challenges posed by the notion of pharmacological futility and instead address how one logically undertakes an "iterative mindset" – perhaps even with the hope that doing so may avert future futility. "Iterative thinking" is rather like playing chess, in which one anticipates the varied possible consequences of any given move and plans accordingly. Consider the chessmanship of the following example (Clinical Vignette 8.2).

Clinical Vignette 8.2

Alice was a 36-year-old euthyroid woman with major depression unresponsive to several adequate and appropriate pharmacotherapy trials. For the moment, ignore the specific drugs that were previously chosen and accept on faith that she officially falls within the category of true treatment-resistant depression (TRD). Alice has never had a manic or hypomanic episode or been psychotic, there is no family history of bipolar disorder, no substance use comorbidity, and good adherence. Imagine that her treating psychiatrist has proposed, as viable next steps, the options of (a) a trial of lithium augmentation of her existing antidepressant medication versus (b) a monoamine oxidase inhibitor (MAOI) trial versus (c) a trial of olanzapine–fluoxetine combination (OFC) versus (d) a trial of esketamine. Assume that electroconvulsive therapy (ECT) has been discussed as a "biggest gun" option but that Alice is not so keen to try that just yet, and that Alice asked about repetitive transcranial magnetic stimulation but her psychiatrist has skepticism about its relative impactfulness. Chessmanship, or perhaps jigsaw-puzzling, makes the sequencing of these choices nonarbitrary, and contingent on their mutual or sequential compatibilities, as depicted in Figure 8.1.

Rather than arbitrarily itemize the viable options, consider how one might flow to the next in ways that account not only for patient preference (say, reserving for later those drugs with particularly disdained possible adverse effects, undesired lifestyle modifications, or degree of invasiveness) but also their relative compatibilities from a pharmacokinetic (e.g., half-life) and pharmacodynamic (e.g., risk for serotonin syndrome or additive pressor effects) perspective.

Figure 8.1 How iterative treatment decisions can fit together. Abbreviations: ECT, electroconvulsive therapy; OFC, olanzapine-fluoxetine combination; MAOI, monoamine oxidase inhibitor; rTMS, repetitive transcranial magnetic stimulation; SGA, second-generation antipsychotic.

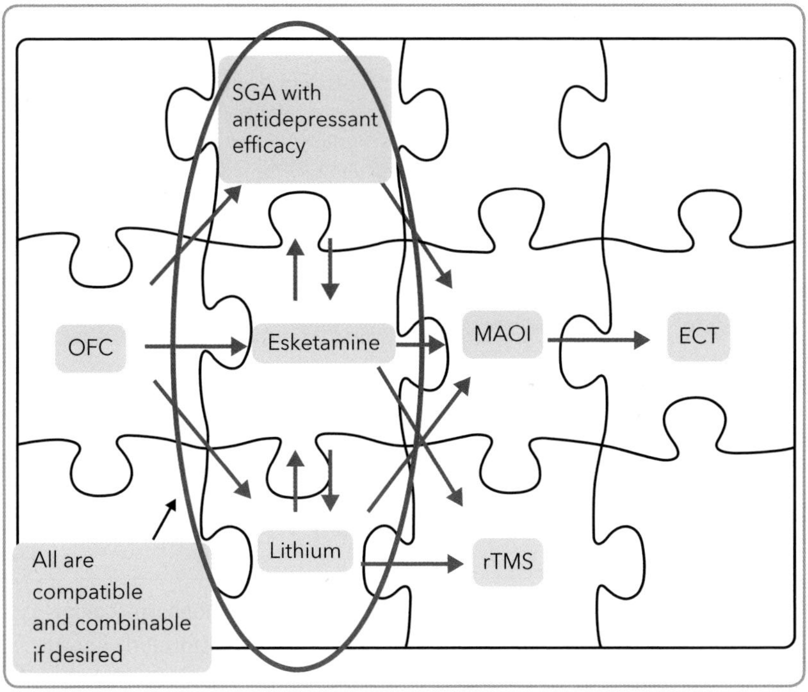

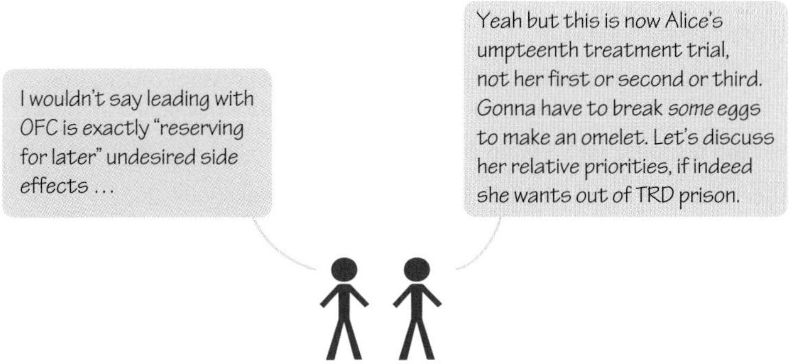

As Figure 8.1 depicts, if OFC were tried next but failed, it would entail a 5-week washout (due to the long half-life of fluoxetine plus its active metabolite norfluoxetine) before an MAOI could be introduced, in order to avoid the risk for serotonin syndrome. That *might* make it more desirable to reserve OFC for after, rather than before an MAOI trial, unless Alice's strong preference was not to forgo aged meats and cheeses, in which case we maintain her autonomy and sequence OFC first, building in potential "bridge" options (an adjunctive second-generation antipsychotic medication with antidepressant efficacy (e.g., quetiapine), esketamine, lithium, or pramipexole) that are compatible with both OFC (during its washout) and an MAOI (during its wash-in, if we end up moving to an MAOI), as well as with each other, as possible adjuncts if not outright successes each in their own right.

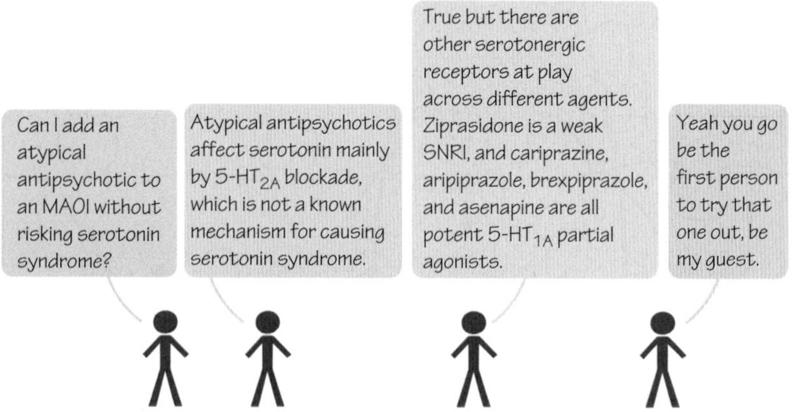

Ⓓ ITERATIVE PHARMACOTHERAPY IN MAJOR DEPRESSION

One of the more common clinical scenarios in iterative psychopharmacology involves decision-making for persistent depressive disorders (formerly known separately as dysthymic disorder and chronic major depression). By what thought process do prescribers choose second, third, or later pharmacotherapy options?

Appreciate the following:

- The probability of efficacy for any first-tried antidepressant medication in major depression is only about 30–40% (i.e., about 10% better than the placebo response rate) (Khan et al., 2017)
- Effect sizes are small (about 0.30 or less (Turner et al., 2008, 2022))
- About 40% of depressed patients will prematurely discontinue an antidepressant (higher among ethnic minorities (Olfson et al., 2006))
- The likelihood for remission after an initial failure declines with successive trials (see Figure 8.2)

On top of that, consider that in STAR*D the likelihood of remission for any given prospectively conducted antidepressant trial decreased as a function of the number of previous failed treatments, as shown in Figure 8.3. It may seem hard to be guided by much more than desperation when faced with more than one or two unsuccessful treatment efforts.

Figure 8.2 Sequential remission rates across successive antidepressant trials in Sequenced Treatment Alternatives to Relieve Depression (STAR*D; Rush et al., 2006)

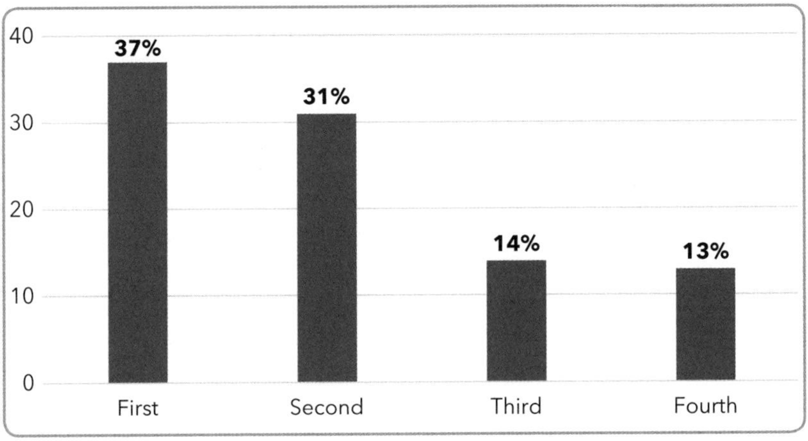

Figure 8.3 Declining likelihood of remission after failure of previous antidepressant trials in STAR*D (Rush et al., 2006)

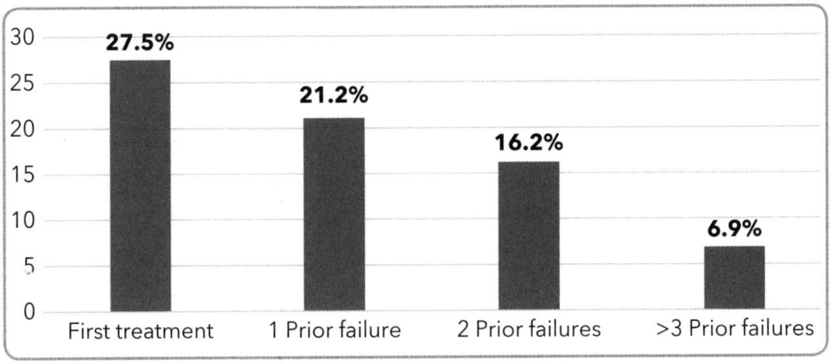

Nevertheless, if we hope to make iterative pharmacology a nonrandom enterprise, we search for factors that make the decision-making process less arbitrary when choosing a second or later antidepressant after an initial failure. Turning to the empirical literature, we are aware of only one post hoc analysis of a large database examining statistical predictors of remission from a second antidepressant trial after failure of a first trial. In the STAR*D major depression trial, Rush et al. (2008) found that major depressive disorder nonremitters after

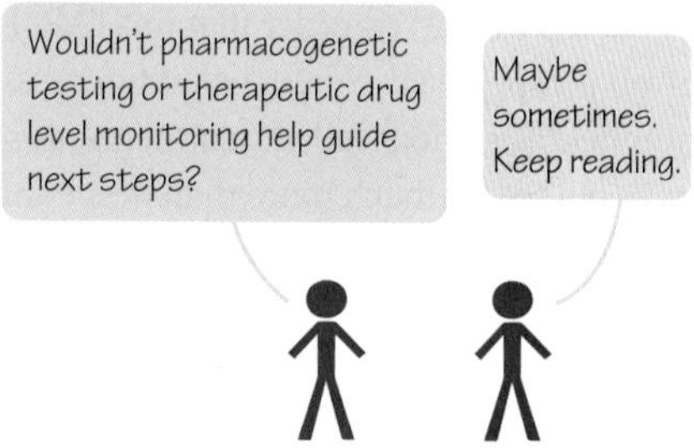

an *initial* trial of citalopram who later remitted with *other* antidepressants were more often white, employed, cohabiting or married, privately insured, intolerant, or responsive (but not "remitted") with citalopram, and had no history of suicide attempts; they also had no anxiety features or signs of melancholia, and their depressive symptoms were more moderate than severe. That description may offer some guidance around the prototype remitter in STAR*D after a first antidepressant failure, but it does not exactly give us a police artist's sketch of the suspect we are looking for.

Intuitively, it makes sense to think that the usual mélange of poor prognostic signs would predict suboptimal outcomes across successive antidepressant trials, while the only changing variable would be the specific agent chosen. In the case of a monoaminergic antidepressant medication, that might be the idea of moving from an SSRI to a serotonin–norepinephrine reuptake inhibitor (SNRI) or other "broader-spectrum" option (such as a tricyclic or MAOI), although at the same time we know that the overall difference in response rates between an SSRI and SNRI is only a modest 6% (Papakostas et al., 2007). Unlike infectious disease doctors, who might simply progressively broaden the "spectrum" of activity across successive antibiotics in the face of a treatment-resistant infection, the effect sizes across most monoaminergic antidepressant medications are not drastically different from one another. And, as noted above within this section, those effect sizes themselves tend to be quite modest in comparison to placebo (Turner et al., 2008, 2022).

The proposition that no particular antidepressant medication is head-and-shoulders superior to another in treating major depressive disorder may leave some readers perplexed, but in fact this observation points us instead toward factors other than efficacy per se that bear on effectiveness – that is, patients' acceptability of one drug relative to another, their likelihood of sustained adherence, tolerability, effects on specific target symptoms, and a variety of other endpoints that ultimately may boost enthusiasm for one treatment option over another – particularly when previous interventions have either shown little or no efficacy or caused substantial problems with tolerability.

This discussion now brings us to a more directed focus on iterative pharmacotherapy decision-making, the use of pro/con lists, and the case of Emma (Clinical Vignette 8.3).

Clinical Vignette 8.3

Emma was a 50-year-old teacher with bipolar II disorder who had a rapid cycling illness course several years ago but not since. In the past year, she had an approximate 9-week depression followed by 3 months of euthymia, now relapsing into a significant depressive episode with passive suicidal thoughts. She reports classical anhedonic features alongside cognitive complaints involving inefficiency when planning lectures and "blanking out" or failing to remember details that she knows during class. She oversleeps but does not overeat. She is euthyroid. Her most recent depression failed to improve significantly after 4 weeks taking lurasidone 20–40 mg/day. Presently, she is adherent to a medication regimen of lamotrigine 200 mg/day, sertraline 200 mg/day, and levothyroxine 25 mcg/day. She reports a moderate degree of depressive symptom severity (Patient Health Questionnaire-9 score = 14) and no current hypomanic symptoms. During a prior depressive episode several years ago, she felt that escitalopram made her feel suicidal. Her psychiatrist, Dr. Bennet, is contemplating next steps.

Tip

Rapid cycling, as a course specifier, has been shown to "phase in" and "phase out" at varying time points in the course of bipolar disorder (Coryell et al., 2003); it is not an all-or-none permanent illness descriptor.

The brief history we are given might prompt thinking along subdiagnostic lines – are her "blank out" periods dissociative phenomena? Flares of social anxiety? Unrecognized alcohol binges? Absence seizures? Can we fashion a credible diagnosis of adult ADHD to explain her cognitive complaints, versus the attentional and executive functioning deficits that may simply be inherent to bipolar disorder? Or iatrogenic cognitive dulling? For now, let us assume nothing too exotic. If we accept that her existing core pharmacology is reasonable, let us simply first explore the initial viable options and their pros and cons in Table 8.1, with an eye toward deciding if we should raise an existing drug in her regimen, switch out something old for something new altogether, or augment her current pharmacology with an addition.

E OUTLIERS AND BLIPS

How do finance managers differentiate "blips" from more meaningful trends when they make decisions to buy versus sell versus hold an account? One hopes to avoid the *affect heuristic* (see Chapter 7) as a purely emotional-reactive influence on decisions about when to alter an existing, established course of

Table 8.1 Pros and cons of intervention options for Emma's bipolar depression

Options	Pros	Cons
Could increase lamotrigine from 200 to 300 mg/day	300 mg/day dose *might* be more efficacious than 200 mg/day	No evidence base from which to infer that 300 mg would convert a depression nonresponse to a response; may get additive nonspecific central nervous system side effects at high doses
Could add lithium to her lamotrigine	"LamLit" is an evidence-based treatment shown to be superior to lithium alone for acute bipolar depression (van der Loos et al., 2009)	Lithium per se has a fairly small effect size in bipolar depression ($d = 0.24$) and is not a rapid remedy. It likely also would not help her cognitive complaints
Could reinstitute lurasidone	Lack of improvement after 4 weeks may not necessarily rule out the possibility of a response; could consider higher doses and longer duration	4 weeks at 20–40 mg/day is probably an adequate trial to gauge at least signs of responsivity, making this a less enthusiastic option
Could try another second-generation antipsychotic medication with known efficacy in bipolar depression	Quetiapine, olanzapine-fluoxetine combination (OFC), cariprazine, or lumateperone are all evidence-based options for bipolar depression; lumateperone has favorable data in both bipolar I and II depression	Quetiapine's strong antihistaminergic properties make it less attractive in the setting of baseline cognitive complaints. Data with OFC or cariprazine apply only to bipolar I depression; OFC has substantial metabolic liability and the latter, along with lumateperone, has minimal adverse metabolic effects, but both are unstudied in treatment-resistant bipolar depression
Could add pramipexole	Evidence-based in treatment-resistant bipolar depression; may help cognition	It is not a rapid remedy; studies are mainly preliminary; risk of nausea, sedation
Could try ketamine/esketamine	Possible rapid intervention, generally well-tolerated with little risk	It is a hassle to go for in-person regular insufflation and monitoring visits

treatment. The inclination to "act" in reaction to what may be a transient or momentary vicissitude in psychiatric symptoms stands at odds with the maxim of identifying and treating trends, rather than mere fluctuations in the course of a condition that may be inherently volatile. Persistent variability, or unstably unstable patterns, tend to invite intervention more than expectable, transient fluctuations or a waxing and waning course that fundamentally does not pose a major disruption to an overall pattern of consistency. We might similarly think of an "outlier" event. Someone with well-controlled panic disorder who experiences a rare panic attack does not necessarily need major revision to their treatment regimen if it is fundamentally reducing the frequency of events. How best to interpret the clinical significance of an event – a panic attack, a day of depressed mood, a night of insomnia – depends very much on the broader context in which a symptom occurs (missed dose? stressful event? new medication?), including the possibility that a rare outlier event could simply be random "noise" rather than a "signal."

F ARTICULATING THE PROS AND CONS OF ONE TREATMENT VERSUS ANOTHER

Ingeniously simple, one of the most powerful things we can ever say to a distressed and puzzled patient for whom two or more viable treatment options exist is, "Why don't we list the pros and cons of each option?" Doing so makes the abstract concrete, articulates an explicit thought process and rationale behind each choice, emphasizes to the patient the fact that they are able to *exercise* choice (i.e., a reminder of their own agency and empowerment), and underscores the shared decision-making that goes into key clinical decisions. It also helps to set the stage for identifying their own priorities (efficacy? sparing of adverse effects? cost? speed of onset?) and expectations, which may in turn prompt converting a pro–con list into a decision-analytic matrix, as described further below.

The pro–con list for Emma in Table 8.1 winnows down the universe of possible options to those that are most viable and evidence-based, providing her and her prescriber with a roadmap for making iterative choices based on the treatment goals they identify as having the highest priorities.

F.1 Thinking It Through

Let us now dive even deeper into Table 8.1, starting with the simplest approach, that of working with (or maximizing) Emma's existing treatments. Should her lamotrigine dose be increased? From an evidence-based standpoint, nobody has ever done a controlled trial taking relapsing bipolar depressed patients already on 200 mg/day of lamotrigine and randomizing them to either an increased dose

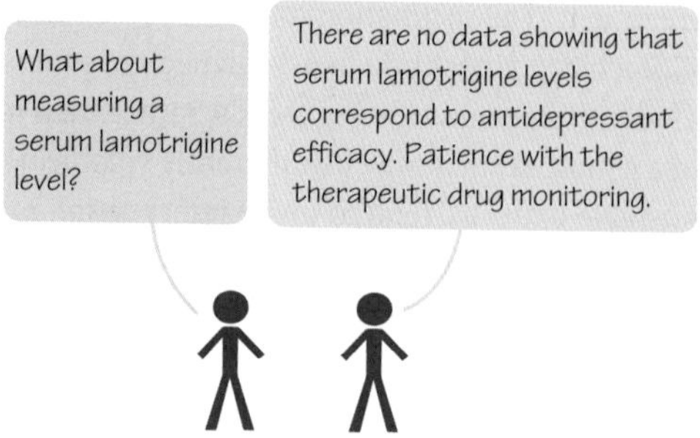

of 300 mg/day or remaining on 200 mg/day. That would be the most compelling scientific means by which to answer the question of whether a 50% dosage increase in lamotrigine would expectably be beneficial. In the existing clinical trials database, for acute bipolar depression, 200 mg/day was the maximum studied fixed dose. A more preliminary flexibly dosed randomized trial in treatment-resistant mood disorder patients from the National Institute of Mental Health (NIMH) found that "response" in major depression occurred at a mean dose of 275 mg/day. What about higher doses? The evidence base here is limited to the industry-sponsored relapse prevention trials of lamotrigine (and only in bipolar I disorder), where a dose of 200 mg/day or 400 mg/day was no different for prophylactic purposes. Keep in mind that the scenario for Emma involves converting an outright nonresponse to a response, rather than fine-tuning a partial response. It is a rather tall order to expect a lamotrigine dose of 300 mg/day to convert a nonresponse at 200 mg/day to a response. Both conceptually and empirically, there is little precedent to make us think that a lamotrigine dosage boost beyond 200 mg/day would produce a dramatic effect in the setting of acute/relapsing depression. But that does not mean this would be a bad idea – just, an understudied one.

How about augmenting her lamotrigine with lithium ("LamLit")? As noted in the pro–con chart, this pairing is certainly an evidence-based option. How impactful is it? Well, we can actually go back to the original article by van der Loos et al. (2009) and, because the authors provide the mean and standard error for changes in depression symptom scores for the drug and placebo groups, we can calculate for ourselves a between-group effect size (Cohen's *d*) from the values shown in Box 8.2.

Box 8.2

Parameters to calculate an effect size for "LamLit" in bipolar depression (van der Loos et al., 2009)

	Mean	Standard error (SE)
Lamotrigine (n = 64)	−15.38	1.32
Placebo (n = 60)	−11.03	1.36

Using a handy online calculator, we determine that the effect size is a whopping 3.25. That is gigantic! As in, why would anyone ever want to use lithium alone to treat bipolar depression when the effect seems so profoundly amplified by lamotrigine co-therapy? (Well, it is just one preliminary study, so before we go and put lamotrigine in the drinking water, we should ideally have at least one or two larger replication trials before over-generalizing about an *expectable* synergy or deduce a broad principle.) On the downside for lithium, it likely won't do much for Emma's cognitive complaints, and the original study did not show separation from lithium monotherapy until week 6 (though perhaps that was an artifact of having added lamotrigine to lithium, with a consequent titration period, rather than the reverse as would be the case for Emma who is already taking lamotrigine). If it is pro-cognitive effects Emma seeks, we have several specific options. Unfortunately for her, lurasidone was not so beneficial in her particular case – even though in clinical trials it was shown to improve overall cognitive function in people with bipolar disorder, perhaps through its antagonistic effects at the 5-HT_7 serotonin receptor (Yatham et al., 2017).

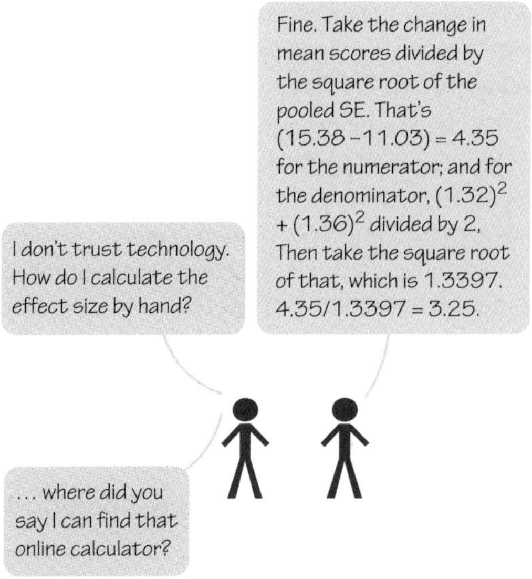

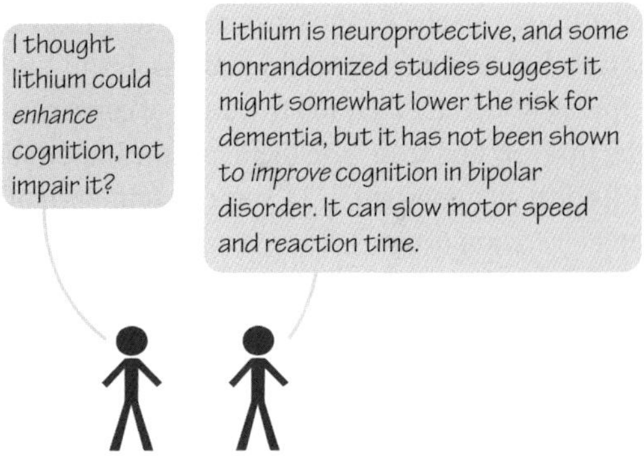

How about a pro-dopaminergic drug, would that help her cognitively? Would bupropion count? Perhaps (since it is a putative norepinephrine–dopamine reuptake inhibitor), but its database in bipolar depression is rather weak – its addition to lithium was shown to be no better than adding a placebo to lithium in the NIMH Systematic Treatment Enhancement Program for Bipolar Disorder program (Sachs et al., 2007). Other, perhaps more potent pro-dopaminergic options for bipolar depression would include cariprazine (as a dopamine D_2/D_3 partial agonist), pramipexole (as a D_2/D_3 full agonist; see Burdick et al., 2012), or simply adding a formulation of amphetamine.

Can we weight the relative options, that is, assign some indicator of our relative degree of confidence or enthusiasm for each? And what about Emma's input? Suppose our main interest is efficacy with a large effect size, but what if her number one priority is speed of onset … or absence of weight gain … or a pro-cognitive effect? Our goal then becomes brokering a match between the viable options and their pro–con lists relative to her wants. Rather like a realtor showing three top contender homes to a prospective client, the decision-making process involves aiming to assure that the buyer understands as best as possible that (a) they have options, which are (b) nonrandom, and (c) each comes with both attractive and unattractive elements. In other words, there is no perfect solution.

F.2 Constructing a Decision-Analytic Matrix

One way to navigate the above options is to construct a **decision-analytic matrix** with scores assigned to each relevant parameter, converting the decision trees described in Chapter 7 (Section L) into more powerfully driven personalized algorithms Chapter 7. The fancy name for this process of complex decision-making is called an **analytic hierarchy process**. Let us have both Emma and Dr. Bennet separately identify their top five areas of concern about a treatment choice along the first row and then have them rate the importance of each component as a 1 ("not at all important"), 2 ("somewhat important"), 3 ("moderately important"), or 4 ("very important"). Then, let us rate subsequent rows based on how well each treatment option is felt to perform for each parameter of interest, as 1 ("performs not very well"), 2 ("performs somewhat well"), 3 ("performs moderately well"), or 4 ("performs very well"). Let us also attach equal weightings to both Emma's and Dr. Bennet's separate "wish lists," and look first at Table 8.2.

Table 8.2 Decision-analytic matrix for Emma

Emma's wish list						
	Fast onset	**No weight gain**	**Cognitive benefit**	**Cost**	**Minimal hassle**	**Weighted total score**
How important is this feature?	3	4	3	2	3	
LamLit	1	2	2	4	2	**39**
Add stimulant	4	4	3	3	4	**55**
Esketamine	3	4	3	2	2	**44**
Bupropion	2	4	3	4	4	**51**
Cariprazine	2	3	2	2	4	**40**

To obtain the weighted scores in the final column, multiply the performance score of each treatment option (row) by its relative importance score (values in the shaded row). And the winner is … adding a stimulant, followed by adding bupropion, all by a sizable margin over the low-scorers (29% more enthusiasm than with LamLit and 27% more than with cariprazine). Does this mean that a stimulant is necessarily the *best* option, or the one most likely to work? Of course not! It means, with some quantitative oomph, that a stimulant would very unambiguously come closer to meeting Emma's wish list (by 20%) over picking esketamine, even though esketamine may be better established from clinical trials specifically for treatment-resistant depression. So, then, should we try to talk Emma out of a stimulant and tell her that her wish list overvalues features that make esketamine seem less likely to help her than it may be? No! All the options listed in the decision matrix are reasonable ones, and that is precisely the reason why we undertook this exercise. There is no "right" answer – only answers that conform better or less well to the criteria the customer says are important to her.

But now suppose, deep down in our hearts, we felt that Emma was making a regrettably misinformed decision and has her priorities all mixed up. Now we come to Dr. Bennet's wish list, and his decision matrix, shown in Table 8.3.

Table 8.3 Decision-analytic matrix for Dr. Bennet

Dr. Bennet's wish list						
	Fast onset	**No weight gain**	**Little or no titration**	**Large clinical effect**	**Patient likely to follow through**	**Weighted total score**
How important is this feature?	3	3	2	4	4	
LamLit	1	2	2	4	3	**41**
Add stimulant	4	4	3	3	4	**58**
Esketamine	3	4	3	4	3	**55**
Bupropion	2	4	3	3	3	**48**
Cariprazine	2	3	2	2	4	**43**

Dr. Bennet and Emma both prioritize speed of onset and absence of weight gain but Dr. Bennet places a premium on magnitude of clinical effect and expectations about adherence, while Emma's vote depends more on cost and minimally perceived hassle. They converge in favoring a stimulant, but for Dr. Bennet esketamine is a close second, although Emma's second choice (bupropion) is his third. They will likely have little trouble negotiating how to proceed because even though their priorities and expectations from pharmacotherapy are not entirely in sync, they each independently are arriving at decisions that are closely enough aligned. In other words, even if they were worlds apart in their respective priorities, the shared decision-making process ultimately renders that divergence a non-issue if they nevertheless ultimately agree on the same action plan, even if that happens for different reasons.

Tip

Colorfully controversial psychiatrist Thomas Szasz differentiated "institutional" psychiatry (involving clinical decisions imposed on an individual, with a potentially coercive, authoritarian stance) from "contractual" psychiatry (in which an individual freely and autonomously pursues help for mental health conditions).

If Dr. Bennet and Emma both liked the same restaurant but not the identical items on the menu, nobody suffers. What if they really could not agree on the same restaurant? The brokerage task is easier if they can both agree they are hungry and prefer vegetarian food than if their wishes were more disparate. If their choices (not necessarily their priorities) were highly incongruent, the decision-making process would likely then enter into the realm of Dr. Bennet's appraisal of Emma's **capacity to express an informed choice**, as summarized in Chapter 4, Section G. To continue the restaurant analogy for another moment, if Dr. Bennet perceived Emma as favoring the high-fat, simple carbohydrate option and he were her diabetologist, he would want to determine if she realizes, or is unable to comprehend, the ramifications of her choice. So long as Dr. Bennet thinks Emma grasps the concepts that enter into the decision-making process, she is essentially free to do to herself whatever she wants – no matter how much Dr. Bennet may think her choices are poor – provided her decisions do not pose imminent self-harm. Dr. Bennet might use his motivational interviewing skills (see Chapter 3, Table 3.1) to see if he can persuade Emma to adopt an alternative point of view. If Emma and Dr. Bennet are operating under a "contractual" psychiatry model in which she freely seeks his input, they are each welcome to reject the other's opinion and go their separate ways if they

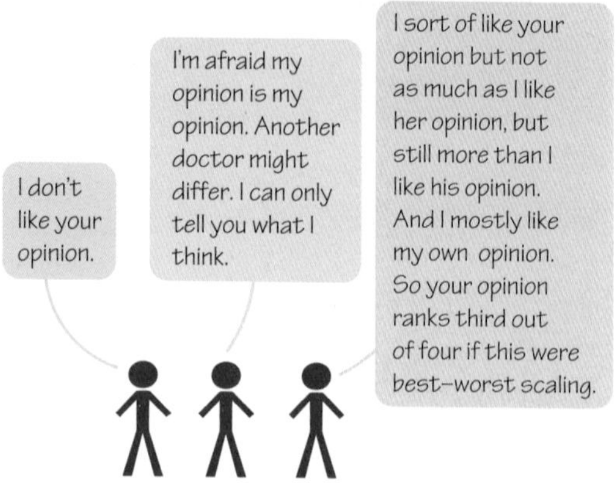

cannot find common ground. In an "institutional model," as might occur during involuntary treatment, Emma's autonomy and input are accorded less weight and the outcome may not be at all to everyone's mutual satisfaction. The decision-making process for Dr. Bennet comes to the proverbial fork in the road, with different pathways beyond, as illustrated in Figure 8.4.

Figure 8.4 Dr. Bennet's fork in the road

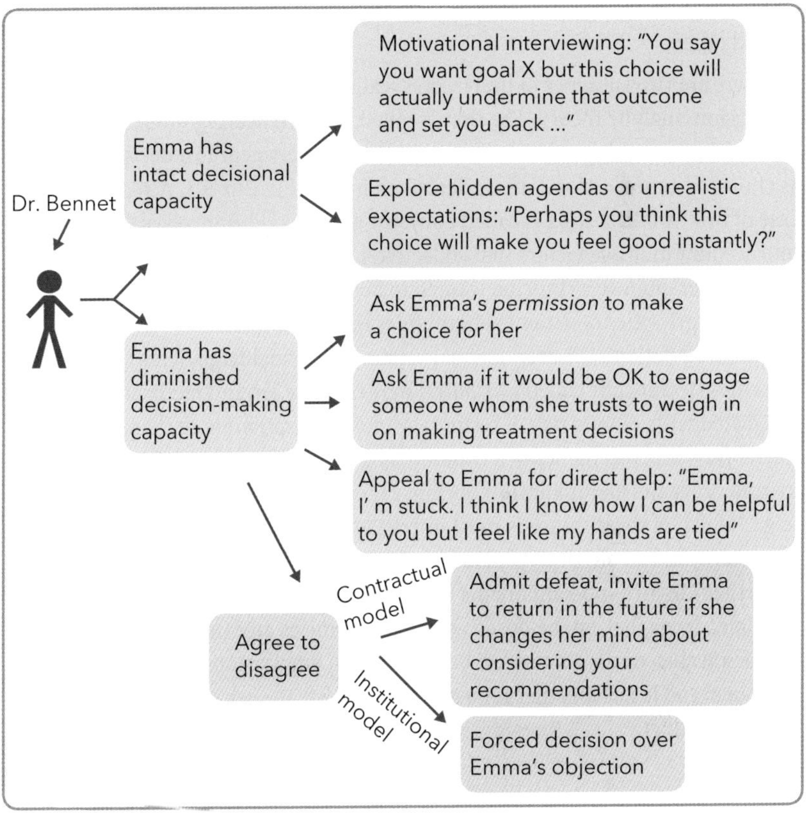

G BEST-WORST SCALING

Best–worst scaling is a type of decision-analytic process that applies when a decision-maker is faced with three or more viable choices. The decision-maker may identify the most-favored and least-favored choices from among several options, but then finds himself making pairwise comparisons of all "middle ground" choices relative to the least- and most-preferred extreme options. The complexity of such pairwise decisions increases when there are many choices available. (Consider, for example, choosing from among the limited antipsychotic medication options for treatment-resistant psychosis as opposed to the multitude for first-episode psychosis.) Moreover, the magnitude of difference between pairwise choices may not be equivalent among all possible combinations. So, for example, clozapine versus olanzapine may represent a less drastic comparison (since both have been studied in treatment-resistant psychosis, and have rather similar metabolic risk profiles) than, say, clozapine versus chlorpromazine (where few if any data support the efficacy of chlorpromazine in that particular setting). Or the decision-maker could be fairly neutral about some options and less so toward others.

There are two subtypes of best–worst scaling worth noting in the world of decision-analytic theory. The first is called **Maxdiff scaling** – relevant for hierarchically ranking a series of features that are pertinent to a decision, such as choosing a medication. This is described in detail in Box 8.3. A second special case of best–worst scaling is called **conjoint analysis**. This involves taking into account multiple factors that collectively bear on an ultimate decision. As an example, suppose a clinician wanted to better understand the hierarchical treatment priorities of patient subgroups (say, ever-hospitalized versus never-hospitalized patients, or ever-suicidal versus never-suicidal patients). Treatment priorities (technically called *attributes*) may coalesce around medications associated with a lower risk of relapse or rehospitalization more than drug tolerability. The mechanics of a conjoint analysis involve either asking a patient to rank order the hierarchical importance they accord to a list of attributes (e.g., "which of these things is most important to you?", then the next-most important, and so on) or to generate their own list. They may then be asked to further identify subcomponents (called *levels*) or a particular attribute (for example, drugs that can be dosed once daily, come as an extended-release form, are dissolvable, or do not need to be taken on an empty stomach). Putting all the attributes and levels together for a given patient creates what is called a *concept*, or ideal product.

Box 8.3

What is MaxDiff scaling?

MaxDiff scaling, also known as maximum difference scaling, is a mathematical term developed in decision theory that is used to describe a special case of best-worst case scaling, in which a decision-maker tends to be guided by the maximum difference in their preferences between two viable choices. In essence, decision-makers must score their relative preferences for all options that lie between their most-favored and least-favored choices. Return to Table 8.2 as an example but now, instead of according coefficients of importance to each criterion listed, let us rank order Emma's and Dr. Bennet's respective preferences based on their

Box 8.3 (cont.)

perceived relative importance, ranging from most (1) to least (5), as follows:

Emma's rankings	Criteria	Dr. Bennet's rankings
2	Fast onset	2
1	Lack of weight gain	1
4	Cognitive benefit	5
5	Cost	4
3	Minimal hassle	3

When Dr. Bennet and Emma address the same criteria, they are fairly aligned - other than that Dr. Bennet may be more cost-conscious than Emma, and/or more skeptical about the likelihood that the viable medication choices will produce a cognitive benefit.

H ITERATIVE PHARMACOTHERAPY IN PSYCHOTIC DISORDERS

The concept of iterative pharmacotherapy is somewhat more limited in the case of primary psychotic than mood disorders. With the singular exception of clozapine, no one antipsychotic medication exerts a markedly larger effect size than another, although subtle differences may exist: for example, a meta-analysis of head-to-head comparisons among second-generation antipsychotic medications in schizophrenia found that olanzapine was superior to aripiprazole, quetiapine, risperidone, and ziprasidone, while risperidone was more efficacious than quetiapine or ziprasidone (Leucht et al., 2009). Augmentation strategies – such as adding lithium or mood-stabilizing anticonvulant drugs to a second-generation antipsychotic medication – also have a very limited and at times ambiguous database, as has been reviewed in detail elsewhere (see Goldberg and Stahl, 2021). Our present goal, rather than to re-review the evidence base for efficacy across antipsychotic medications, specific augmentation strategies, or novel therapeutics, is to identify factors that might aid the clinician in recognizing key decision points. These can be summarized in the decision tree depicted in Figure 8.5.

Tip

Clozapine is the only known effective medication for treatment-resistant schizophrenia, with a response rate of 60–70% (Wahlbeck et al., 1999).

Figure 8.5 Decision tree for iterative pharmacotherapy in primary psychotic disorders

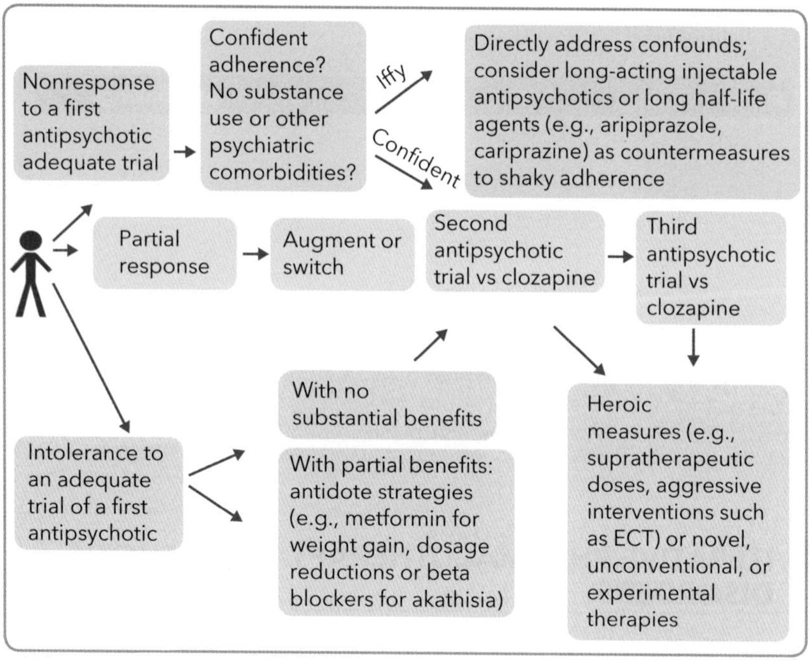

The core concepts reflected in Figure 8.5 might be summarized as follows:

- Differentiate nonresponses from partial responses from drug intolerances
- Assure adequate dosing/duration of an initial antipsychotic drug
- Keep in mind that more than half of schizophrenia patients are non- or poorly adherent to oral antipsychotic medications and that a substantial proportion of prescribers express low confidence in gauging adherence (Semahegen et al., 2020)
- Gauge drug response based on identifiable targets of treatment (e.g., delusional intensity, formal thought disorder, negative symptoms, agitation/aggression, cognition, interpersonal functioning)
- Discuss long-acting injectable formulations as an option when poor adherence is suspected or obvious
- Decisions about choosing "big gun" agents – namely, olanzapine or clozapine – should enter into clinical conversations sooner than later and hinge on illness severity and degree of impairment
- Combinations of antipsychotic medications are sometimes worthwhile to fine-tune partial responses and might capitalize on expected benefits from specific agents (such as anxiolytic or sedative properties from more antihistaminergic antipsychotics)

- ECT is a sometimes a worthwhile novel/heroic measure for severe psychosis (not just catatonia), even in the absence of mood symptoms
- Clozapine remains unrivaled in its magnitude of effect among antipsychotic medications – as further discussed in Box 8.4 – but response may take many months to fully judge

Tip

Avoid combining antipsychotics with "tight" D_2 binding affinities to avoid adverse neurological effects; favor augmentation of "loose" dopamine D_2 binders such as clozapine or quetiapine.

Box 8.4

When should clozapine enter iterative pharmacotherapy for psychotic disorders?

Clozapine is the sole drug with US Food and Drug Administration approval for treatment-resistant schizophrenia, and its manufacturer's product label calls out its potential to reduce suicidal acts in people with schizophrenia. The burden posed by its metabolic, hematologic, and other end-organ potential adverse effects has traditionally made its use reserved for nonresponse to several (at least two) other antipsychotic medications. The OPTiMiSE trial (Kahn et al., 2018) in first-episode schizophrenia or schizophreniform disorder argued that clozapine should be a viable option after only *one* failed antipsychotic trial, on the grounds that switching from a first antipsychotic (amilsulpride) to olanzapine was generally not effective whereas clozapine was. Similar findings suggest that in even moderately refractory schizophrenia patients, clozapine outperforms risperidone based on discontinuation due to lack of efficacy, although patients may be more likely to discontinue clozapine due to intolerance (Schooler et al., 2016). Collectively, these reports suggest that clozapine should not be thought of as a "last-line" treatment option – but the risk-benefit analysis must factor in concerns about tolerability, feasibility, suicidality, chronicity, and *degree* of treatment resistance, as well as viability of alternatives on a case-by-case basis.

I KNOWING *WHICH* ONE VARIABLE AT A TIME TO CHANGE FIRST

As much as the principle of changing only one variable at a time is often indispensable for hypothesis-testing, there are times when we might change two (or more) variables simultaneously – not with caution thrown to the winds so much as with an awareness of when the effects of the concomitant variables being changed are unlikely to produce conflictual results or confusion about which drug is likely causing what effect. Chaos sometimes descends upon iterative pharmacotherapy trials when patients abruptly stop multiple medications at once and then seek guidance and direction for how to regain equilibrium. Often, simply restarting the ensemble of a halted regimen delivers a suitable solution, but consider instances in which the patient wishes for a more selective remedy, and becomes choosy about what medications from a regimen they think they should or should not resume. We traverse these issues in the case of Danny (Clinical Vignette 8.4).

Vocabulary

Ceteris paribus means "holding other things constant" and is often invoked in economic decision analyses

Clinical Vignette 8.4

Danny was a 47-year-old divorced attorney with persistent depressive disorder (formerly chronic major depression), obsessive-compulsive traits, and prominent affective instability with low distress tolerance. He had been functioning with reasonably good stability (defined by maintaining his job with minimal interpersonal skirmishes, dating occasionally, and maintaining financial responsibility). Nevertheless, he projected an overall sense of dismay and chagrin that life had given him a raw deal and was in a weekly psychotherapy, which he felt "did little for him." For several years he had been taking lamotrigine 200 mg/day, vilazodone 20 mg/day, and lithium 600 mg/day, with normal renal and thyroid functioning. Irked by the prospect of remaining on medicines indefinitely, he rather arbitrarily and summarily chose to abruptly stop his lithium and lamotrigine and within 2 weeks experienced a range of somatic complaints (dizziness, light-headedness, malaise, fatigue, loss of appetite) as well as depressed mood. He called his psychiatrist, Dr. Gilmore, in a panic. A search by Dr. Gilmore of the medical literature found a handful of published case reports of withdrawal phenomena associated with abrupt lamotrigine discontinuation and the decision was made to resume it at his usual dose of 200 mg/day. A retitration from zero was opted against on the grounds that he had been taking lamotrigine for over 3 years and the likelihood of developing a serious cutaneous reaction was near nil this far out from his initial exposure to the drug (even in the absence of empirical evidence about abrupt restarts, and despite the manufacturer's recommendation to retitrate from the beginning in patients who have been off the drug for more than 5 days). Within a few days he felt "somewhat better but not 100%." Reluctant to restart lithium because of concerns about its long-term safety, he asked Dr. Gilmore, if a higher lamotrigine dose might yield a more robust improvement, or if vilazodone could instead be increased.

Tip

Significant rashes associated with lamotrigine usually occur between weeks 2 and 8, and seldom after week 15.

I.1 Clinical Reasoning

Let us consider Danny as an *n*-of-1 trial. The essence of the problem he presents is a somewhat blurred amalgam of possible discontinuation/somatic symptoms from the abrupt cessation of two core medicines in his regimen. If only Danny had stopped one at a time, and done so prospectively, ideally not in a sequential crossover design but better yet with several cloned versions of himself. Short of that level of fastidiousness, we are left having to "post hoc" our way through the data Danny gives us, confounded by the question of whether the symptoms he reported after stopping lithium and lamotrigine were simply an abrupt relapse of depression. Supporting the latter interpretation are observations from the literature that abrupt lithium cessation in bipolar disorder patients can increase the rate of depression relapse more than five-fold as compared to gradual cessation (Faedda et al., 1993), as well as the general impression in the literature that true "withdrawal" from lamotrigine is not a common event, if it even exists. From one perspective, the most straightforward way to clarify things is to break Danny's situation into separate components, akin to how an investigator might frame the aims and hypotheses of a grant proposal designed to empirically answer a question in pursuit of generalizable knowledge:

Hypothesis 1: This was a rapid depression relapse caused by abrupt lithium cessation, possibly compounded by coincident lamotrigine cessation; lithium resumption should resolve the problem

Hypothesis 2: Lamotrigine and lithium had been yielding synergy and the simultaneous cessation of both led to a depressive relapse; resumption of both would resolve the problem

Hypothesis 3: This is an example of rare lamotrigine discontinuation/withdrawal syndrome and resumption of lamotrigine alone should resolve the problem

Danny, however, wishes to elaborate on this paradigm with additional queries:

Hypothesis 4: Pushing lamotrigine dosing higher than 200 mg/day might yield a faster resolution of his relapse/withdrawal and possibly compensate (or otherwise avert the need) for adjunctive lithium

Hypothesis 5: Vilazodone dosed higher than 20 mg/day might produce an overall greater mood benefit that would avert the need for resuming lithium, assuming lamotrigine alone served as a mood stabilizer and assuming that vilazodone was delivering some degree of mood benefit

There are a few too many "what ifs" in this overall situation to arbitrarily capitulate to Danny's plea for staying off lithium without sacrificing important knowledge that will help us discern what has been helping and what may be irrelevant. If one wished to test Hypothesis 3, some meaningful period on resumed full-dose lamotrigine would really be the only way to rule in or rule out the possibility of a discontinuation/withdrawal phenomenon. On the other hand, if Danny's main priority is to "feel well again" as soon as possible, the best rationale would be simply to retrace his pharmacological footsteps and resume the same regimen he previously took (i.e., lithium 600 mg/day plus lamotrigine 200 mg/day), down to wearing the same socks and underwear (i.e., lithium 600 mg/day plus lamotrigine 200 mg/day), expecting to reattain euthymia and no somatic complaints, and then one could readily and electively embark on the other "experiments" at hand – namely:

Hypothesis 6: Higher-dose lamotrigine could replace lithium to sustain (rather than attain) euthymia

Hypothesis 7: Higher-dose vilazodone could replace lithium to sustain (rather than attain) euthymia

Raising the lamotrigine dose only a few days after resuming it deprives us of any real opportunity to form conclusions about the possible pharmacodynamic value of a dose above what had been his stable dose.

The practicalities and demands of real life preclude turning Danny into seven *n*-of-1 trials and making him a human laboratory. Danny's level of distress and urgent quest for relief also make it difficult for the clinician treating him to frame the above possible explanations for his symptoms as testable hypotheses from which generalizable inferences can be drawn. A byproduct of faulty clinical reasoning, should Danny simply spontaneously improve, could be that Dr. Gilmore may conclude, without solid evidence, that perhaps abrupt lamotrigine cessation *did* cause a withdrawal syndrome, and carry this hypothesis forward as if it were factual into her clinical practice – maybe even publish a letter to the editor about her novel observation.

What actually ultimately happened to Danny is in some ways less pertinent than how we go about deducing likely cause-and-effect relationships among the relevant variables, and how our assumptions influence our decision points. If Dr. Gilmore preferred the most conservative approach, she might favor simply putting Danny back on the exact regimen that last corresponded to a state of wellness, and save the hypothesis-testing perhaps for future undertakings if and when she and Danny both think it is wise and worthwhile to test one hypothesis at a time. From a decision-making standpoint, the most essential elements for Dr. Gilmore likely entail:

- Focusing on sustaining her therapeutic alliance with Danny (i.e., curiosity and interest in his decision to stop his medications – being not at all judgey). Clearly Danny wanted her to know he was unhappy with the status quo and voted with his feet
- Responding to Danny's sense of chaos with a sense of calm competence, like a parent comforting a distraught child injured after breaking a vase – "we can fix this together, but let's not go crazy together about what to do"

- Recognizing, herself, the most plausible and sensible explanation that will most expediently mend Danny's injury (though it is tempting to Dr. Gilmore to explore Hypothesis 3, and she must set aside the conflict of interest posed by her desire to make a novel observation and publish a new finding)
- An awareness that if a first plan of action fails to ameliorate the problem, Dr. Gilmore has back-up plans in mind for how to pursue a successive course of action, perhaps informed by the other hypotheses above

This discussion now brings us to some conceptual aspects about back-up plans.

J BACK-UP PLANS AND BACK UPS TO THE BACK-UP PLANS

Well-crafted back-up plans can separate adequate from extraordinary clinicians. With no crystal balls available to know with certainty the result of any one decision, the best any practitioner can do is spell out the logic and rationale for the available options and go through with the patient, as shown throughout this chapter, the relative pros and cons and identify priorities and intended goals. Here is where the magic can happen: if Plan A fails, we can turn to Plans B and C. In Emma's case, we already know what her and her doctor's second and third preferences would be (see Tables 8.2 and 8.3) if a stimulant was unsuccessful. We can forecast this for her. We can even help encourage her to embark on a first plan knowing that if it does not work out, for whatever reason, we know exactly what to do next (barring any new information that might arise from the results of Plan A – for instance, were a stimulant to unmask a diathesis for psychosis). The secret "pearl" of wisdom in this exchange is to make it as clear as possible to Emma that a roadmap exists, courtesy of her own input in its construction, for knowing exactly what to do if the best-laid intentions and plans are unsuccessful. The one thing we can promise her is a rationale and a plan.

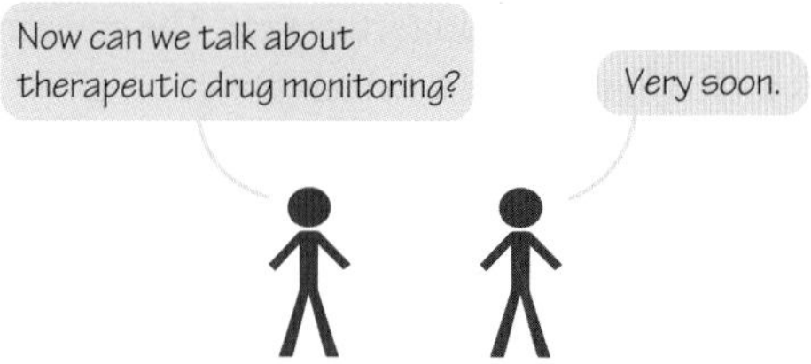

K HOW IS THE CLINICIAN'S OWN WORKING MEMORY?

Working memory means holding facts in mind that are necessary in order to make an executive decision, for which the "best" decision is predicated on a collation of inter-related details. Our best clinical example comes from baseball. The runner on second needs to decide if he is going to steal third base. What bits of information go into that decision? Stealing third is a much wiser proposition if the batter has a full count, there are already two outs, the batter has a low strikeout rate, the pitcher and runner are matched in handedness, and a hit-and-run play is on; extra credit for noticing rainy conditions that make it harder to grip the baseball. That is a lot of information to hold in mind and coalesce before making a go/no-go decision. Picture a prescriber integrating an analogous conglomeration of clinical facts about a given patient with as much fluidity and coherence in order to be the Rickey Henderson of psychopharmacology. Swift action alone could lead to disaster in the absence of proper planning. While on the topic of neurocognitive performance, one hopes the astute base-running psychopharmacologist is fairly able to block out the distraction of background noise – that is, information that is not so directly relevant to the decision at hand. For Rickey, that may be "overriding" bad advice from the third base coach or the grandstands, or noticing a balk from the pitcher. For the prescriber, the decision to use a dopamine partial agonist over a full antagonist is probably not terribly influenced by the patient's having a family history of panic disorder, a personal history of peripheral neuropathy, or comorbid trichotillomania – all interesting details, but not so germane to the immediate decision task at hand.

Trivia

Rickey Henderson, nicknamed "The Man of Steal," holds the Major League Baseball all-time record for stolen bases (1406).

Besides focused attention and intact working memory, Rickey also needs good running shoes and protective gear. The equipment of good psychopharmacology is no less fundamental, which brings us, at last, to laboratory tests – no replacement for clinical wisdom, but a helpful accessory.

L HOW DOES THERAPEUTIC DRUG MONITORING OR PHARMACOGENETICS FIT INTO ITERATIVE PHARMACOTHERAPY?

All laboratory tests should be ordered for the purpose of answering a specific question, or testing a hypothesis. Therapeutic drug monitoring (TDM) and pharmacogenetics are both examples of tools that can be relevant to understanding pharmacokinetics and pharmacodynamics – but clinicians do not always appreciate where and how, like any other tool, they should or should not be deployed. For a comprehensive discussion of each, we would refer the reader elsewhere (Goldberg and Stahl, 2021; Meyer and Stahl, 2021). A handful of drugs have known therapeutic windows, above or below which efficacy and/or tolerability may be suboptimal. Common examples include lithium (bipolar mania and relapse prevention), divalproex (bipolar mania), all tricyclic antidepressants and bupropion (major depression), and clozapine (schizophrenia), among others. There are also more experimental approaches with using TDM to inform decisions about optimizing dosages of other antidepressant (e.g., venlafaxine) or second-generation antipsychotic medications (e.g., olanzapine). Dosing perseverance generally makes sense, as tolerability permits, before augmenting or changing drugs if a meaningful therapeutic drug level of an initial agent has not been achieved. Likewise, further dosage optimization before making iterative changes makes sense when low drug levels could reflect malabsorption (e.g., celiac disease), pharmacokinetic interactions (e.g., co-therapy with cytochrome P450 inducers; impaired distribution due to poor protein binding), or ultra-rapid-metabolizer phenotypes.

Pharmacogenetic testing – discussed further in Chapter 9, Section K – is a useful means to affirm suspicions about ultra-rapid-metabolizer phenotypes for patients taking drugs that are substrates of relevant Phase I or Phase II metabolic enzymes. Poor-metabolizer phenotypes can also account for nonresponses to a "pro-drug" that requires conversion to an active metabolite (such as venlafaxine, dependent on cytochrome P450 2D6 (CYP2D6) degradation to form desvenlafaxine; or risperidone, also dependent on CYP2D6, for its conversion to 9-hydroxyrisperidone).

M RECOGNIZING PHARMACOLOGICAL FUTILITY AND ALTERNATIVES TO PHARMACOTHERAPY

Declarations of pharmacological futility happen throughout all of medicine, and psychiatry is no special exception. In the eventual course of iterative pharmacotherapy, it is sometime inevitable that no drug intervention yields a meaningful improvement for a severe or complex clinical problem. At what point should clinicians engage patients in a frank discussion about the likelihood that further pharmacological efforts are unlikely to yield a benefit, rather than continue further iterations ad infinitum? Certainly, well before such a decision point, one has searched far and wide for remediable explanations for poor response to iterative pharmacotherapy. Apart from obvious confounds such as poor adherence or unrecognized psychotoxic effects from substance use or other medical and psychiatric comorbidities, consider the following cases of mistaken identity:

- Antidepressant failure when perceived depression actually reflects negative symptoms of schizophrenia
- Mood stabilizer or second-generation antipsychotic medication failure when the perceived "mood swings" of bipolar disorder, or paranoia associated with schizophrenia, more accurately represent, respectively, the affective lability or micropsychotic distortions of borderline personality disorder

- Odd, idiosyncractic thinking and poor interpersonal relatedness thought to reflect schizophrenia instead derives from autism or a related developmental disability
- Inattention or distractibility that is presumed to reflect adult ADHD, which actually represents mild cognitive impairment as the prelude to major neurocognitive disorder

There are also certain negative prognostic factors, such as early childhood trauma, or severe comorbid personality disorders, that can seemingly render almost any psychopharmacology a fruitless endeavor. Psychiatrists and other mental health practitioners who treat highly treatment-refractory patients may find themselves struggling, sometimes unwittingly, with the realization of futility after numerous appropriate and adequate pharmacotherapy trials, and despite the cleverest of pharmacodynamic combinations or use of agents that lack a known superior alternative (such as clozapine). Denial of futility may take the form of doubled-down perseverance, analogous to the last clinician willing to disengage from a futile cardiac resuscitation. Herein, however, lies the difference between futility and defeat: acknowledging medical humility by acceptance of limitations is not synonymous with defeat. We would propose that the "decision tree" at this point may take one of four routes, as shown in Figure 8.6.

Figure 8.6 A decision tree when facing pharmacological futility

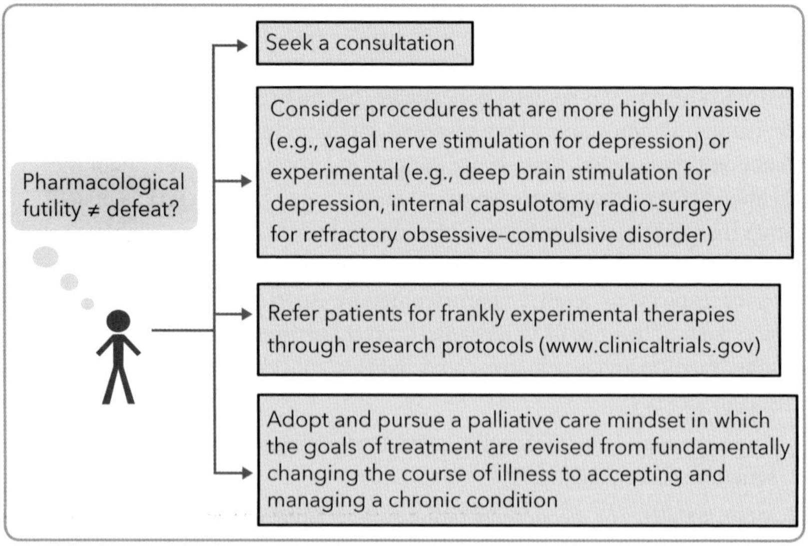

The pros and cons of each option are considered in Table 8.4.

Table 8.4 Pros and cons of clinical options when facing pharmacological futility

Option	Pros	Cons
Seek a consultation	• A fresh pair of eyes can sometimes catch a missed diagnosis (e.g., somatic symptom disorder or psychosis) or truly viable but not-considered pharmacotherapy option • Consultants can help authoritatively affirm that the care has been proper and perhaps exemplary, and that further pharmacotherapy is indeed unlikely to be productive • Chess experts can help distinguish "check" from "checkmate"	• Affirming the impression of pharmacological futility may not be what either the patient or the referring clinician wants to hear • Futility may be misconstrued as being synonymous with abandoning hope if pharmacotherapy is the only known "tool" • Consultants afraid of disappointing stakeholders, or appearing not "expert" enough, may disingenuously propose untried medications that have little to no likelihood of benefit
Invasive procedures	• Represent the most heroic, aggressive interventions	• Possible unknown risks and hazards
Research protocols	• Can provide access to options that might not otherwise be available • The structure of a study protocol brings with it additional support resources and engages a team approach • Usually no cost to patient	• Appropriate study protocols may not exist • Inappropriate study protocols may simply further foster unrealistic expectations • There may be little or no provision for sustained aftercare when the study ends • Patients with a history of extensive nonresponses to many prior treatments may be deemed ineligible for study inclusion
Palliative care mindset	• Strives to maintain hope by not abandoning the patient ("I have nothing more to offer you" becomes "I do not think more medicines are likely to change your condition so let's instead focus on ways to help you better cope, accept, and manage this problem")	• May be misconstrued as defeat or "proof" that the situation is indeed hopeless

Table 8.4 (cont.)

Option	Pros	Cons
Palliative care mindset	• Dispels magical thinking about unlikely success from further pharmacological remedies • Spares the patient exposure to inappropriate, expensive, or otherwise unsubstantiated/sensational options that might capitalize on their sense of desperation and vulnerability • Introduces the concept that psychotherapy may exert greater utility as the primary treatment modality • Does not negate the possibility that future therapeutics may someday emerge and could be tried with caution rather than magical expectations	• Would be erroneous to pursue if past treatments were in fact inadequate, inappropriate, or intolerable rather than ineffective • Runs the risk of failing to identify new viable pharmacotherapies or other new treatments as technology advances

TAKE-HOME POINTS

- Pharmacological decision points about altering an existing medication regimen depend on recognizing the context of a current presentation relative to past treatment outcomes, severity, chronicity, urgency, tolerability, priorities, and related factors that influence the best next steps
- Recognize the viable options and alternatives for any given treatment decision; articulate their pros and cons, alternatives, and relative priorities for both the patient and the clinician. Consider devising simple decision-analytic matrices both to define relative priorities as well as to delineate back-up plans if a first planned intervention fails
- Enlist patients as active partners in the decision-making process, as feasible, once viable options have been identified
- Recognize pharmacological endpoints when continued use of a drug or strategy seems ineffective; reassess diagnostics and clinical factors (such as nonadherence or inadequate dosing) that might attenuate a drug's optimal effect or otherwise prompt interest in deviating from an original plan by changing medications or dosages
- Clinical problems for which true pharmacological futility seems apparent demand adopting a new approach, which might include seeking an outside consultation, intensifying non-pharmacological/psychosocial strategies, and otherwise striving to maintain a sense of hope without repeating the same behaviors but expecting different results

References

Burdick KE, Braga RJ, Nnadi CU, et al. Placebo-controlled adjunctive trial of pramipexole in patients with bipolar disorder: Targeting cognitive dysfunction. J Clin Psychiatry 2012; 73: 103–112

Coryell W, Solomon D, Turvey C, et al. The long-term course of rapid cycling bipolar disorder. Arch Gen Psychiatry 2003; 60: 914–920

Faedda GL, Tondo L, Baldessarini RJ, et al. Outcome after rapid versus gradual discontinuation of lithium treatment in bipolar disorders. Arch Gen Psychiatry 1993; 50: 448–455

Goldberg JF. When further pharmacotherapy is futile. J Clin Psychiatry 2018; 80: 18ac12276

Goldberg JF, Stahl SM. Practical Psychopharmacology: Translating Findings from Evidence-Based Trials into Real-World Clinical Practice. Cambridge: Cambridge University Press, 2021.

Khan A, Fahl Mar K, Faucett J, et al. Has the rising placebo response impacted antidepressant clinical trial outcome? Data from the US Food and Drug Administration 1987–2013. World Psychiatry 2017; 16: 181–192

Kahn RS, Winter Van Rosum I, Leucht S, et al. Amisulpride and olanzapine followed by open-label treatment with clozapine in first-episode schizophrenia and schizophreniform disorder (OPTiMiSE): A three-phase switching study. Lancet Psychiatry 2018; 5: 797–807

Leucht S, Komossa K, Rummel-Kluge C, et al. A meta-analysis of head-to-head comparisons of second-generation antipsychotics in the treatment of schizophrenia. Am J Psychiatry 2009; 166: 152–163

Meyer JM, Stahl SM. The Clinical Use of Antipsychotic Plasma Levels. Cambridge: Cambridge University Press, 2021

Olfson M, Marcus SC, Tedeschi M, et al. Continuity of antidepressant treatment for adults with depression in the United States. Am J Psychiatry 2006; 163: 101–108

Papakostas GI, Thase ME, Fava M, et al. Are antidepressant drugs that combine serotonergic and noradrenergic mechanisms of action more effective than the selective serotonin reuptake inhibitors in treating major depressive disorder? A meta-analysis of studies of newer agents. Biol Psychiatry 2007; 62: 1217–1227

Rohsenow DJ, Tidey JW, Miranda R, et al. Olanzapine reduces urge to smoke and nicotine withdrawal symptoms in community smokers. Exp Clin Psychopharmacol 2008; 16: 215–222

Rush AJ, Trivedi MH, Wisniewski SR, et al. Acute and longer-term outcomes in depressed outpatients requiring one or several treatment steps: A STAR*D report. Am J Psychiatry 2006; 163: 1905–1917

Rush AJ, Wisniewski SR, Warden D, et al. Selecting among second-step antidepressant medication monotherapies: Predictive value of clinical, demographic, or first-step treatment features. Arch Gen Psychiatry 2008; 65: 870–880

Sachs GS, Nierenberg AA, Calabrese JR, et al. Effectiveness of adjunctive antidepressant treatment for bipolar depression. N Engl J Med 2007; 356: 1711–1722

Schooler NR, Marder SR, Chengappa KNR, et al. Clozapine and risperidone in moderately refractory schizophrenia: A 6-month randomized double-blind comparison. J Clin Psychiatry 2016; 77: 628–634

Semahegen A, Torpey K, Manu A, et al. Psychotropic medication non-adherence and its associated factors among patients with major psychiatric disorders: A systematic review and meta-analysis. Syst Rev 2020; 9:17

Turner EH, Matthews AM, Linardatos E, et al. Selective publication of antidepressant trials and its influence on apparent efficacy. N Engl J Med 2008; 358: 252–260

Turner EH, Cipriani A, Furukawa TA, et al. Selective publication of antidepressant trials and its influence on apparent efficacy: updated comparisons and meta-analyses of newer versus older trials. PLoS Med 2022; 19(1): e1003886

van der Loos ML, Mulder PG, Hartong EG, et al. Efficacy and safety of lamotrigine as add-on treatment to lithium in bipolar depression: A multicenter, double-blind, placebo-controlled trial. J Clin Psychiatry 2009; 70: 223–231

Wahlbeck K, Cheine N, Essali A, et al. Evidence of clozapine's effectiveness in schizophrenia: A systematic review and meta-analysis of randomized trials. Am J Psychiatry 1999; 156: 990–999

Yatham LN, Mackala S, Basivireddy J et al. Lurasidone versus treatment as usual for cognitive impairment in euthymic patients with bipolar I disorder: A randomised, open-label, pilot study. Lancet Psychiatry 2017; 4: 208–217

9 Hierarchical and Complex Pharmacotherapy Decision-Making

LEARNING OBJECTIVES

- ☐ Recognize the importance of a hierarchical approach to iterative pharmacotherapy – with contingency planning – for chronic or recurrent psychiatric disorders
- ☐ Understand the pharmacokinetic and pharmacodynamic parameters that influence medication changes and cross-tapers
- ☐ Describe tenets of the chronic illness model when facing possible pharmacological futility
- ☐ Recognize logical rules that govern the rationale, safety, and efficacy of purposeful (versus haphazard) combination pharmacotherapy regimens
- ☐ Discuss strategies for, and circumstances that warrant, psychotropic drug deprescribing
- ☐ Describe the role of pharmacogenetic testing to answer specific clinical questions that can inform individualized treatment rules when crafting patient-specific treatment decision trees

In preceding chapters, we have focused mainly on how to think through clinical problems that are often ambiguous or have multiple viable solutions, each with their respective pros and cons. We have deliberately refrained from offering specific recommendations about "what to do" in a given situation when no single best answer may exist. When that happens, the clinician's task involves framing testable hypotheses and applying a reasoning process to arrive at a sensible individualized treatment regimen (ITR) for a given patient based on their unique clinical profile. Our goal has been to steer readers away from one-size-fits-all protocol-driven care and replace that approach with a more decision-analytic patient-specific iterative strategy, where nodes along a decision tree are determined by the personalized characteristics of a given individual.

Yet, instances obviously arise in which clinicians rightfully seek more specific guidance about the "best" (or least-worst) course of action for certain complex situations, beyond simply reciting the pros and cons of all viable alternatives. In this chapter we will now slightly reverse course and focus more on "what to do," by considering the features that make one viable option more or less compelling than another. Once again, let us begin by recapitulating the concept of iterative rather than definitive "one-and-done" approaches to clinical decision-making, particularly in the case of treating more complex forms of psychopathology.

A TAKING A HIERARCHICAL TRIAGE APPROACH TO ITERATIVE THERAPEUTICS

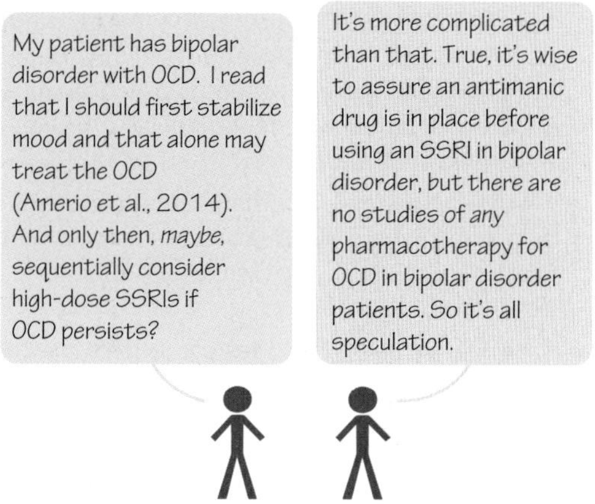

In Chapter 1 (Section E) we noted that most patients with complex psychiatric conditions often have more than one diagnosable disorder, and clinicians must discern a relative hierarchy of symptoms and related features to interpret clinical data (e.g., using a RIME (see Table 1.5) evaluative approach (Pangaro, 1999)). Let us now apply the same triaging to decision-making about therapeutic interventions. How do we decide what to treat first, or does sequencing even matter? Does one identified ailment take precedence over another? When does it make sense to consider the treatment of one disorder as a prerequisite for treatment of a comorbidity? And when does the treatment of one disorder affect the manifestations and treatment of a co-occurring condition (as when one might prioritize treatment of depression with poor concentration before speculating about the role for stimulants to treat "comorbid" attentional problems)?

Sometimes "urgency" takes obvious precedence – acute delirium, catatonia, and physiological withdrawal all demand stabilization before one can properly assess "underlying" conditions. Psychosis with paranoid ideation may cry out for immediate treatment but it may not be clear if the driving force is an underlying primary psychotic disorder, a toxic delirium, or severe posttraumatic stress disorder – for which the core treatments (both pharmacological and psychosocial) all differ. In the absence of empirical studies on hierarchical treatment of comorbidities, we would offer a few tips, as summarized in Box 9.1.

Perhaps the greatest challenge when crafting hierarchical treatments is knowing whether, and which, disorders rightfully "take precedence" over others. There are no simple solutions to this conundrum, because it can be hard if not impossible to know with certainty when any one given disorder might "drive" another, or if treatment for one condition will reliably alleviate symptoms of the other. Consider the common case of coexisting depression and anxiety – a scenario in which monoaminergic antidepressant medications tend to have

Box 9.1

Tips for triaging iterative interventions for comorbid conditions

- Acute intoxication/withdrawal states and active alcohol or substance use disorders tend to preclude the new diagnosis or treatment of other psychiatric disorders. A sequential approach that prioritizes abstinence (and clearance of the potential psychotoxic effects of psychoactive substances) is usually necessary to formulate a reasonable assessment and treatment plan
- Medically unstable conditions that can manifest with psychiatric symptoms (e.g., hypothyroidism) require correction before one can reasonably pursue separate treatments for a presumptive freestanding psychiatric disorder
- Prominent trauma histories can pose a psychiatric wildcard and manifest with a wide range of symptoms including emotional instability, psychosis, dissociation, and cognitive complaints; often, behaviorally oriented interventions that target trauma (e.g., exposure-based therapies) may be prerequisites in order to leverage consequent affective, behavioral, or cognitive symptoms
- "Parsimonious" interventions that target multiple domains - such as noradrenergic antidepressant medications for both pain and depression, or gabapentinoids for both anxiety and neuropathy - may help to simplify decision-making when feasible
- Solicit patients' own preferences for identifying hierarchical treatments - they themselves may be more concerned about one symptom constellation than another, or one treatment modality relative to another

lower overall response rates than when depression occurs without anxiety (Fava et al., 2008). Box 9.2 illustrates the uncertainty of this paradigm. If we think depression takes precedence over (or drives) anxiety, then we spare no effort to deploy aggressive interventions with the largest effect sizes for depression. On the other hand, if we think anxiety is more the driver, dunking the patient in a vat of clonazepam should, in theory, render their depression more responsive to depression-specific interventions once the right hierarchical sequence of targeted interventions has been deduced. Right? At least in principle?

Well, at least in principle, this idea makes sense and is a reasonable conceptual framework for devising a hierarchical treatment approach. In practice, of course, little is known about whether solitary treatment of anxiety before treatment of depression works better than a tandem approach (in part lies the dilemma that many treatments for anxiety *are* antidepressants; and that some monoaminergic antidepressant medications – such as vilazodone (Thase et al., 2014) – may have particularly robust anxiolytic properties). At the very least, though, clinicians must recognize forms of "comorbid" psychopathology that could impede efforts

Box 9.2

Depression and/or anxiety: Which drives which?

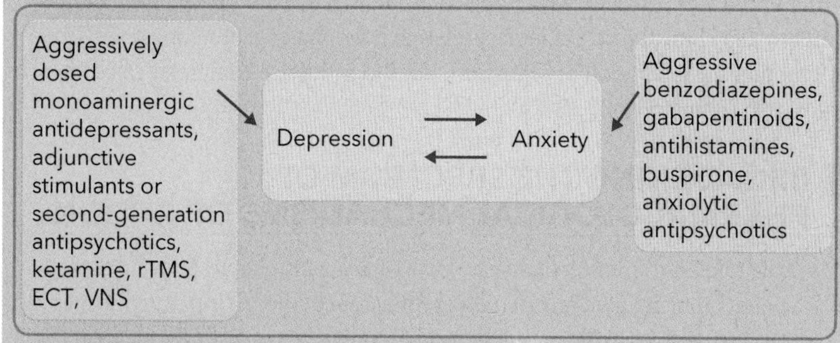

Abbreviations: ECT, electroconvulsive therapy; rTMS, repetitive transcranial magnetic stimulation; VNS, vagus nerve stimulation

to make headway with a presumptive "primary" psychiatric diagnosis such as major depression, bipolar disorder, schizophrenia, or an anxiety disorder.

Consider also the question of whether there may be instances in which the treatment of major depression might be better when pharmacotherapy and psychotherapy are *sequenced* rather than begun concurrently – akin to the way oncologists might advise neoadjuvant chemotherapy to shrink the size of a solid tumor before then surgically debulking or irradiating it. It is certainly a plausible hypothesis that hard-to-treat forms of depression might benefit from pharmacotherapy before psychotherapy in order to optimize someone's capacity to exercise cognitive flexibility, improve attentional processing, and enhance motivation and drive as prerequisites to tackling the work of, say, a cognitively based therapy that addresses distorted attitudes and beliefs.

In actuality, the combination of cognitive–behavioral therapy (CBT) plus antidepressant pharmacotherapy (specifically, escitalopram or duloxetine) was studied in a group of 112 outpatient major depression patients who initially did not remit after treatment with either that pharmacotherapy regimen alone or CBT alone;

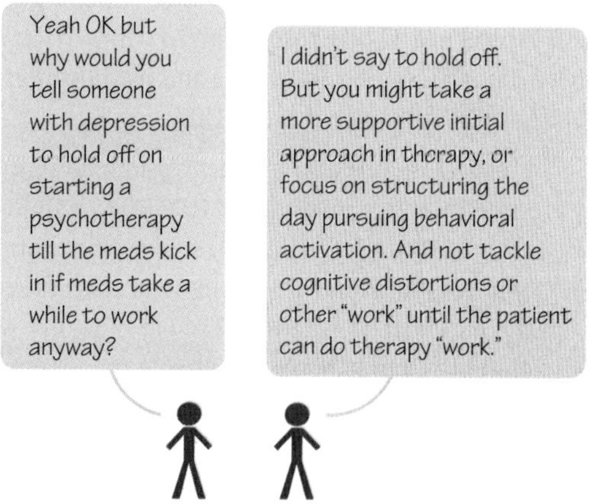

the sequence of introducing CBT after pharmacotherapy or pharmacotherapy after CBT produced similar outcomes (Dunlop et al., 2019). What about patient preference for one modality versus another? In the initial phase of that randomized clinical trial, patients' preference for pharmacotherapy or CBT did not predict the likelihood of remission, but did influence completer rates in each study arm (Dunlop et al., 2017).

B BROADENING THE SPECTRUM OF PHARMACOLOGICAL MECHANISMS OF ACTION

It is often taken for granted that successive pharmacotherapies may be more efficacious if they involve broadening the presumed underlying drug mechanisms of action – analogous to using increasingly broad-spectrum antibiotics for treatment-resistant infections, or increasingly broad-spectrum antiarrhythmics for hard-to-treat cardiac arrhythmias. While there is obvious conceptual appeal in crafting a pharmacotherapy "dirty drug" regimen that "hits more receptors" or putatively invokes multiple neurotransmitter systems, the actual empirical database on favoring an ever-increasing broadened spectrum of mechanistic action is not so well established. For example, one can readily move beyond a single-monoaminergic (e.g., a selective serotonin reuptake inhibitor (SSRI) or noradrenergic tricyclic medication) approach through drug combinations that involve complementary receptor binding (such as mirtazapine (a serotonin 5-HT_{2A} and 5-HT_3 antagonist) plus alpha-2 autoreceptor and heteroreceptor antagonist) combined with a serotonin–norepinephrine reuptake inhibitor (SNRI)) – although the actual database with this mechanistically attractive combination has so far shown only modest response. In the Sequenced Treatment Alternatives to Relieve Depression (STAR*D) study, response to mirtazapine plus venlafaxine was only 13.7% (McGrath et al., 2006); in another study of initial venlafaxine nonresponders, mirtazapine augmentation produced a 50.7% response (as compared to 76.9% after switching to imipramine; Navarro et al., 2019), and in a 12-week randomized comparison no differences were found between adjunctive mirtazapine and placebo after incomplete response to an SSRI or SNRI (Kessler et al., 2018).

In recurrent/chronic major depression, no significant differences in outcome were seen in a large randomized trial (the Combining Medications to Enhance Depression Outcomes (COMED) study) when comparing escitalopram alone versus in combination with bupropion versus the combination of mirtazapine plus venlafaxine (Rush et al., 2011). Even monoamine oxidase inhibitors (MAOIs) – arguably, highly broad-spectrum triple-monoaminergic enhancers – performed poorly in the STAR*D trial, with only a 6.9% response rate (McGrath et al., 2006), although suboptimal dosing (as well as the passage of several previous treatment failures) may have contributed to this unexpectedly low degree of improvement.

Does this mean one should *not* consider broadened-spectrum pharmacotherapies as a factor in the decision tree after initial inadequate responses? Certainly not! For one thing, studies such as those mentioned above are not without their methodological critique. In STAR*D, for example, the mean dose of tranylcypromine used was only a rather modest 36.9 mg/day, likely diminishing responsivity. (Consider that in *highly* treatment-resistant depression, the evidence base using tranylcypromine sometimes favors aggressive and heroic dosing as high as 170 mg/day (!) – very much not for the faint of heart (Amsterdam and Berwish, 1989).) Additionally, remember the pitfalls of thinking that one size fits all. There may very well be patient-specific characteristics that can help to define treatment plans for distinct patient subgroups with a unique likelihood of response to aggressive or broad-spectrum pharmacotherapy.

Let us dive a bit deeper into the last point and reconsider the notion of machine-based learning as discussed in Chapter 6 (Section J). Chekroud and colleagues (2016) used data from STAR*D and COMED (the above-noted studies) to develop a machine learning (ML) algorithm to generate predictors of drug response. They identified 25 variables that produced a 64.6% accuracy

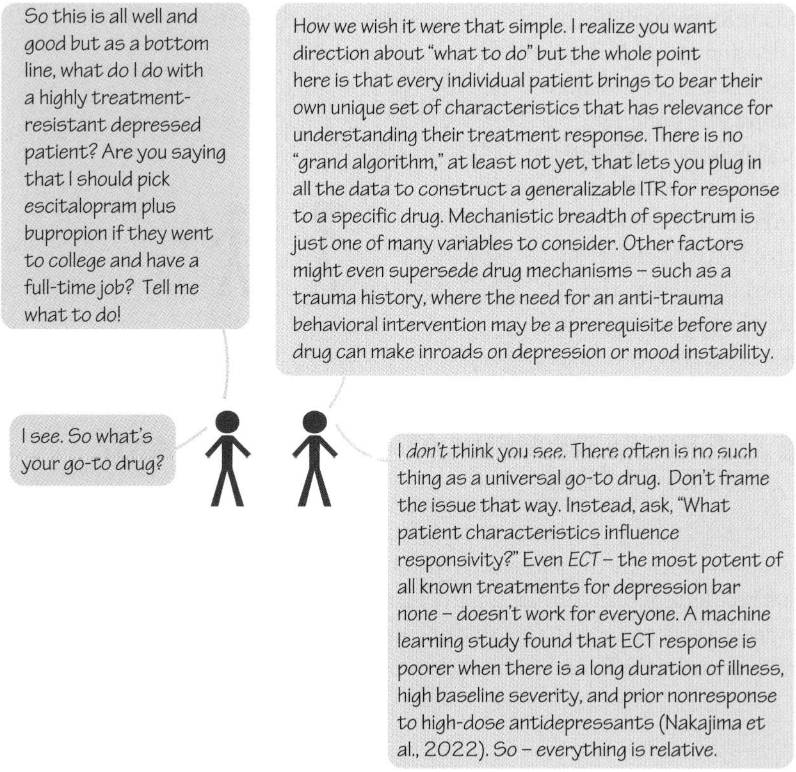

in predicting response to escitalopram or escitalopram plus bupropion. Importantly, rather than identifying any one single predictor variable for response, the ML approach brought together a collection of features to define the ITR. Among the pertinent 25 variables were both demographic features (e.g., race, education, employment status) and clinical characteristics (e.g., overall depression severity and subcomponents such as lethargy/fatiguability, agitation, somatic anxiety, sleep parameters, and trauma history). Once again, the decision-analytic approach might usefully consider not simply whether a drug mechanism has a "broad" or "narrow" mechanistic spectrum but, as importantly, for what profile of patient a "broader" spectrum drug might be especially useful.

There is enormous value in outlining an iterative treatment plan with built-in contingencies. As we have described in earlier chapters, from an engineering standpoint, identifying "back-up plans" and failsafe strategies in the event of a first option failing is logical. It acknowledges the multiple factors that influence treatment response, and the frequent need for successive approximations when trying to solve a problem. Moreover, it reflects the wisdom of adopting a Bayesian-analytic approach – recognizing how prior probabilities in a decision tree yield data that shape them into more informative posterior probabilities (see Chapter 6, Section J), making successive steps far from a random trial-and-error enterprise when earlier steps in a patient-specific algorithm fail.

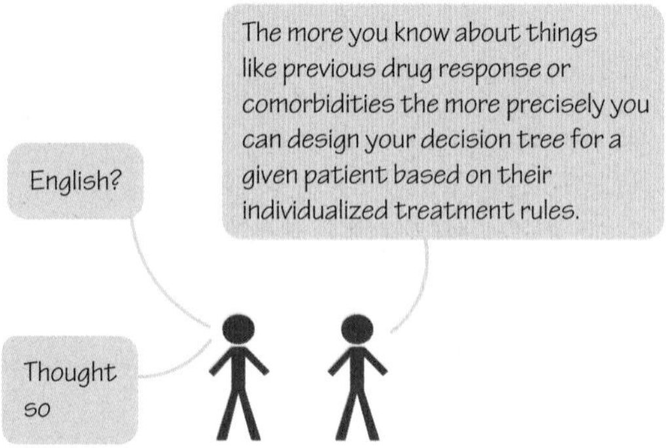

C THE RULES OF MEDICATION SWITCHES AND CROSS-TAPERS

When is a cross-taper necessary or advisable, when can an abrupt switch be made, and what are the pharmacodynamic and pharmacokinetic parameters that best inform such decisions, particularly when empirical data on switching strategies may be absent? The fundamental rules that dictate such decisions can be summarized in Table 9.1.

Table 9.1 Points of consideration when switching from one pharmacotherapy to another

Issue	Comments
Half-life of outgoing drug	Outgoing drugs with a long half-life may pose a greater risk for additive adverse effects in combination with a newly added agent. Also, drugs with a long half-life such as fluoxetine, aripiprazole, or cariprazine will auto-taper and not necessarily require dose reductions or imposed taper-downs; they can usually just get stopped abruptly with no ill effects
Concern for rebound, withdrawal, or discontinuation effects from stopping an outgoing drug too quickly	Short half-life serotonergic drugs (e.g., sertraline, paroxetine, venlafaxine, duloxetine) may be prone to discontinuation effects, often remediable by switching briefly to a long-half-life drug (e.g., fluoxetine). Abrupt cessation of short-half-life antipsychotic medications (e.g., risperidone, ziprasidone) carries an approximate eight-fold risk for inducing withdrawal symptoms (including nausea, vomiting, diarrhea, abdominal pain, headache, restlessness) (Brandt et al., 2020). Abrupt cessation of alpha-1 agonists such as clonidine can cause rebound hypertension
Mechanistic incompatibilities or contradictory actions at the same target	The best-known example is probably the potential for adverse drug interactions with MAOIs (i.e., hypertensive crises or serotonin syndrome). Clinicians may often combine drugs with pharmacodynamically opposing effects (e.g., stimulants with sedative-hypnotics) but that may be to purposefully offset adverse effects of an otherwise beneficial agent, and there is no conflictual or contradictory mechanism of action
Competition for receptor binding	A debated topic! See Box 9.3
Drug effect on seizure threshold	At least in principle, anticonvulsants or other medications that raise the seizure threshold warrant taper-offs rather than abrupt cessation unless they are being replaced by other medications that similarly raise the seizure threshold
Discontinuing a drug with no planned replacement	The original studies of abrupt versus gradual lithium discontinuation in bipolar disorder involved no new drug being introduced to replace outgoing lithium. One would *presume* that rapid versus gradual lithium cessation bears less on outcome if it is followed by immediate replacement (e.g., with divalproex or a second-generation antipsychotic medication)

Box 9.3

What is the net effect of drugs that compete for the same receptors?

This remains a burning question with more speculation than data to inform decision-making. It is reasonable to ask whether two (or more) agents that compete for binding at the same ligand – say, two different dopamine D_2 antagonists, or a D_3 partial agonist (such as cariprazine) plus full agonist (such as pramipexole), have complementary or additive pharmacodynamic effects or, rather, interfere with receptor access for each respective agent, leading to a net *reduction* in potential efficacy. (Think of the game musical chairs; two people cannot simultaneously occupy the same seat … sharing is pharmacokinetically awkward). Empirically, clinicians prescribe such combinations all the time without necessarily knowing if the net effect of such "competitive" binding is additive, synergistic, or effect-cancelling. The fancy term for clarifying such interactions is called **isobolographic analysis**. Adding a full competitive agonist to an antagonist at the same receptor site could at least theoretically reverse the effects of the antagonist – but then, adding the ergoline D_2 agonist bromocriptine to risperidone as an antidote for hyperprolactinemia does not seem to override its antipsychotic efficacy. When two drugs compete for the same receptor, the outcome depends on both dose and affinity. Low receptor occupancy by one can be overwhelmed by high occupancy/high dose by another (i.e., mass action). A low-affinity drug (e.g., most atypical and conventional antipsychotic medications) can be displaced by a high-affinity one (e.g., aripiprazole). A high-affinity ligand (e.g., cariprazine at the D_3 receptor) displaces atypical antipsychotic drugs that have lower D_3 binding affinities (or even endogenous dopamine itself). The net effect thus depends on the doses of the competing drugs and their relative receptor affinities.

A final consideration regarding pharmacodynamic compatibility involves brain real estate, or location, location, location. Stimulants and antipsychotics, for example, exert opposing action at dopamine receptors but do so in different brain regions (antipsychotic medications predominantly block dopamine in mesolimbic tracts while stimulants are agonists for dopamine receptors in mesocortical regions).

Doesn't cyproheptadine, often used for iatrogenic sexual dysfunction, essentially nullify the effects of a serotonergic antidepressant?

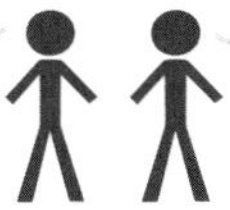

No. Cyproheptadine is a potent 5-HT_1 and 5-HT_2 antagonist. It can be used to treat serotonin syndrome. It's not an "anti-serotonergic" drug, it just blocks binding at specific receptors.

ECT, clozapine, lithium … those are really treatments of last resort, right?

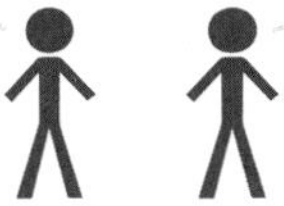

There's really no reason to think that way. They are examples of interventions whose effects may be optimal when begun sooner rather than later in a patient who doesn't respond to "simpler" treatments. So, for instance, lithium prophylaxis seems to work better when begun within the first few manic episodes (Gelenberg et al., 1989). In schizophrenia, clozapine seems to be appropriate after only one failed antipsychotic trial (Kahn et al., 2018), and even ECT response declines with an increasing number of failed antidepressant trials during an index depressive episode, as noted above (Nakajima et al., 2022).

Some medications require careful planning and consideration before they can be implemented through an iterative decision tree. For example, when anticipating the potential need for an MAOI, it makes little sense to precede that option with a long-half-life antidepressant medication such as fluoxetine (with its active metabolite norfluoxetine having a half-life of 7–15 days) or vortioxetine (with a 66-hour half-life) that will first need a five-half-life washout. Other drugs require timing and preparation for reasonably anticipating results (for example, a clozapine trial in refractory schizophrenia may take many months; a trial of vagus nerve stimulation for multi-treatment-resistant depression may take 12 months or more to see a response (Aaronson et al., 2017)).

> **Tip**
>
> Don't confuse "half-life" with an extended-release (XR) drug formulation. XR drug formulations typically have the same half-life as an immediate-release formulation but involve slower absorption and less variable maximum and minimum concentrations.

D NONRESPONSE TO AN SSRI FOR DEPRESSION: NOW WHAT?

We hope it is apparent that there is no definitive or far-and-away best "next step" after a nonresponse to an adequate trial of an SSRI for major depression. The STAR*D trial amply demonstrated that an iterative approach (augmenting with bupropion or buspirone or CBT, or switching to a different antidepressant class) yielded no clear superiority of one strategy over another. Does this mean iterative psychopharmacology really is a trial-and-error free for all? Hopefully not, when one is aware of the empirical literature and individualized patient-specific characteristics that make one option relatively more or less compelling than another.

What do the data show? After nonresponse to one adequate SSRI trial, the probability of response to a(ny) different SSRI is about 40–70% (Thase and Rush, 1997). Does it matter which SSRI was used first? That is hard to say, because the literature regarding comparative trials is complicated and there are many apples-to-oranges studies (i.e., patients may not necessarily be evenly matched on severity, chronicity, past treatments, comorbidities, or other baseline characteristics that likely influence both treatment choice and outcome). On top of that, if potential differences between two generally effective treatments are only small or modest, a very large sample size becomes necessary in order to detect small effect sizes – and, are small effect size differences between two treatments really all that clinically meaningful? Probably not, inasmuch as the effect sizes across all SSRIs for major depression are fairly comparable and their confidence intervals overlap (meaning there are no significant differences in primary outcome measures of a depression rating scale score). On the other hand, one network meta-analysis of 15 head-to-head SSRIs argued that escitalopram was overall more effective than other SSRIs with respect to response and remission rates in major depression (Darab et al., 2020) – perhaps (?) because it has the highest affinity among existing SSRIs for the serotonin transporter. *Maybe*. We still need to consider patient-specific factors that impact treatment response, as well as safety and tolerability.

Tip

Decisions to switch agents versus augment after an initial incomplete response in major depressive disorder are not hard and fast, and depend in part on patient preference. A rule of thumb is to augment partial responses and switch after a frank nonresponse but, among partial responders, outcomes are not vastly different between switching versus augmentation strategies (Connolly and Thase, 2011).

Let us consider the hierarchical sequence of operations to map out in the decision tree for the case of Dionne presented in Clinical Vignette 9.1.

We should acknowledge at the outset that persistence of depression despite numerous adequate pharmacotherapy trials, and especially 18 ECT treatments and esketamine, bodes poorly from a prognostic standpoint. For decision-planning purposes, it may be useful to stage Dionne's illness using, say, the Maudsley staging model as shown in Table 9.2, from which summed scores (up to "15") have been normed to reflect either "mild" (3–6), "moderate" (7–10), or "severe" (11–15) levels of treatment resistance.

Clinical Vignette 9.1

Dionne was an obese 83-year-old woman with multi-drug-resistant persistent depressive disorder (formerly known as chronic major depression), as well as nonresponse to 18 unilateral electroconvulsive therapy (ECT) treatments. She had a myocardial infarction at age 74 treated with coronary artery stenting. She now presents for consultation while taking duloxetine 120 mg/day and bupropion XL 150 mg/day, having previously taken adequate trials of two SSRIs, venlafaxine plus mirtazapine, and augmentations with aripiprazole and quetiapine. Her current Montgomery-Åsberg Depression Rating Scale (MADRS) score is 36 (severe depression). She has prominent apathy, anhedonia, and many negative attitudes and self-perceptions, with passive suicidal ideation but no prior attempts. There is no substance use disorder and no other psychiatric comorbidities. What would be a reasonable hierarchically iterative treatment plan for Dionne?

Table 9.2. Maudsley staging model in depression*

Dimension	Specification	Score	Dionne's score
Duration	Acute (<12 months)	1	
	Subacute (13–24 months)	2	3
	Chronic (>24 months)	3	
Baseline symptom severity	Subsyndromal	1	
	Syndromal - mild	2	4
	Syndromal - moderate	3	
	Syndromal - severe without psychosis	4	
	Syndromal - severe with psychosis	5	
Past treatment failures	1-2 antidepressants	1	
	3-4 antidepressants	2	3
	5-6 antidepressants	3	
	7-10 antidepressants	4	
	>10 antidepressants	5	
Antidepressant augmentations	Not used	0	
	Used	1	1
ECT	Not used	0	
	Used	1	1
Total score		≤15	12

* Modified from Fekadu et al. (2009).

Dionne's Maudsley staging score of 12 places her in the "severe" category of treatment resistance. This does not mean that we necessarily consign Dionne to palliative psychiatry within the land of acceptance and commitment therapy – but it does mean that we must offer an honest appraisal of her condition and the low probability of success with any next treatment intervention. In the here and now, Dionne is experiencing a chronic condition that will need management under the "chronic illness" model, as described in Box 9.4.

But there are therapeutic stones that remain not yet turned over. It would make sense to deprescribe the ineffective duloxetine plus bupropion, particularly given that bupropion will increase her duloxetine levels via its cytochrome P450 2D6 (CYP2D6) inhibition and, additionally, duloxetine is itself a CYP2D6 inhibitor, potentially further delaying its own metabolism. Let us hope Dionne is normotensive. One could gradually reduce her dose of duloxetine with the hope of minimizing discontinuation symptoms. Alternatively, one could replace her duloxetine with fluoxetine as a strategy to prevent SNRI discontinuation effects (Schatzberg et al., 2006), which then subsequently invites the opportunity to augment it with olanzapine for possible synergy from that unique pairing (i.e., olanzapine–fluoxetine combination (OFC)).

But then what about Dionne's obesity? How does that influence the pros and cons of OFC, given its propensity to cause weight gain and metabolic dysregulation? In the clinical-trials database examining olanzapine augmentation after an inadequate response to an SSRI, SNRI, or bupropion, OFC was associated with an 11-point reduction from based MADRS scores within the first week, which was significantly better than seen with fluoxetine alone (Thase et al., 2007). In other words, signs of potential efficacy might very well become apparent fairly quickly, and long before the potential for significant iatrogenic weight might ensue: if OFC were efficacious and deemed worthy of retaining, there are a wide range of viable strategies to help stave off or mitigate potential weight gain; if OFC showed no hint of benefit within the first few weeks, the concern becomes moot as there would be no reason to continue it.

> **Tip**
>
> There are parameters to help anticipate the likelihood of significant weight gain with olanzapine. Patients who gain more than 4–5 pounds in the first 3 weeks are highly likely to gain more than 20 pounds by week 26 with continued treatment (Lipkovich et al., 2008).

In an ideal world we would choose options that are only weight-neutral, but in the setting of severe treatment resistance, the real-world risk–benefit analysis involves the reality that Dionne has relatively few evidence-based options. One could arbitrarily pick only pharmacotherapies with known antidepressant value that are weight neutral, but few such treatment options satisfy the simultaneous criterion of known efficacy in treatment resistance as well as weight neutrality. Well, then, what *are* the viable weight-neutral options for treatment-resistant depression? Could Dionne try replacing her bupropion and duloxetine with bupropion plus dextromethorphan? That is certainly a relatively weight-neutral option, and worthy of consideration, but there is only limited evidence for its efficacy specifically in treatment-resistant depression. On the other hand, real-world clinical experience with this compound in treatment-resistant depression patients may be more optimistic than seen in small clinical trials, making this more of a viable but unpredictable option.

How about repetitive transcranial magnetic stimulation (rTMS)? Once again, searching the medical literature on PubMed comes to the rescue (at least for us, if not for Dionne herself). A meta-analysis of 29 rTMS studies found that a high degree of treatment resistance, older age, and a long duration of the current episode collectively predicted poor response to rTMS (Dumas et al., 2012) – diminishing our enthusiasm for plain vanilla rTMS for Dionne.

How about *theta-burst* rTMS? The so-called Stanford Accelerated Intelligent Neuromodulation Therapy (SAINT) rTMS protocol for treatment-resistant depression involves administering 10 sessions daily for 5 days (a total of 18,000 pulses). In its original clinical trial with 22 unipolar and bipolar depressed-phase subjects, theta-burst rTMS produced a remarkable remission rate of 86.4% despite a mean Maudsley staging score of 10.86 (Cole et al., 2020). Although septuagenarians were not enrolled in that protocol, Dionne's odds have just begun to improve a little.

Our take-away for Dionne is, once again, an amalgam of ITRs that must include a blend of possible untried biological interventions as well as psychosocial approaches that address coping with a chronic medical condition.

Box 9.4

The chronic illness management model for psychiatry

The notion of pharmacological futility is delicate in psychiatry - even though, in every other area of medicine, there is acknowledgment that there comes a point when the limits of existing technology have been reached and the goals of treatment then shift from efforts toward disease modification to disease management. Efforts in this model, which draw on elements from palliative care, include the following:

- Deprescribing drugs with no obvious benefit
- Differentiating acceptable from unacceptable residual symptoms or drug side effects
- Focusing on strategies to manage rather than eliminate symptoms
- Conceptualizing pharmacotherapy as an adjunct to psychotherapy as the primary treatment modality
- Honing coping skills
- Maintaining hope while simultaneously gently redirecting unrealistic expectations or magical thinking about dramatically transformative effects of new or untried treatments, in the setting of high treatment resistance
- Maintaining a focus on quality of life and the pursuit of reasonable goals

E RISKY BUSINESS: AGGRESSIVE DRUG COMBINATIONS FOR HARD-TO-TREAT CONDITIONS

Consider a treatment-resistant major depressive disorder patient with a Maudsley staging score > 11 – or the analogous degree of treatment resistance in any other disorder besides depression. As we move farther down the hierarchical decision tree for such a patient, one can choose iterative interventions that have demonstrated efficacy in the setting of prior treatment nonresponses, or that have particularly large effect sizes, and hope for the best with cautious optimism. One could also concoct extensive polypharmacology regimens that are rationale-based and capitalize on complementary receptor profiles, nonredundant mechanisms, and theoretical pharmacodyamic synergies (even if empirical data on specific multi-drug regimens are lacking). Risks, obviously, include additive adverse effects (e.g., sedation) or previously unrecognized drug interactions; it never hurts to run a pharmacokinetic interaction check before assembling a conglomerate of multiple medications. Several examples are presented in Table 9.3.

Table 9.3 Examples of rationale-based heroic combination pharmacotherapy regimens

Clinical Scenario	Concoction
Major depressive disorder-treatment-resistant depression	Combining an SSRI or SNRI ± bupropion ± mirtazapine ± buspirone ± esketamine ± lithium[a] ± a second-generation antipsychotic medication ± a(ny) stimulant ± thyroid hormone ± pramipexole ± L-methylfolate
Treatment-resistant psychosis	Clozapine[b] as the "base" treatment ± a dopamine partial agonist (e.g., aripiprazole, brexpiprazole, cariprazine) ± lamotrigine (known adjunctive value with clozapine; Tiihonen et al., 2009) ± topiramate (reviewed by Sommer et al., 2012) ± sulpride (reviewed by Sommer et al., 2012)[c]
Treatment-resistant anxiety	Serotonergic antidepressant medication ± high-dose buspirone ± second-generation antipsychotic with anxiolytic properties ± pregabalin or gabapentin ± mirtazapine ± antihistaminergic anxiolytic medication (e.g., hydroxyzine)

[a] While adjunctive lithium added to antidepressant medications has demonstrated an approximate three-fold increased likelihood of response in major depressive disorder (Nelson et al., 2014), other mood stabilizers lack this claim; lamotrigine, for example, has only negative randomized controlled trial data in major depressive disorder (Barbosa et al., 2003; Barbee et al., 2011).

[b] Beware aggressive dosing of clozapine; serum clozapine levels > 350 ng/mL are considered to be a therapeutic threshold in schizophrenia, but blood levels > 838 ng/mL are likely to be futile and have a substantially increased risk of toxicity (Remington et al., 2013; Meyer, 2014).

[c] A quantitative literature review disputed the potential value of *any* adjunctive therapies to clozapine in refractory schizophrenia, noting favorable results from single trials have not been replicated (Sommer et al., 2012).

F MORE ON THE PROS AND CONS OF RISK-BENEFIT ANALYSES

Everything that we can prescribe – including placebos – can have adverse effects, making risk–benefit analyses an indispensable component of both shared decision-making and iterative decisions among therapeutic options. Consider another example of the risk–benefit decision-making process, when the benefits are not so obvious, as described in Clinical Vignette 9.2.

Clinical Vignette 9.2

Jason was a 28-year-old man diagnosed with persistent depressive disorder (formerly known as chronic major depression) who had incomplete or transient responses to initial trials of escitalopram, sertraline, bupropion, and venlafaxine. His symptoms had historically been severe and included periods of suicidal ideation with several suicide gestures, but no hospitalizations. His psychiatrist, Dr. Tremante, switched venlafaxine to desvenlafaxine to avoid its CYP2D6 metabolism and Jason's Patient Health Questionnaire-9 (PHQ-9) score reduced from 20 to 14. When aripiprazole 5 mg/day was then added to desvenlafaxine his PHQ-9 score fell to below 10 and remained in the low single digits for several years. On a routine follow-up visit, Dr. Tremante noticed occasional tongue sweeps and lip pursing, conducted an Abnormal Involuntary Movement Scale (AIMS) exam yielding a score of 5, and diagnosed Jason with tardive dyskinesia (TD). Should Jason continue the aripiprazole with adjunctive use of a vesicular monoamine transporter type 2 (VMAT2) inhibitor to treat his TD? Or should he discontinue the aripiprazole on the grounds we do not know if he really needs it indefinitely as an adjunct for nonpsychotic depression - regardless of whether or not a VMAT2 inhibitor should now be added?

The risk–benefit decision process would be more straightforward for Jason if he had a history of worsening depression after cessation of aripiprazole; this is an unknown for him, but obviously, if it were the case, the benefit of relapse prevention would favor its continuation over the risk of worsening TD, particularly when TD is treatable. But with no such prior knowledge, we must weigh the risk–benefit analysis with fewer data. If Jason favored a shared decision-making approach and asked what the optimal duration of adjunctive aripiprazole is for

Tip

Stopping an antipsychotic medicine when TD newly emerges may not necessarily improve TD symptoms, which could progress even after a dopamine-blocking drug is stopped. The decision to add a VMAT2 inhibitor is therefore based on the persistence of TD symptoms, regardless of clinical decisions about whether ongoing use of an anti-dopaminergic drug is warranted.

relapse prevention in nonpsychotic depression, the answer is nobody knows. One can only present the pros and cons, the shared unknowns, and the testable hypotheses of pursuing aripiprazole cessation versus continuation, regardless of adding a VMAT2 inhibitor.

G SYMPTOM CLUSTERS: CAN THEY, AND SHOULD THEY, GUIDE MEDICATION DECISIONS?

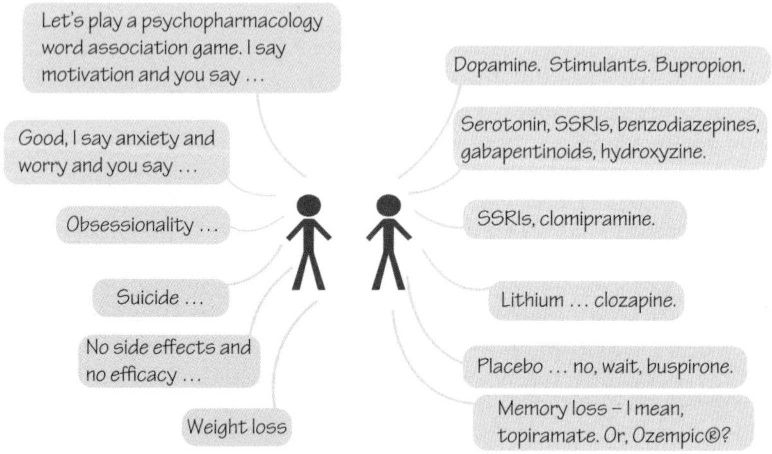

For better or worse, and rightly or wrongly, psychopharmacologists tend to become entrained in the mindset of associating particular medications with special relevance for certain symptoms or symptom clusters. How much does urban legend, or Pavlovian conditioning, operate more persuasively than findings from the empirical literature when clinicians, say, opt to avoid bupropion in anxious-depressed patients, or think of fluvoxamine sooner than other SSRIs when they hear the words "obsessive–compulsive"? Or duloxetine over other noradrenergic agents for "pain." It is hard to say with empirical confidence that particular symptoms or symptom clusters make for slam-dunk decisional nodes when choosing from among viable treatment options. The data here are limited, many come from post hoc or hypothesis-generating rather than hypothesis-testing studies, of which few are replicated, most are underpowered, and they rarely control for relevant confounding factors. (For example, on the latter point, MAOIs are sometimes regarded as being especially useful for depression with high mood reactivity, or atypical depression as a broader construct, but such observations historically have not controlled for potentially linked confounders such as early age at onset and chronicity, comorbid anxiety, or a more familial pattern of transmission, any of which might in turn be a more proximal influence over treatment outcome.)

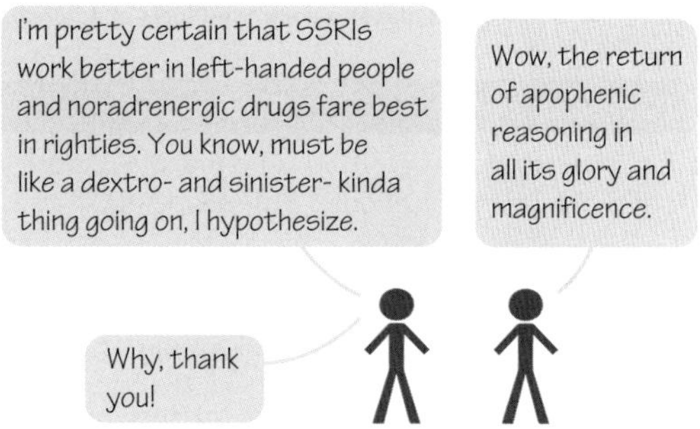

Nevertheless, for hypothesis-generating purposes, it is reasonable for clinicians not only to maintain an awareness of the literature on symptom clusters and treatment outcomes but, in addition, to contemplate symptom patterns they themselves identify in connection with treatment responses or nonresponses and then test the falsifiability of those hypotheses. Be curious but also be skeptical, and beware of falling into traps that could be apophenic (see Chapter 7, Section C) or otherwise involve invalid or misinterpreted clinical constellations.

What does the literature regarding symptom clusters tell us with respect to pharmacotherapy outcomes, and the role of that knowledge for purposes of iterative decision-making? Unfortunately, not nearly as much as we would hope. One study comparing "anxious" versus "melancholic" versus "atypical" presentation of major depression found no discernible differences in treatment response rates with sertraline, escitalopram, or venlafaxine XR – although, notably, most patients had amalgams of depressive symptom cluster subtypes, with few manifesting "pure" presentations of only one of these three clinical profiles (Arnow et al., 2015).

Let us now consider several representative examples of challenging clinical scenarios in which decision-making hinges on specific knowledge about differential pharmacodynamic effects of several or more candidate treatments.

H REFRACTORY OCD

Are there any rules of the road for choosing iterative pharmacotherapies for refractory OCD? Starting with an SSRI, and anticipating the need for high doses, is Psychopharmacology 101. How high, exactly, does one go with dosing? OCD nonresponders to up to 16 weeks of 200 mg/day of sertraline who were then randomized either to continue or further titrate upward to a maximum of 400 mg/day revealed significantly greater improvement in Yale–Brown Obsessive–Compulsive Scale and Clinical Global Impressions scores in the latter versus former group (Ninan et al., 2006).

What are evidence-based augmentation strategies in OCD when it responds inadequately to optimized dosing of a serotonergic antidepressant? Findings from a systematic review of adjunctive pharmacotherapy randomized trials by Albert et al. (2018) are summarized in Table 9.4.

Table 9.4 Summary of placebo-controlled trials of adjunctive pharmacotherapy for treatment-resistant OCD[a]

Decisional option	Findings
Second-generation antipsychotic medications	Aripiprazole: 2 positive trials (dosing of 10–15 mg/day) Risperidone: 4 positive trials (mean dosing of 0.5–2.25 mg/day across trials) Haloperidol: 1 positive trial (mean dose 6.2 mg/day) Olanzapine: 1 positive trial (mean dose 11.2 mg/day), 1 negative trial (mean dose 6.1 mg/day) Quetiapine: 2 positive trials (mean doses 91 and 100 mg/day each), 4 negative trials (mean dosing 142–215 mg/day across trials) [b]
Lamotrigine	1 positive trial (mean dose 100 mg/day)
Topiramate	1 positive trial (dose range 100–200 mg/day), 2 negative trials (dose range 50–400 mg/day)
Memantine	1 positive trial (dose range 5–10 mg/day)
Pindolol	1 positive trial (mean dose 7.5 mg/day)

[a] Based on review findings of Albert et al., 2018.

[b] In one trial, placebo was superior to quetiapine.

This review also found no differences from placebo using lithium, buspirone, inositol, paliperidone, desipramine, gabapentin, clonazepam, naltrexone, and riluzole. From an evidence-based standpoint, risperidone tends to lead the pack (and was even shown to be superior to aripiprazole in one head-to-head comparison of 41 subjects as noted by Albert et al. (2018)). Importantly, however, what do the findings in Table 9.4 mean for purposes of constructing a decision tree for someone like Molly, a 31-year-old woman whose significant OCD symptoms (involving contamination fears that lead her to wash her hands more than 20 times a day and avoid public transportation or social interactions) responded poorly to sertraline 300 mg/day, then clomipramine 150 mg/day, and then duloxetine 120 mg/day? She asks if one SSRI is really so different from another in treating OCD and, after we scour PubMed, we tell her that sertraline has shown a higher remission rate than fluoxetine in one head-to-head comparison (Bergeron et al., 2002), and that five head-to-head comparisons of fluoxetine or fluvoxamine found comparable efficacy to clomipramine but poorer tolerability with clomipramine (Pigott and Seay, 1999). This exercise is not helping Molly in the shared decision-making process.

Adjunctive aripiprazole 5–10 mg/day previously caused Molly to have akathisia and insomnia, making her leery of trying other second-generation antipsychotic medications. She has worked diligently in CBT and tried to use exposure therapy with response prevention techniques. She is hesitant to pursue rTMS for OCD because of the time commitment and her skepticism about the efficacy of the procedure despite its US Food and Drug Administration approval. There are no untreated psychiatric or substance use disorder comorbidities. Molly is becoming demoralized about her predicament.

Molly really has two options: we can comb through the evidence-based options in Table 9.4 and discuss the pros and cons (and her potential reluctances) in a shared decision-making paradigm and hope to persuade her to (re)consider a different adjunctive second-generation antipsychotic medication such as risperidone (and we will be ultra-vigilant for akathisia) or memantine, or we can try to be more persuasive about rTMS. Above all, we do not want to let ourselves get contaminated by her demoralization.

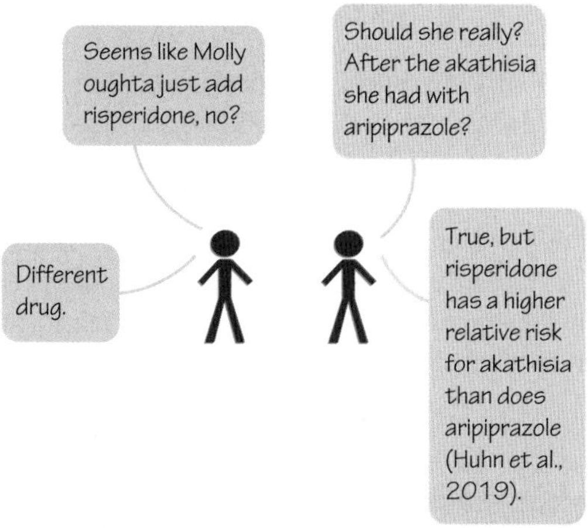

Alternatively, we could also propose more experimental options. For example, some studies have shown efficacy with intravenous clomipramine in OCD patients unresponsive to oral clomipramine (Koran et al., 1997; Fallon et al., 1998) – though, as Molly said, "and then what?" for relapse prevention purposes. Molly is skeptical. If we go to www.clinicaltrials.gov and search the terms "obsessive–compulsive disorder" we find an array of ongoing experimental treatment protocols which may offer relevant further options for Molly's care. The clinician's role is to help Molly sort through and find the least imperfect option from among those that are viable.

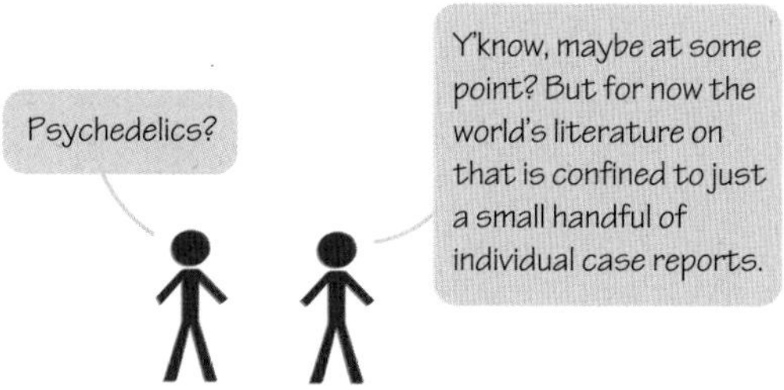

I STIMULANT TOLERANCE DURING TREATMENT FOR ADHD

A PubMed search of the terms "stimulant" + "tolerance" + "attention deficit–hyperactivity disorder" reveals no studies that identify the prevalence of long-term loss of efficacy due to pharmacological tolerance of stimulants in attention deficit–hyperactivity disorder (ADHD), although tolerance is a well-recognized complication of long-term stimulant treatment, occurring in 60% or more of patients during long-term use (Handelman and Sumaya, 2022). There is also surprisingly little empirical study of specific interventions to counteract tolerance, leaving it to clinicians to devise their own strategies based mainly on rationale.

Dosage increases of a particular stimulant are probably the most common initial strategy to overcome pharmacological tolerance to stimulants, although the literature in this area is mostly anecdotal. The two predominant classes of stimulants are methylphenidate- and amphetamine-based drugs. If tolerance develops to one class, is there a rationale for switching to the other? We again can find no empirical literature to test that hypothesis. Pharmacological strategies, and their rationales, for ADHD in the setting of tolerance to optimized stimulants are presented in Table 9.5.

Table 9.5 Pharmacological strategies in ADHD relevant to managing stimulant tolerance

Intervention	Rationale
Stimulant dosage increases	May buy time but an eventual return of tolerance may often be an inevitability
Stimulant holiday	Popularly endorsed strategy that may facilitate architectural receptor remodeling, although few controlled trials exist
Add atomoxetine	Norepinephrine reuptake inhibitor; but no adjunctive therapy trial data available
Add viloxazine	Norepinephrine reuptake inhibitor; but no adjunctive therapy trial data available (and beware of its potent CYP1A2 inhibition)
Add bupropion	Putative norepinephrine-dopamine reuptake inhibitor. Favorable placebo-controlled data in adult ADHD dosed up to 400 mg/day (Wilens et al., 2001)
Add an alpha-2 agonist (clonidine or guanfacine)	Nightly dosing may help symptoms of insomnia and autonomic hyperarousal if present (though beware daytime sedation) via *pre*synaptic (autoreceptor) alpha-2A agonism, while daytime pro-attentional effect derives from *post*synaptic alpha-2A agonism increasing noradrenergic tone in prefrontal cortex. Favorable augmentation trials of alpha-2 agonists plus stimulants are limited to studies in pediatric ADHD populations
Add modafinil	Robust evidence base in children and adolescents with ADHD, but failed to achieve regulatory agency approval due to the occurrence of severe cutaneous reactions

J BAD, BAD, BAD INSOMNIA

Insomnia is notoriously often a symptom in search of a diagnosis. Sometimes insomnia is just insomnia, (that is, International Classification of Diseases, 10th revision, Code 51.01), and not the manifestation of any number of other disorders for which the differential diagnosis list is long and includes a litany of both psychiatric and medical conditions, circadian rhythm disturbances, as well as primary sleep disorders. From a decision-analytic perspective, before we clobber someone with one soporific agent after another, let us do due diligence to assure we are not unwittingly attempting to treat sleepless mania with "Z"-drugs, missing alcohol withdrawal by plying antihistamines, discounting chronic pain, or ignoring sleep apnea or a parasomnia.

For the treatment of primary insomnia, there is a relatively finite number of viable pharmacological strategies, as summarized in Table 9.6. It is also worth

Table 9.6 Sleep aids: the diversity of pharmacological strategies

Putative mechanism	Clinical examples
Antihistamines	Mirtazapine (increases deep sleep, reduces rapid-eye-movement sleep), quetiapine (effect size = 0.05), diphenhydramine, doxepin (effect size = 0.30), hydroxyzine, trazodone (also $5HT_{2A}$ and alpha-1 antagonism are thought to promote hypnotic effects; effect size = 0.52)
Short-acting benzodiazepines	Alprazolam, triazolam (effect sizes of about 0.83)
Intermediate- or long-acting benzodiazepines	Clonazepam, lorazepam, temazepam (effect sizes range from 0.58 to 0.67)
Benzodiazepine analogs, or gamma-amino butyric acid (GABA)-A receptor positive allosteric modulators ("Z"-drugs)	Zaleplon (effect size = 0.19), zolpidem (effect size = 0.45), eszopiclone (effect size = 0.51)
Gabapentinoids	Pregabalin (promotes sleep maintenance; Roth et al., 2014); gabapentin (promotes sleep efficiency and slow wave sleep; Lo et al., 2010)
Dual orexin receptor antagonists (DORAs)	Daridorexant (effect size = 0.23), suvorexant (effect size = 0.31), lemborexant (effect size = 0.36)
Alpha agonists	Clonidine, guanfacine (downregulation of sympathetic tone is thought to produce hypnotic effects)
Melatonin/analogs	Melatonin (effect size = 0.13), ramelteon (effect size = 0.12)

Note: effect sizes are standardized mean differences (SMDs) relative to placebo as reported (and noted for agents where data are available) by De Crescenzo et al. (2022).

noting that for the treatment of insomnia in patients with major depression, adjunctive CBT for insomnia during treatment with an SSRI or SNRI has shown superiority to antidepressant pharmacotherapy alone (Manber et al., 2016).

How might hierarchically iterative prescribing, or deprescribing, capitalize on our knowledge of complementary drug mechanisms and likely pharmacodynamic effects when it comes to difficult-to-treat forms of insomnia? Consider Clinical Vignette 9.3.

Clinical Vignette 9.3

Alicia was a 43-year-old woman with schizoaffective disorder that was well controlled with a longstanding regimen of aripiprazole 15 mg/day and divalproex 1,000 mg/day. She took gabapentin 300 mg once daily and amitriptyline 50 mg daily for sciatica as well as trazodone 150 mg at night for insomnia paired with eszopiclone 3 mg at night. For the past month she has had middle-of-the-night awakenings with up to 45 minutes to fall back asleep, followed by next-day fatigue. Her sleep regimen appeared to be effective until recently and she can identify no recent changes in her life, new conflicts at work or in her relationships, medical illnesses (her sciatica is fairly well controlled), or changes to her medications that might account for her worsening insomnia. How might one proceed?

The above history, ruling out likely pharmacokinetic, pharmacodynamic, or psychosocial explanations for Alicia's sleep disruption, lays out a fairly compelling narrative to support the diagnosis of primary insomnia (as opposed to insomnia secondary to a current mood episode or other, broader active psychiatric problem). One could approach her existing insomnia regimen somewhat arbitrarily: change the eszopiclone to a different "Z"-drug with the hope it may be more effective; perhaps raise the trazodone with the same hope; one could add a sleep aid from another class (such as ramelteon or a DORA, as noted in Table 9.6). Parsimony tends to favor the simplest strategies that involve the fewest sweeping changes and might even capitalize on agents that have more than one relevant pharmacodynamic target. Enter gabapentin, which prolongs Stage 3 sleep and could therefore be particularly relevant at higher doses as a strategy to sustaining sleep continuity. Is it necessarily the best option for Alicia? There probably is no best option. But it possesses sleep-architecture properties that are attractive and pertinent to her unique clinical profile of poor sleep continuity, and therefore offers a nonrandom, rationale-based augmentation strategy.

K LABORATORY TOOLS TO INFORM PHARMACOTHERAPY DECISIONS: THE ROLE OF PHARMACOGENETICS

The use of biomarkers to guide or predict treatment responses in psychiatry remains an elusive field in which most endeavors (such as patterns of resting-state functional connectivity on brain MRI in major depression, or quantitative EEG findings in major depression) remain highly experimental and less well established for commercial than investigative use. Pharmacogenetics is perhaps the best-recognized laboratory tool that has begun to make the transition from bench to bedside. We touched briefly on this topic in Chapter 8, Section L. Let us now elaborate on this discussion by describing instances and clinical examples in which pharmacogenetic testing can yield information relevant to decisional nodes when constructing an ITR. As a caveat, nobody knows exactly what proportion of the variance in psychotropic drug response is explainable by genetic versus nongenetic factors, with estimates of the genetic contribution ranging widely in the literature from 20% to 95%. That leaves plenty of room for positioning pharmacogenetic data alongside other known factors that affect treatment outcomes (such as chronicity, age at onset, substance use, comorbidities, psychosocial supports, trauma histories, renal function, medication adherence, drug–drug interactions, and on and on).

Combinatorial pharmacogenetics involves identifying a series of genetic variants (called polymorphisms) that are considered candidates for influencing the synthesis, metabolism, or function of some gene product involved in neurotransmission. A polymorphic variant in one gene is known as a single nucleotide polymorphism (SNP) and if that gene product is functional (meaning that it is involved in a key synthetic or metabolic pathway involving brain structure or function), we describe it as a candidate gene for its possible association with some physiological effect. Relevant candidate genes for association studies could be enzymes involved in Phase I hepatic metabolism (e.g., variants of cytochrome P450 isoenzymes whose activity may be ultra-rapid (producing ultra-rapid metabolizer phenotypes) or unusually slow (producing poor metabolizer phenotypes)). Other candidate genes might be variants for neurotransmitter receptors (such as the serotonin transporter gene, SLC6A4) or enzymes involved in the synthesis or degradation of key neurotransmitters (such as catechol-*o*-methyltransferase, responsible for the degradation of dopamine). Like any medical test, the decision to obtain a pharmacogenetics panel

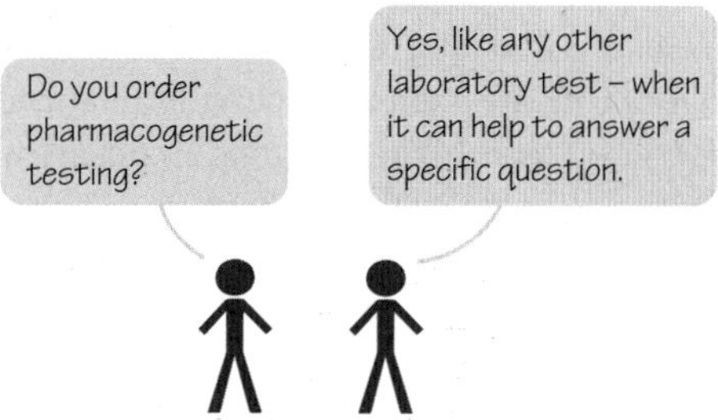

should be for the purpose of answering a question that bears on a particular outcome. To the extent such data can be fundamental to constructing an individualized treatment decision tree, we offer some examples in Clinical Vignettes 9.4 and 9.5.

Clinical Vignette 9.4

Monica was a 32-year-old woman with a history of significant and disabling recurrent major depression with a previous suicide attempt, who ultimately was successfully treated with fluoxetine at a dose of 60 mg/day, following nonresponses to escitalopram 40 mg/day and duloxetine 120 mg/day. She opted to discontinue her medication in order to become pregnant and conceived after about 6 months. Her depression recurred in the first trimester. If she were to resume fluoxetine, should we assume her target dose would again be 60 mg/day?

Monica presents a useful opportunity to use pharmacogenetics for a specific purpose. We can hypothesize that she is a likely CYP2D6 ultra-rapid metabolizer based on the need for a high fluoxetine dose during her last depression, particularly after high doses of escitalopram (a CYP2C19 and CYP3A4 substrate) and duloxetine (a CYP1A2 and CYP2D6 substrate) did nothing for her. But wait, there is more: her pregnancy will likely lead to even more accelerated metabolism of fluoxetine, if she restarts it, due to rising estrogen levels inducing her cytochrome P450 system in general. This means that she may very well need a gigantic dose of fluoxetine during pregnancy. Why not just give her that on the presumed CYP2D6 hypothesis alone? Or could we not just measure fluoxetine blood levels to guide her dosing? (No, not really: plasma fluoxetine levels have shown no correlation with relapse risk in major depression (Brunswick et al., 2002).) And for that matter, why not pick some other drug that avoids CYP2D6 altogether and be done with this issue? Well, Monica has already had two antidepressant medication nonresponses, so going out and picking some random drug other than fluoxetine (that Bayesian posterior probability is looking good on her personal decision tree, is it not?) is utterly risky business. Plus, we would just as soon not expose a pregnant patient to higher than necessary doses of any psychotropic drug – but at the same time, suicide is a leading cause of death during the perinatal period. If Monica is in fact a CYP2D6 poor metabolizer by pharmacogenetic testing, based on her posterior probabilities, a strong argument can be made for choosing fluoxetine as the preferred pharmacotherapy and bringing her dose back to 60 mg/day as soon as feasible, since pharmacokinetically it would be tantamount to a much lower usual dose.

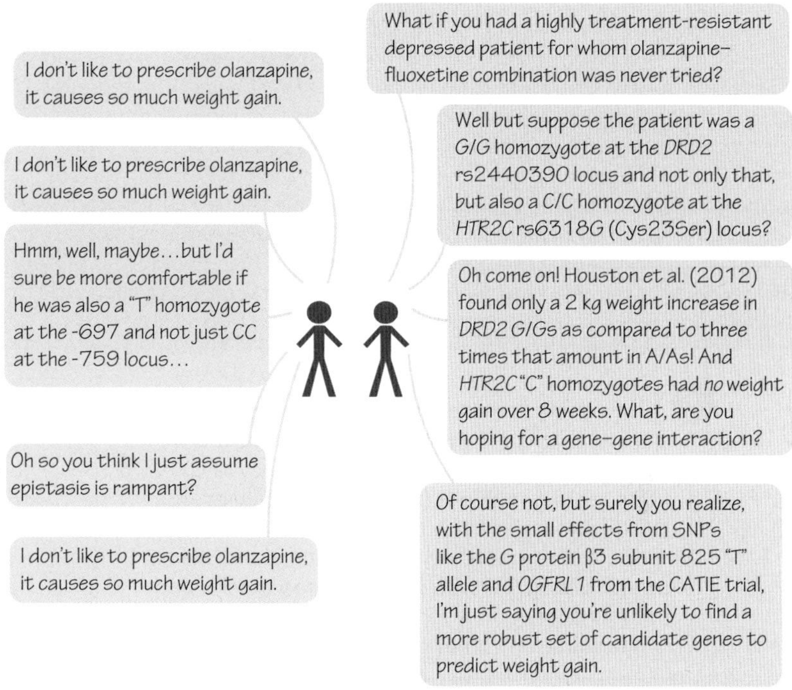

Translation

Patients who take olanzapine often gain significant weight, but there are a handful of identified pharmacogenomic predictors of weight gain, particularly two variants in genes that code, respectively, for the dopamine D_2 receptor (encoded by the *DRD2* gene) and the serotonin 5-HT_{2C} receptor (which is encoded by the *HTR2C* gene). In prospective studies, each of these were found to attenuate the magnitude of iatrogenic weight gain from olanzapine. Our colleague expresses skepticism about the magnitude of the observed effects on weight mitigation and proposes another candidate gene variant about which he has more confidence, to which his comrade bristles. A veiled accusation is then made that perhaps one of these gene variants could be eclipsing the effects of the other, a remark met with great skepticism in light of the rather modest effects seen with a number of other candidate genes vis à vis iatrogenic weight gain.

Clinical Vignette 9.5

Omari was a 21-year-old African American young man of Ethiopian ancestry with schizophrenia unresponsive to aripiprazole 10 mg/day. He was switched to risperidone 1 mg/day cautiously dosed upward due to concerns about sensitivity to extrapyramidal adverse effects. At 4 mg/day he showed neither improvement nor worsening, and no evidence of extrapyramidal symptoms. He was switched to risperidone long-acting injectable (initially 25 mg intramuscularly every 2 weeks and then 50 mg every 2 weeks) based on concerns that he was nonadherent to oral risperidone. He still demonstrated neither an improvement in global psychopathology (Positive and Negative Symptoms Scale total scale score = 73 (moderately ill; see Chapter 6, Table 6.10)) nor signs of extrapyramidal side effects (Simpson-Angus scale score = 0). Concern was raised about the possibility that he was a CYP2D6 ultra-rapid metabolizer, which was confirmed by pharmacogenetic testing. His condition stabilized after a switch to ziprasidone, which is primarily metabolized by aldehyde oxidase and to a lesser degree by CYP3A4.

TIP

African blacks of Ethiopian heritage have a disproportionately high allelic frequency of CYP2D6 ultra-rapid genotypes (about 29%; Aklillu et al., 1996) as compared to most European-ancestry populations – meaning they are at higher risk for metabolizing CYP2D6 substrates too quickly and might consequently fare better with an agent that is metabolized by other catabolic pathways.

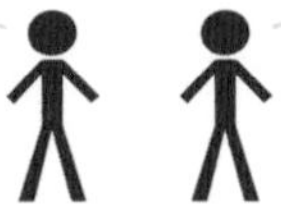

Abbreviations

3A4 and 1A2 are CYP variants. UGT is the Phase II hepatic metabolic enzyme uridine diphosphate glucuronosyltransferase, and the suffixes (i.e., 1A1, 1A4, 2B15) are the names of genes that encode UGT enzyme subtypes.

L FUN WITH SNPS

Certain single candidate genes, or collections of genes, have been examined in exploratory fashion as influencing a possible drug response. These are relatively experimental findings from candidate gene association studies, mostly unreplicated and underpowered, often more hypothesis-generating than hypothesis-testing, and thus not quite so ready for "prime time" implementation as a standard of care approach. Nonetheless, there are some intriguing hypotheses raised in the examples presented in Table 9.7, and future studies may eventually help to affirm these preliminary observations. For now, consider these as a teaser for hypothesis generation.

Table 9.7 Examples of possible candidate gene variants that may inform pharmacotherapy outcomes

Disease state	SNP(s) of interest	Implications
Stimulant response in ADHD	*COMT* (catechol-o-methyltransferase gene)	1.4-fold better response in high-activity Val/Val variant carriers (Myer et al., 2018)
Naltrexone response in alcohol use disorder	*OPRM1* (mu-opioid receptor gene)	May be better in Asp40 allele carriers than Asn40Asn homozygotes (Hartwell et al., 2020)
Atomoxetine augmentation of sertraline in major depression	*5-HTTLPR* (serotonin transporter gene)	Better response in S/S (short allele) homozygous variants (Reimherr et al., 2010)
Lithium response in bipolar disorder	*GSK-3β* (glycogen synthase kinase 3β gene)	May be better in "C" allele carriers of -50 T/C variant (Pagani et al., 2019)
	XBP1 (X-box binding protein 1)	May be better in "C" allele carriers of -116 C/G variant (Pagani et al., 2019)
	NTRK2 (neurotrophic tyrosine receptor kinase 2)	May be better in T/T (dominant) homozygotes of the C/T variant (Pagani et al., 2019)
	BDNF (brain-derived neurotrophic factor)	May be better in Val/Met carriers of the Val66Met variant (Pagani et al., 2019)

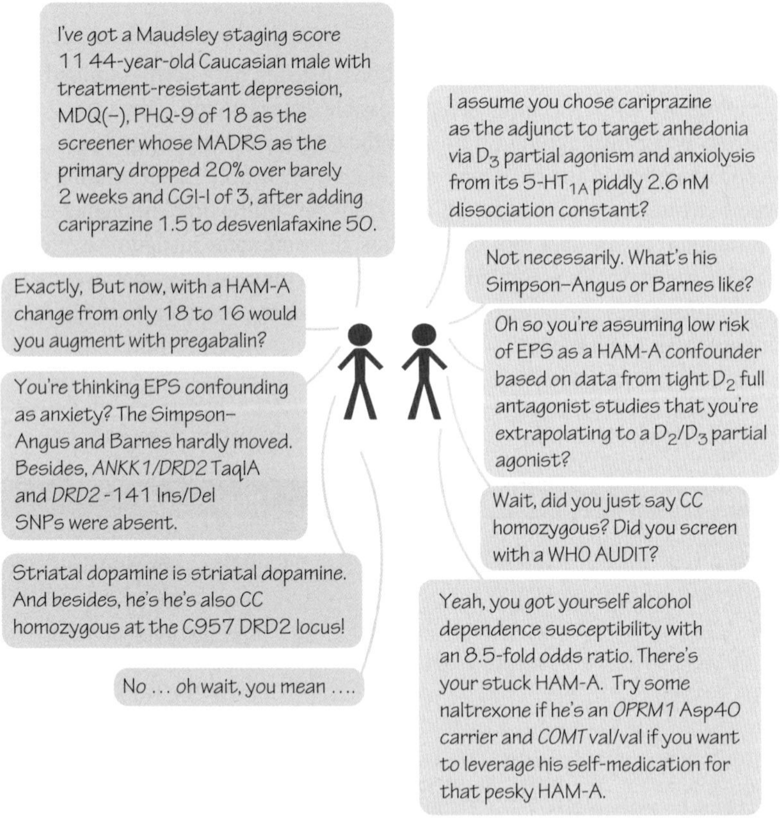

Translation

A middle-aged man with moderately severe unipolar depression who didn't get better after two antidepressants plus a tricyclic now shows a glimmer of depression improvement after 2 weeks on an SNRI plus atypical antipsychotic medication but little change in anxiety. It seems unlikely that extrapyramidal symptoms (EPS) like akathisia are mimicking anxiety. He's genetically less predisposed to akathisia from antipsychotics than most people (based on his *DRD2* TaqIA polymorphism status – a polymorphism located within the ankyrin repeat and protein kinase domain-containing protein 1 gene (*ANKK1*)). Additionally, presence of the A1 minor allele in that gene has been associated with heavy alcohol use (Noble, 2000). And yet another variant of the *DRD2* gene, called *C957T*, has also been associated with heavy alcohol use in men when the "C" rather than "T" allele is present, with an odds ratio of 8.5 (Swagell et al., 2012). Together, this information prompts the idea of performing an alcohol screen (the WHO-AUDIS) to judge if alcohol use is likely keeping his anxiety scores high. If he drinks heavily, he might be an especially good candidate for naltrexone depending on his genotype at a known mu-opioid receptor candidate gene (*OPRM1*), and if he has a particular variant in the *COMT* gene (which encodes catechol-o-methyltransferase) that makes him break down dopamine faster than normal.

M (MORE ON) THERAPEUTIC DRUG MONITORING AS A DECISIONAL TOOL

One obtains a serum drug level for several reasons, as summarized in Box 9.5. It is especially useful to rely on therapeutic drug monitoring (TDM) when an established therapeutic reference range exists for a given compound; and it may be a dicier proposition when serum levels of the drug of interest do not follow linear pharmacokinetics, in which case blood levels may be less informative about predicting drug efficacy (as has been shown with fluoxetine blood levels; Amsterdam et al., 1997). Some drugs may have a threshold therapeutic minimum blood level without necessarily following a linear dose–blood level response curve (such as clozapine; see the footnote in Table 9.3). Key points regarding the utility of TDM as a decisional support tool in pharmacotherapy are summarized in Box 9.5.

Box 9.5

Reasons for therapeutic drug monitoring

- To aid decisions about medication adherence
- To assure the absence of toxicity states
- To determine if a drug is being converted to its active metabolite products (e.g., venlafaxine to *o*-desmethylvenlafaxine; amitriptyline to desipramine and nortriptyline)
- To judge whether drug dosing has achieved a therapeutic window (e.g., nortriptyline, lithium), or a minimum threshold therapeutic level (e.g., clozapine) has been achieved
- To gauge whether there is room to increase a dose in the presence of ongoing symptoms

N THE ART OF DEPRESCRIBING

Deprescribing – a term originating in the geriatric literature – refers to the systematic elimination of medications that are ineffective, mechanistically redundant, or contradictory with other components of a regimen, or otherwise inappropriate to the diagnosis or target symptoms of interest. Particular attention on this topic has been paid in the literature to vulnerable populations such as children and dementia patients. There is little question that instances of pharmacological hoarding can arise and the role for spring cleaning has its place for the sake of hygiene. But, on another level, extensive medication regimens may sometimes simply represent the stigmata of pharmacological desperation when attempting to leverage symptoms or other problems for which pharmacotherapy may simply not be very effective. When one considers that, in major depression, the probability of achieving response or remission declines rather exponentially with every successive nonresponse, and the effect sizes of most monoaminergic antidepressant drugs is relatively modest (Cohen's *d* effect sizes in the range of 0.3–0.4), there are times when medications become added to a regimen in a less-than-elegant manner simply because persistent symptoms fail to diminish despite numerous appropriate earlier interventions. Clinicians often face the following dilemma: do they declare that an existing regimen is categorically ineffective and therefore discontinue it, gambling that a new treatment will work better? Or do they hedge their bets and favor retaining an existing regimen, on the belief that there may be at least some degree of partial benefit, and deprescribing before replacing could put the patient at risk for decompensating.

PHARMACOLOGICAL JENGA®

Who cannot appreciate the game Jenga®, in which the objective is to serially remove blocks from an intact standing tower in order to determine which fateful block, once removed, leads to the collapse of the tower. Much as the winner of Jenga® must possess not only nerves of steel but also the insight and common sense to know when *not* to tamper with an important structural component, so too does the wise psychopharmacologist recognize when deprescribing of a medication amounts to de-cluttering and when it is instead an invitation to structural collapse. Some Jenga® players try to slyly make tentative moves at dislodging a tower block when they are not entirely sure if it is or is not an essential component of the ensemble. A small wiggle that reverberates may or may not be forgiving enough to leave the structure intact if the piece is gently nudged back into place. Call that the slow dosage reduction approach to gauging relapse potential. Bold, sweeping removals of a component are daring maneuvers, although prominent and persistent symptoms inescapably leave one doubting the necessity of a structural component – unless things were to go from bad to worse upon swift removal of a perceived "irrelevant" element. One must be quite certain about the utter lack of usefulness and relevance of a component before pulling it from the tower.

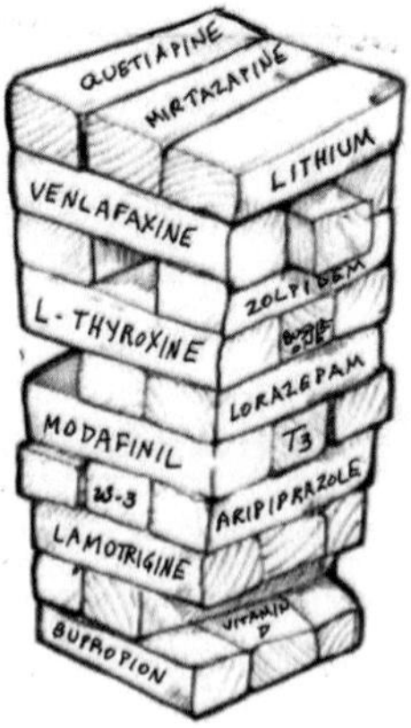

Are there Jenga® rules for deprescribing psychotropic drugs? We would propose those we have created in Box 9.6 as a means to prevent, or at least minimize, the risk of structural collapse.

Box 9.6

Rules of pharmacological Jenga®

- Gauge, as best as possible, the probability that the component of a regimen being considered for removal is *definitely irrelevant*, *probably irrelevant*, or *possibly irrelevant*. "Definites" can probably be dispatched more rapidly (all else being pharmacokinetically equal) than "probables" or "possibles," inasmuch as slow removals preserve the opportunity to put things back the way they were if the situation becomes wobbly
- Anticipate the potential interactive effects of removing one component relative to those remaining. Eliminating a drug that induces or inhibits the metabolism of the remaining components may require dosage compensation (e.g., doubling a lamotrigine dose if concurrent divalproex becomes removed)
- Do not remove a component of the regimen until enough time has elapsed to judge relevance (that is, an adequate trial) – unless poor tolerability supersedes the completion of an adequate trial
- Once stability is reached, *do not breathe on the regimen* for at least 6 months – the time frame in which recovery is generally measured – without a very compelling reason (e.g., poor tolerability of an existing regimen component) before proposing to play Jenga®
- The mechanics of removing a component within a regimen may very well be different depending on whether that component is being replaced by a new component. New components are often unvetted in a given patient; hence, recognize that the "new" piece may take time before you can judge its usefulness, and making a "swap" is in some ways trickier than the simple elimination of a defunct or ineffective component with no needed replacement
- When in doubt, *do not pull it out*

TAKE-HOME POINTS

- Recognize clinical situations in which the sequence of interventions has hierarchical importance because of the impact of one treatment on a system-wise clinical presentation
- Always have a Plan B and Plan C and quite possibly Plans D, E, and F
- When making changes to a medication regimen, understand the impact of half-lives, effects on seizure threshold, potential for withdrawal states, and pharmacokinetic interactions between incoming and outgoing medications in order to anticipate the need for cross-tapers versus safe direct switch-overs
- Cautiously deprescribe medications for which lack of efficacy is definite or highly probable
- Integrate concepts from palliative psychiatry and the chronic medical model for patients with high levels of treatment resistance, for whom the goals of treatment may revolve more around disease management than disease modification

References

Aaronson ST, Sears P, Ruvuna F, et al. A 5-year observational study of patients with treatment-resistant depression treated with vagus nerve stimulation or treatment as usual: Comparison of response, remission, and suicidality. Am J Psychiatry 2017; 174: 640–648

Aklillu E, Persson I, Bertilsson L, et al. Frequent distribution of ultrarapid metabolizers of debrisoquine in an Ethiopian population carrying duplicated and multiduplicated functional CYP2D6 alleles. J Pharmacol Exp Ther 1996; 278: 441–446

Albert U, Marazziti D, Di Salvo G, et al. A systematic review of evidence-based treatment strategies for obsessive–compulsive disorder resistant to first-line pharmacotherapy. Curr Med Chemistry 2018; 25: 5647-5661

Amerio A, Odone A, Liapis CC, et al. Diagnostic validity of comorbid bipolar disorder and obsessive-compulsive disorder: A systematic review. Acta Psychiatr Scand 2014; 129: 343–358

Amsterdam JD, Berwish NJ. High dose tranylcypromine for refractory depression. Pharmacopsychiatry 1989; 22: 21-25

Amsterdam JD, Fawcett J, Quitkin FM, et al. Fluoxetine and norfluoxetine plasma concentrations in major depression: A multicenter study. Am J Psychiatry 1997; 154: 963-969

Arnow BA, Blasey C, Williams LM, et al. Depression subtypes in predicting antidepressant response: A report from the iSPOT-D trial. Am J Psychiatry 2015; 172:743–750

Barbee JG, Thompson TR, Jamhour NJ, et al. A double-blind placebo-controlled trial of lamotrigine as an antidepressant augmentation agent in treatment-refractory unipolar depression. J Clin Psychiatry 2011; 72: 1405–1412

Barbosa L, Berk M, Vorster M. A double-blind, randomized, placebo-controlled trial of augmentation with lamotrigine or placebo in patients concomitantly treated with fluoxetine for resistant major depressive episodes. J Clin Psychiatry 2003; 64: 403–407

Bergeron R, Ravindran AV, Chaput Y, et al. Sertraline and fluoxetine treatment of obsessive–compulsive disorder: Results of a double-blind, 6-month treatment study. J Clin Psychopharmacol 2002; 22: 148–154

Brandt L, Bschor T, Henssler J, et al. Antipsychotic withdrawal symptoms: A systematic review and meta-analysis. Front Psychiatry 2020; 11: 569912

Brunswick DJ, Amsterdam JD, Fawcett J, et al. Fluoxetine and norfluoxetine plasma concentrations during relapse-prevention treatment. J Affect Disord 2002; 68(2–3): 243–249

Chekroud AM, Zotti RJ, Shehzad Z, et al. Cross-trial prediction of treatment outcome in depression: A machine learning approach. Lancet Psychiatry 2016; 3: 343–350

Cole EJ, Stimson KH, Bentzley BS, et al. Stanford Accelerated Intelligent Neuromodulation Therapy for treatment resistant depression. Am J Psychiatry 2020; 177: 716–726

Connolly KR, Thase ME. If at first you don't succeed: A review of the evidence for antidepressant augmentation, combination, and switching strategies. Drugs 2011; 71: 43-64

Darab MG, Hedayati A, Khorasani E, et al. Selective serotonin reuptake inhibitors in major depression disorder treatment: An umbrella review on systematic reviews. Int J Psychiatry Clin Pract 2020; 24: 357–370

De Crescenzo F, D'Alò GL, Ostinelli EG, et al. Comparative effects of pharmacological interventions for the acute and long-term management of insomnia disorder in adults: a systematic review and network meta-analysis. Lancet 2022; 400 (10347): 170–184

Dunlop BW, Kelley ME, Aponte-Rivera V, et al. Effects of patient preferences on outcomes in the predictors of remission in depression to individual and combined treatments (PReDICT Study). Am J Psychiatry 2017; 174: 546–556

Dumas R, Padovani R, Richieri R, et al. Repetitive transcranial magnetic stimulation in major depression: Response factor. Encephale 2012; 38: 360–368

Dunlop BW, LoParo D, Kinkead B, et al. Benefits of sequentially adding cognitive-behavioral therapy or antidepressant medication for adults with nonremitting depression. Am J Psychiatry 2019; 176: 275–286

Fallon BA, Liebowitz MR, Campeas R, et al. Intravenous clomipramine for obsessive–compulsive disorder refractory to oral clomipramine: A placebo-controlled study. Arch Gen Psychiatry 1998; 55: 918–924

Fava M, Rush AJ, Alpert JE, et al. Differences in treatment outcome in outpatients with anxious versus nonanxious depression: A STAR*D report. Am J Psychiatry 2008; 165: 342-351

Fekadu A, Wooderson S, Donaldson C, et al. A multidimensional tool to quantify treatment resistance in depression: The Maudsley staging method. J Clin Psychiatry 2009; 70: 177–184

Gelenberg AJ, Kane JM, Keller MB, et al. Comparison of standard and low serum lithium levels for maintenance treatment of bipolar disorder. N Engl J Med 1989; 321: 1489-1493

Handelman K, Sumaya F. Tolerance to stimulant medication for attention deficit hyperactivity disorder: Literature review and case report. Brain Sci 2022; 12: 959

Hartwell EE, Feinn R, Morris PE, et al. Systematic review and meta-analysis of the moderating effect of rs1799971 in OPRM1, the mu opioid receptor gene, on response to naltrexone treatment of alcohol use disorder. Addiction 2020; 115: 1426-1437

Houston JP, Kohler J, Bishop JR, et al. Pharmacogenomic associations with weight gain in olanzapine treatment of patients without schizophrenia. J Clin Psychiatry 2012; 73: 1077-1086

Huhn M, Nikolakopoulou A, Schneider-Thoma J, et al. Comparative efficacy and tolerability of 32 oral antipsychotics for the acute treatment of adults with multi-episode schizophrenia: A systematic review and network meta-analysis. Lancet 2019; 394: 939–951

Kahn RS, Winder van Rossum I, Leucht S, et al. Amisulpride and olanzapine followed by open-label treatment with clozapine in first-episode schizophrenia and schizophreniform disorder (OPTiMiSE): A three-phase switching study. Lancet Psychiatry 2018; 5: 797–807

Kessler D, Burns A, Tallon D, et al. Combining mirtazapine with SSRIs or SNRIs for treatment-resistant depression: The MIR RTC. Health Technol Assess 2018; 22: 1-136

Koran LM, Sallee FR, Pallanti S. Rapid benefit of intravenous pulse loading of clomipramine in obsessive–compulsive disorder. Am J Psychiatry 1997; 154: 396–401

Lipkovich I, Jacobson JG, Hardy TA, et al. Early evaluation of patient risk for substantial weight gain during olanzapine treatment for schizophrenia, schizophreniform, or schizoaffective disorder. BMC Psychiatry 2008; 8: 78

Lo H-S, Yang C-M, Lo HG, et al. Treatment effects of gabapentin for primary insomnia. Clin Neuropharmacol 2010; 33: 84–90

Manber R, Buysse DJ, Edinger J, et al. Efficacy of cognitive–behavioral therapy for insomnia combined with antidepressant pharmacotherapy in patients with comorbid depression and insomnia: A randomized controlled trial. J Clin Psychiatry 2016; 77: e1316–1323

McGrath PJ, Stewart JW, Fava M, et al. Tranylcypromine versus venlafaxine plus mirtazapine following three failed antidepressant medication trials for depression: A STAR*D report. Am J Psychiatry 2006; 163: 1531–1541

Meyer JM. A rational approach to employing high plasma levels of antipsychotics for violence associated with schizophrenia: Case vignettes. CNS Spectr 2014; 19: 432–438

Myer NM, Boland JR, Faraone SV. Pharmacogenetics predictors of methylphenidate efficacy in childhood ADHD. Mol Psychiatry 2018; 23: 1929–1936

Nakajima K, Takamiya A, Uchida T, et al. Individual prediction of remission based on clinical features following electroconvulsive therapy: A machine learning approach. J Clin Psychiatry 2022; 83: 21m14293

Navarro B, Boulahva I, Obach A, et al. Switching to imipramine versus add-on mirtazapine in venlafaxine-resistant major depression: A 10-week randomized open study. J Clin Psychopharmacol 2019; 39: 63–66

Nelson JC, Baumann P, Delucchi K, et al. A systematic review and meta-analysis of lithium augmentation of tricyclic and second generation antidepressants in major depression. J Affect Disord 2014; 168: 269–275

Ninan PT, Koran LM, Kiev A, et al. High-dose sertraline strategy for nonresponders to acute treatment for obsessive–compulsive disorder: A multicenter double-blind trial. J Clin Psychiatry 2006; 67: 15–22

Noble EP. The *DRD2* gene in psychiatric and neurological disorders and its phenotypes. Pharmacogenomics 2000; 1: 309–333

Pagani R, Gasparini A, Ielmini M, et al. Twenty years of lithium pharmacogenetics: A systematic review. Psychiatry Res 2019; 278: 42–50

Pangaro LN. A new vocabulary and other innovations for improving descriptive in-training evaluations. Academic Med 1999; 74: 11

Pigott TA, Seay SM. A review of the efficacy of selective serotonin reuptake inhibitors in obsessive–compulsive disorder. J Clin Psychiatry 1999; 60: 101–106

Reimherr F, Amsterdam J, Dunner D, et al. Genetic polymorphisms in the treatment of depression: speculations from an augmentation study using atomoxetine. Psychiatry Res 2010; 175(1–2): 67–73

Remington G, Agid D, Foussias G, et al. Clozapine and therapeutic drug monitoring: Is there sufficient evidence for an upper threshold? Psychopharmacol (Berl) 2013; 225: 505–518

Roth T, Arnold LM, Garcia-Borreguero D, et al. A review of the effects of pregabalin on on sleep disturbance across multiple clinical conditions. Sleep Med Rev 2014; 18: 261–271

Rush AJ, Trivedi MH, Stewart JE, et al. Combining medications to enhance depression outcomes (CO-MED): Acute and long-term outcomes of a single-blind randomized study. Am J Psychiatry 2011; 168: 689–701

Schatzberg AF, Blier P, Delgado PL, et al. Antidepressant discontinuation syndrome: Consensus panel recommendations for clinical management and additional research. J Clin Psychiatry 2006; 67 (Suppl 4): 27–30

Sommer IE, Begemann MJH, Temmerman A, et al. Pharmacological augmentation strategies for schizophrenia patients with insufficient response to clozapine: A quantitative literature review. Schiz Bull 2012; 38: 1003–1011

Swagell CD, Lawford BR, Hughes IP, et al. DRD2 C957T and TaqIA genotyping reveals gender effects and unique low-risk and high-risk genotypes in alcohol dependence. Alcohol Alcoholism 2012; 47: 397–403

Thase ME, Rush AJ. When at first you don't succeed: Sequential strategies for antidepressant nonresponders. J Clin Psychiatry 1997; 58 (suppl 13): 23–29

Thase ME, Corya SA, Osuntokun O, et al. A randomized, double-blind comparison of olanzapine/fluoxetine combination, olanzapine, and fluoxetine in treatment-resistant major depressive disorder. J Clin Psychiatry 2007; 68: 224–236

Thase ME, Chen D, Edwards J, et al. Efficacy of vilazodone on anxiety symptoms in patients with major depressive disorder. Int Clin Psychopharmacol 2014; 29: 351–356

Tiihonen J, Wahlbeck K, Kiviniemi V. The efficacy of lamotrigine in clozapine-resistant schizophrenia: A systematic review and meta-analysis. Schizophr Res 2009; 109(1–3): 10–14

Wilens TE, Spencer TJ, Biederman J, et al. A controlled clinical trial of bupropion for attention deficit hyperactivity disorder in adults. Am J Psychiatry 2001; 158: 282–288

10 Prioritizing the Components of Any Decision-Making Model

LEARNING OBJECTIVES

- ☐ Recognize factors that govern patient candidacy for specific psychiatric interventions
- ☐ Articulate the roles for structured psychotherapy modalities when constructing patient-specific treatment decision trees
- ☐ Know the basic pharmacodynamic properties of commonly used psychotropic medications and the rationales and evidence bases that support or refute their utility in specific clinical situations
- ☐ Understand the goodness-of-fit between one potential therapeutic intervention relative to another for a given patient's clinical presentation
- ☐ Understand the concept of "proportion of explained variance" and its relevance for accounting for the features of a given patient's clinical presentation
- ☐ Identify endpoints for a psychiatric treatment versus the indications for indefinite treatment
- ☐ Differentiate pharmacological futility from the loss of hope within a psychiatric palliative model of care

A THE SINGLE MOST IMPORTANT FACTOR IN CLINICAL DECISION-MAKING

If we had to pick the single most important factor that goes into clinical decision-making in psychiatry, it would not be anything related to pharmacology, psychotherapy, genetics, Maudsley staging scores, or any other kinds of historical illness characteristics, but rather, it would be determining the appropriate level of care needed for a given individual patient. Why is that, given the many breakthroughs in neuroscience and our understanding of psychopharmacology? Nobel prizes have been awarded for elucidating the intricacies of second messenger signal transduction in neurons, but not for the intricacies of deducing the merits of an intensive outpatient program versus a partial hospital program. Or for knowing when a multidisciplinary "team" approach is wiser than being seen by an individual practitioner. For all the attention heaped upon presumptive brain mechanisms of psychopathology and the impact of evidence-based treatments thought to modulate brain dysfunction, one cannot escape the psychosocial context in which most mental health conditions arise. Chronic and recurrent mental health conditions often spill into people's daily lives in ways that can be tumultuous, volatile, and precarious. Coping with distress and adversity often can become a primary goal of treatment, and for some difficult-to-treat psychiatric conditions, questing for a medicine to eradicate chronic symptoms may sometimes need relegation to a secondary rather than primary objective. Many treatments in psychiatry are more disease-managing than disease-modifying (meaning, they may lessen the adverse impact of psychiatric symptoms but not necessarily eradicate or prevent them). Consequently, even the best of biological therapies may be no match for the vast problems patients often encounter with coping strategies, managing and tolerating negative affect states, negotiating interpersonal discord, maintaining role functioning, and dealing with feelings of emotional urgency.

Let us draw upon three case examples for better context, as illustrated in Clinical Vignettes 10.1–10.3.

Clinical Vignette 10.1

Veronica was a 20-year-old undergraduate who had longstanding problems related to volatile mood dysregulation, chronic suicidal thoughts, chaotic relationships, and maintaining consistency in her academic efforts and overall functioning. She had several brief psychiatric hospitalizations and multiple emergency department overnight stays during her teenage years for episodes of cutting herself and "feeling suicidal." She participated in several intensive outpatient programs focused around dialectal behavior therapy (DBT) but found it hard to make use of the skills being taught. She had been treated with a litany of psychotropic medications since about age 14, including various combinations of sertraline, fluoxetine, venlafaxine, vilazodone, bupropion, quetiapine, aripiprazole, ziprasidone, risperidone, lurasidone, cariprazine, lithium, lamotrigine, mixed amphetamine salts, and a course of 12 intravenous ketamine treatments, none with any discernible impact on her mood. She had seen several psychiatrists whom she collectively dismissed as "incompetent" or otherwise unhelpful to her, and never formed a meaningful working relationship with any psychotherapist. During her sophomore year of college, she stopped attending classes. A fight after sex with a man she had just met prompted a heavy drinking binge, which caused a blackout that led to an emergency department visit. She was again hospitalized, diagnosed with "ultra-ultra-rapid cycling bipolar disorder," posttraumatic stress disorder (PTSD), attention deficit-hyperactivity disorder (ADHD), and "borderline traits." A recommendation was made for electroconvulsive therapy (ECT) which she refused. She called the emergency services from the inpatient unit to request that an ambulance take her to a different hospital. Ultimately, she left the hospital against medical advice after several days and her mother began calling psychiatrists looking for a new doctor who could offer her a "fresh start."

Of the many striking features about Veronica's case, perhaps the most blatant is that none of the many interventions she previously received had been particularly helpful. Where does one go from here? If Veronica's mother contacted you for an appointment, would you decline to see her, even if for just an evaluation? Or would her story evoke a sense of medical heroism and inspire fantasies of rendering relief through some transformative new intervention? Might pharmacogenetic testing turn her ship around? What about repetitive transcranial magnetic stimulation (rTMS) or vagus nerve stimulation? Pick any medicine that she has not previously taken and call that her fresh start? Try them at supratherapeutic doses. Perhaps a monoamine oxidase inhibitor (MAOI), within the old model of "hysteroid dysphoria" (Klein and Liebowitz, 1982; Kayser et al., 1985). How about a more intensive individual psychotherapy to help her sort out the deep complexities of her life? Maybe a wilderness program? Perhaps a long-term residential treatment program where the goals of treatment would be ... well, elucidated over time based on a shared decision-making model?

Veronica seems destined to rapidly cycle through an ongoing succession of encounters with the mental health system, individual practitioners, programs, emergency departments, and probably more biological interventions in her future without there necessarily being a clear focus on what exactly might "stabilize" her multifaceted condition. The ultimate "parent" node in her personalized decision tree will necessarily involve, first and foremost, identifying the *setting* in which any kind of treatment can reasonably occur. Outpatient treatment by any solo practitioner will likely become consumed by a tsunami of chaos, and any initial rescue fantasies on the part of a well-meaning clinician will likely turn quickly to feelings of helplessness, overwhelm, desperation, and resentment. Psychodynamically minded clinicians will recognize this phenomenon as projective identification – that is, the clinician unconsciously adopts the same kind of intolerably awful feelings that consume Veronica, rather like contracting her infectious disease from close-proximity ministrations. So powerful is Veronica's ailment, the reader may find himself having a visceral reaction to Veronica without even having met her.

Clinical Vignette 10.2

Neal is a 28-year-old software engineer living alone, who has had longstanding periods of depression and a self-described ambivalent attachment style. His periods of depression tend to intensify in the context of ill-fated romantic pursuits – as he himself says, finding himself attracted to women with an avoidant attachment style who ultimately and predictably fill him with separation distress. Despite several years of psychodynamic psychotherapy and the possession of great insight into what he called "the blueprint of [his] operating system," Neal found little relief from symptoms of depression and anxiety. Serial trials of a number of traditional monoaminergic antidepressant medications and augmentation strategies with second-generation antipsychotic medications or lithium yielded little in the way of symptom improvement. After one particularly devastating break-up, his therapist became increasingly worried about his welfare and functioning. Though Neal denied suicidal thoughts, he became increasingly reclusive, ruminative, preoccupied, and inattentive to personal hygiene. Over about 7 months, Neal's psychiatrist successively changed his pharmacology: existing escitalopram was optimized to 40 mg/day, aripiprazole was added (without much benefit, but incurring akathisia at doses beyond 7.5 mg/day) and then switched to quetiapine up to 300 mg/day (producing mainly sedation), then escitalopram was switched to desvenlafaxine (again without distinct change up to 100 mg/day) and then the regimen was changed altogether to olanzapine–fluoxetine combination. Neal's Patient Health Questionnaire-9 (PHQ-9) scores remained in the high teens. He denied substance misuse. His therapist wondered if his ruminative preoccupations reflected either obsessive–compulsive disorder (OCD) or psychosis, to which his psychiatrist asked how either of those diagnoses would change management. He entered an intensive outpatient program without much impact on his symptoms as his treatment team grew increasingly weary and demoralized – which Nick, in turn, picked up on and began to feel the intensified distress of emotional abandonment.

Can projective identification go both ways? Meaning, did Neal begin to experience the exasperation of his psychiatrist and therapist, which then somehow played out to intensify his perception of rejection and emotional abandonment – now by his treaters, whose arms are thrown up in defeat? The fundamental parent node for Neal's decision tree, similar to Veronica's, does involve ensuring the appropriate treatment setting; his therapist, at least, feels overwhelmed because she cannot seem to make inroads in leveraging Neal's distress and she cries out for the psychiatrist to "do more" pharmacologically, or reroute Neal toward a higher level of care. Both are understandable reactions to his ongoing symptoms. But in Neal's case, his clinicians' discomfort in treating him as an outpatient encompasses, on the one hand, the urge to mobilize a broadened team approach (how big a village will it take?) and, on the other hand, the risk of conveying to Neal an implicit message that his problems are too much for any one person to handle, or tolerate, reinforcing his most basic fears.

And lastly, speaking of the idea of *tolerating* psychopathology, consider the case of Angelina in Clinical Vignette 10.3.

Clinical Vignette 10.3

Angelina was a 64-year-old widowed woman living alone who had chronic and persistent depression (as defined by dysthymic disorder in DSM-IV-TR (American Psychiatric Association, 2000)) and elements of generalized anxiety disorder. Though she was involved in many volunteer groups, took adult education classes, and frequently saw her small but stable group of friends, she struggled with feelings of loneliness and isolation, which she identified as the cause of her persistent depressed mood. Her psychiatrist, wondering about the reverse process (could depressed mood curtail her social functioning?), took her through a litany of medications over the course of many years, each of which for one reason or another routinely produced an adverse effect that led to her discontinuing them. Her expectations of medication side effects dominated over any alternative hypotheses that treatment for depression might help. Selective serotonin reuptake inhibitors (SSRIs) or serotonin–norepinephrine reuptake inhibitors (SNRIs) caused her tremors, insomnia or "jitteriness." Adjunctive second-generation antipsychotic medications either contributed to actual weight gain or frightened her with that possibility. Side-effect fears at times verged almost on paranoia, or at least all-or-none rigid thinking: she refused an MAOI for fear of having a stroke. She declined procedures such as rTMS or intranasal esketamine for fear of iatrogenic harm from "being a guinea pig." Angelina found DBT "interesting" but not applicable to her situation. She saw a "solution-focused" therapist, Dr. de Shazer, twice weekly, whose many ideas about strategies to counteract despair and loneliness she summarily rejected. Dr. de Shazer wondered at times if she needed hospitalization for the chronic suicidal ideation that she never acted upon. Her psychiatrist, Dr. Tollerare, noting that Angelina's symptoms seemed ego-syntonic, wondered if Angelina's main treatment goal was simply to have someone listen to her talk about her sense of misfortune but not make suggestions, and accept her wish not to undertake treatments that she deemed to be risky, which might actually alter her condition.

Take Angelina's situation as an example in which she *is* in the right level of care (an individual psychotherapy with adjunctive medication management), but her chronic level of distress and discomfort prompts Dr. de Shazer to wonder if she needs a treatment that provides more structure and intensity. To what end? Angelina is outwardly highly functional, not at all gravely impaired, and poses no imminent risk to her own safety or welfare. She is very unhappy with her life and wants to talk at length about her sense of victimhood from an unfair plight. She periodically drops the *s-bomb* – that psychiatric expletive about self-destruction that creeps out many a practitioner – coupled with being stubbornly unopen to any real dialogue, exploration, or input from a mental health professional, which makes Dr. de Shazer feel devalued and ineffectual. That in turn prompts his questions about a "higher level of care," since he is all about finding solutions, but he presumes that Angelina finds her complaints of suffering as ego-dystonic as he does. But what if – gasp – Angelina is less interested in change than in just having someone listen to her complain and acknowledge her unhappiness? What if the patient's and clinician's goals in that sense are misaligned? Does Dr. de Shazer need a round of acceptance and commitment therapy mixed with some DBT for himself, in order for him to better radically accept that Angelina's real objective may just be to have an audience? Should a dose of psychodynamic thinking be brought in, along the lines of pointing out that perhaps Angelina feels she deserves to suffer and encourage more exploration of why that might be? Or point out the paradox to her that on the one hand she seems to cry continually for help and yet on the other summarily rejects every lifeline sent her way? Is it OK for Dr. Tollerare to just sit with Angelina and be present, like a spotter at the gym, resisting the urge to offer concrete ideas or sound any alarm bells? Or should he reverse course and just carpet-bomb the dickens out of her paranoid rigidity with as much anti-dopaminergic pharmacology as he can muster, because, after all, her misery should not be so ego-syntonic, right? And if she cannot see that, maybe more medications will change that – right?

Let us move beyond alignment of the treatment setting with the goals of treatment and the severity of a clinical condition, with the hope that Veronica, Neal, and Angelina have collectively provided a sufficient illustration and educational experience.

B THE SECOND MOST IMPORTANT FACTOR IN CLINICAL DECISION-MAKING

If we had to pick what we would consider to be the *second* most important factor involving decision-making about therapeutic interventions, it would be the concept of **patient candidacy** for any particular treatment. This concept is ubiquitous throughout medicine but often underappreciated in psychiatry. It bears on the idea that from among what is often a wide field of many possible and potentially appropriate therapeutic options, individual patient characteristics govern someone's candidacy for undertaking a particular intervention with likely success. Cardiac surgeons who evaluate leaky valves tend not to rush to replace them without first considering a given patient's candidacy for the procedure and the expectancy of a successful outcome – taking into account factors such as their age, pulmonary and renal function, obstacles to wound-healing, and the degree of aortic valve calcification, among other considerations. Oncologists determine a specific patient's candidacy for an antineoplastic therapy regimen based on clinical features such as tumor markers, hormonal receptors, and, increasingly, genetic markers. In one sense, this approach to judging patient candidacy is an example of personalized medicine; but in a broader sense, it is also ruling in and ruling out basic features that inform the likelihood of futility before undertaking an intervention. Consider the decision to hospitalize a patient based on forming an estimate of whether hospitalization would yield a meaningful benefit, relative to alternative options, as described in Clinical Vignette 10.4.

Clinical Vignette 10.4

Nick was a 37-year-old single unemployed man supported by disability due to chronic depression. He struggled with chronic suicidal ideation but had never made a suicide attempt, and he had intermittent binge alcohol drinking but never required a formal detoxification, nor was he inclined to pursue treatment for alcohol use disorder. He had multiple brief psychiatric admissions, each typically lasting no more than 2–3 days, for complaints of suicidal ideation. On one occasion he presented to the emergency department and was evaluated by a psychiatry resident who knew him from previous admissions. Though Nick felt that he "needed admission" because he was not "sure" whether he might act on his suicidal thoughts, the resident expressed concern that frequent brief hospitalizations had become a pattern for Nick that had yielded him no real benefit, and felt that a different plan would be more sensible. The more Nick insisted on his wish to be hospitalized, the more the resident spoke about specific alternatives to hospitalization, the use of intermediate levels of care, and possible strategies to help Nick function more effectively in the community. Nick became frustrated, said he was not really interested in such ideas, and demanded to leave, declaring that he was not planning to kill himself but wanted to go look for another hospital that might admit him if the resident was unwilling to.

Nick's situation invites us to consider the goals of his treatment before making a decision about what to do in the context of his emergency department visit. Was he malingering? Perhaps. Was he seeking respite? Maybe. Did he perceive the resident's offer to help him develop a better outpatient plan, rather than use hospitalization as a fall-back solution, as confrontational of his limited coping skills? The resident's impression was that Nick's primary goal was neither to avert an imminent suicide attempt nor to get help in constructing a better plan for managing his life situation. It was not apparent that hospitalization would accomplish any specific therapeutic goal. Might Nick try to hurt himself? Of course he *might*, but is that a high probability? Absent the proverbial crystal ball, an assessment based on Nick's personal history and current presentation suggest that suicidal behavior would be a low-probability event. Nick's preference to go look for a more hospitable hospital speaks more to his future-orientation and capacity to adapt to the environment than a plan to harm himself, and in some respects may even be a wise move for Nick, depending on what Nick's own goals are for himself.

As another, more specific example of gauging patient candidacy for a proposed treatment, let us consider the decision to undertake a brief dynamic psychotherapy. The psychiatrist Peter Sifneos was a pioneer in the development of brief therapies, having devised a specific modality known as short-term anxiety-provoking psychotherapy (STAPP). He articulated criteria by which a patient's suitability and appropriateness for the treatment could be estimated in order to judge a likely successful outcome, as summarized in Box 10.1 (Sifneos, 1979). Factor analyses of these criteria have demonstrated their value in predicting successful outcomes from brief dynamic psychotherapy (Høglend et al., 1992); said differently, prospective patients who do not demonstrate these elements would be regarded as poor candidates for that treatment because it is unlikely to produce clinical improvement in those individuals. (Based more on theoretical than empirical grounds, psychodynamic therapists have long considered a patient's capacity to attain insight into their own lives and make use of interpretive statements as fundamental criteria for anticipating whether that treatment modality is likely to be an appropriate and productive endeavor.) Sifneos himself acknowledged the dilemma created by imposing strict criteria on suitability for this particular form of treatment, noting that over a 4-year period his team at the Massachusetts General Hospital identified no more than 50 appropriate candidates for STAPP.

Note that this approach is essentially an example of sample enrichment – that is, "cherry-picking" candidates for a specific treatment based on a priori expectations of likely success. Critics of enrichment would object to the lack of generalizability of outcomes if this were a clinical trial; proponents of enrichment would extol the same concept; one size does not fit all, nor should there be a reason to assume otherwise.

Box 10.1

Sifneos' criteria for judging suitability for brief dynamic psychotherapy

- A circumscribed focus
- High motivation for change
- Flexible interaction with the evaluation interviewer
- Above-average problem-solving capacity
- A history of mutual give-and-take relationships

C CRITERIA AND INDICATIONS FOR SPECIFIC PSYCHOTHERAPIES

How Sifneos arrived at the precise listing shown in Box 10.1 (and whether it represents a whittling down from a larger list of candidate criteria that were vetted through some empirical process) is unknown. Specific psychotherapy modalities, in general, often tend to reflect distinct psychological processes that underlie the theoretical orientation of that treatment, and presumably should be salient features in a given patient's presentation in order to be regarded as germane. Can everyone equally benefit from family therapy? (After all, is there not always *some* way to construe family dynamics as pertinent to a given psychiatric problem, or the impact of the patient's problems on the family unit?) Or should that modality be reserved primarily for instances in which compelling problems in the family system are prominent or bear directly on the reasons someone seeks treatment? Should cognitive therapy be reserved for clinical problems in which a patient's attitudes and beliefs about themself and their world are clearly faulty? Or is that a sufficiently universal aspect of nearly all psychiatric problems so as to make cognitive approaches equally pertinent to nearly all patients? Trauma-based psychotherapies would presumably be relevant only when specific traumatic events are thought to have contributed to the pathogenesis of a psychiatric problem (say, PTSD), but in a larger sense, who among us is entirely trauma-free, and if a past traumatic experience is only a matter of degree, where and how does one draw the line in determining a direct link between trauma as a *determinant* of psychopathology? What if a trauma-oriented therapist devotes inordinate time to hunting for a presumptive trauma when no salient trauma actually exists?

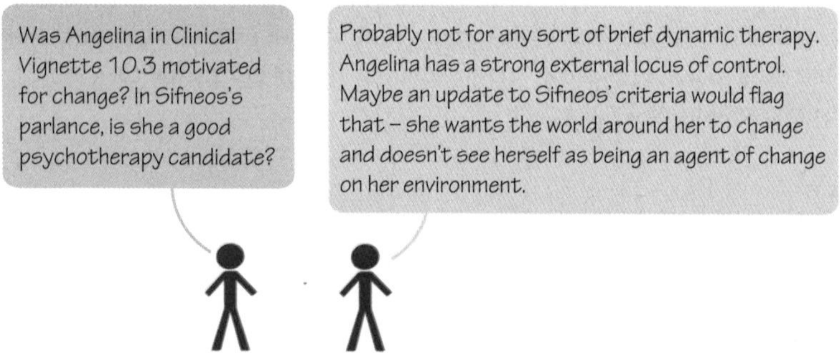

One might also ask what defines an adequate trial of a specific psychotherapy modality, with respect to duration and dose (i.e., frequency and length of appointments). And, if a course of psychotherapy were deemed unsuccessful for a given intended purpose, should the idea of iterative psychotherapy modality trials be considered, in analogous fashion to sequential pharmacotherapies? How does one decide, say, after a suboptimal response to cognitive therapy for depression whether to then prescribe a course of interpersonal therapy for depression? Lastly, are there times when one might consider augmentation strategies in psychotherapy, such as augmenting a long-term dynamic psychotherapy with a course of DBT? (Certainly, in modalities such as DBT itself, individual sessions are augmented with group-based sessions as fundamental to the overall treatment.) Are multiple psychotherapy modalities ever synergistic, or do their nonspecific elements (such as the relationship with the therapist) disrupt the idea of overlapping interventions?

There is not an extensive empirical or evidence-based literature to guide thinking about *differential* psychotherapy indications, or even when a particular psychotherapeutic approach is more appropriate than other types of interventions (e.g., pharmacology; environmental manipulation), aside from patient preference. Randomized comparisons of one psychotherapeutic modality versus another within the same diagnostic group (say, severe personality disorders) have largely not been studied. When considering when and whether to implement a structured psychotherapy within a decision tree, degrees of symptom severity also do not necessarily contraindicate implementing psychotherapy of some form or other, although it is hard to imagine the utility of a meaningful or structured psychotherapy in patients with catatonic mutism, delirium, disorganized psychosis, or profoundly melancholic and vegetative depression, who are largely uncommunicative.

In their text, *What Works for Whom: A Critical Review of Psychotherapy Research*, Roth and Fonagy (2005) describe different schools of thought behind different psychotherapy orientations and discuss the applicability of specific approaches (e.g., psychodynamic, behavioral–cognitive, interpersonal, supportive) to specific diagnoses. While they present an evidence base for the effectiveness of structured psychotherapies, they focus less on the distinctions between different modalities and their relative indications (or contraindications) for patient characteristics (such as attachment styles, attitudes and world views, past experiences, interpersonal dynamics, and functioning per se) than on implementation for psychiatric diagnoses. Consider, in this sense, the situation posed by Marie's depression in Clinical Vignette 10.5.

It is not so clear that Marie's symptoms are factitious (as in Munchausen syndrome) although her parents' apparent reinforcement of illness behaviors and maintaining the sick role is a salient component of her overall problem. Marie does meet diagnostic criteria for both persistent depressive disorder and somatic symptom disorder, but the context in which those diagnoses exist and persist holds relevance to her treatment. No somatic therapies have produced much leverage for her mood, while the idea of trying to extricate Marie from the sick role seems to be at cross-purposes with her engrained injured sense of self. Her parents' fierce resistance to an acceptance and commitment therapy approach, and its threat to divest her of emotional patienthood, suggests that forces are at play which likely go beyond efforts toward basic cognitive techniques such as behavioral activation and psychoeducation about depression. To the extent that

Clinical Vignette 10.5

Marie was a 30-year-old single woman with chronic depression and various medically unexplained physical symptoms, leading to diagnoses of gastroparesis, irritable bowel syndrome, and chronic fatigue syndrome. Her parents brought her to an endless succession of specialists from all disciplines seeking a cure for her physical debilitation. Psychiatrists offered the usual array of antidepressants, second-generation antipsychotics, stimulants, (ar)modafinil, benzodiazepines, and even ECT (the latter producing persistent memory complaints but little change in her depressed mood). The diagnosis of somatic symptom disorder (that is, acknowledged distress involving her physical symptoms and consequent disruption to her functioning) led to cognitive therapy approaches that did not loosen Marie's grip on constant preoccupations with her physical health. She and her parents resisted efforts to redirect her energies toward identifying and pursuing life goals given her predicament (that is, an acceptance and commitment therapy approach). Her therapist, hoping to tap some inner desire within Marie for autonomy and independence, wondered if an environmental change (moving out of her parents' home and into a therapeutic residential setting) might yield benefit. Marie called such suggestions "unempathic" and "a denial of her reality." Her father double-downed on finding more specialists to affirm the marked disability caused by Marie's condition, one of whom wondered about the possibility of Munchausen syndrome by proxy.

anyone on her psychiatric team so much as hints at encouraging Marie toward construing patienthood as an ego-dystonic experience, Marie and her family system bristle and clamp down all the more tightly in opposition.

Should the next step in Marie's decision tree be an umpteenth antidepressant? How about an experimental therapeutic for depression – realizing that enrolling in a clinical trial could reinforce the *idée fixe* that Marie's condition cannot be helped by any conventional methods. That could be a potential foot in the door, inviting an opportunity for change, if it provided a work-around to engage her and her family, rather than battle with them over their collective stronghold on her maintaining the sick role. There is no recognized excellent pharmacotherapy for somatic symptom disorder and, from among structured psychotherapies, mindfulness-based cognitive therapy, mindfulness-based stress reduction, and acceptance and commitment therapies are considered preferred modalities, yielding a medium effect size ($g = 0.51$) in meta-analyses (Maas Genannt Bermpohl et al., 2023). Beyond this, could a skilled family therapist provide value as a primary, rather than ancillary, strategist for defusing the bomb that is Marie's diseasehood? His or her mission, should he or she choose to accept it, would be to somehow call attention to the ways in which Marie gains affirmation or validation from her parents mainly through her suffering and sense of physical impairment and debilitation. Such insight, though probably accurate, might not do much to alter her sense of debilitation so long as it remains ego-syntonic. If Marie ultimately becomes a case of treatment futility, the decision tree will need revision to focus mainly on managing rather than modifying her condition.

Consider two more examples (Clinical Vignettes 10.6 and 10.7) in which the role of pharmacotherapy vis-à-vis psychotherapy enters with some degree of friction into a patient's decision tree.

Clinical Vignette 10.6

Daria was a 37-year-old woman previously in psychotherapy and diagnosed with dysthymic disorder, who was embroiled in an acrimonious divorce. Her children were the focus not only of a bitter custody battle but also were being pitted by one parent against the other amid accusations of parental alienation. She was angry, frustrated, dysphoric, and complained constantly to her therapist that she was fed up and did not know how much longer she could take the stress of the divorce. Her psychiatrist prescribed her a benzodiazepine for anxiety and agitation which she took appropriately, along with sertraline 200 mg/day for the diagnosis of dysthymia. However, apart from depressed mood and a sense of misery with her life circumstances, there were no vegetative signs or other tangible targets for pharmacotherapy. Daria called her psychiatrist with some regularity to report on her frustrations with her estranged husband; her psychiatrist would refer her back to her therapist to hone her skills for managing her distress; the therapist would in turn call the psychiatrist to reiterate how miserable Daria felt, asking if more could not be done pharmacologically.

Should Daria's psychiatrist seize upon the fact that she meets diagnostic criteria for dysthymic disorder and, based on that alone, try dosing sertraline supratherapeutically, or augment it with the usual augmentors, or switch to another antidepressant medication or two or more? Would we expect more aggressive pharmacotherapy *to do more*, in the absence of vegetative signs, coupled with the strong presence of a circumscribed life event, and her sense of victimhood? The psychiatrist will track Daria's mildly elevated PHQ-9 scores and ask about physical symptoms while she wants to talk mainly about the adversarial relationship with her estranged husband. One could hypothesize that more aggressive pharmacotherapy might give Daria a greater sense of agency over her life. The metric for gauging success would then not be her PHQ-9 score so much as the tenor of her complaints about her life circumstances. One could adopt this approach, but if it did not yield the desired effect, what then?

Clinical Vignette 10.7

Daria's cousin, Dahlia, also went through a contentious divorce, where the associated emotional stresses revolved mostly around disputes over money. Dahlia never worked while she was married and was awarded spousal maintenance for 7 years, which then ended. During that time, she continued not to work and did not plan for her financial self-sufficiency in anticipation of the end of her spousal support. She became highly distressed about how she would be able to meet her expenses and take care of herself. She met with a therapist recommended by a friend, who in turn referred her to a psychiatrist for a "med eval." The psychiatrist was struck mostly by lifelong features suggestive of histrionic and dependent personality traits, and resultant anxiety symptoms, which did not clearly constitute an anxiety "disorder." He was lukewarm about the idea of prescribing a benzodiazepine for anxiety and advised that she continue working in psychotherapy as the next step rather than exploring pharmacotherapies for which the targets of drug therapy (emotional distress?) seemed rather amorphous.

One thinks of pharmacotherapy when (a) there are clear target symptoms that define a clinical syndrome, and not just an isolated negative emotion, and (b) there is an impression of brain dysfunction. Medication cannot offset how one copes with the reality of stressful life events, but can address dysfunction in how the brain processes emotional information. Think eyeglasses for myopia, rather than for hazardous road terrain.

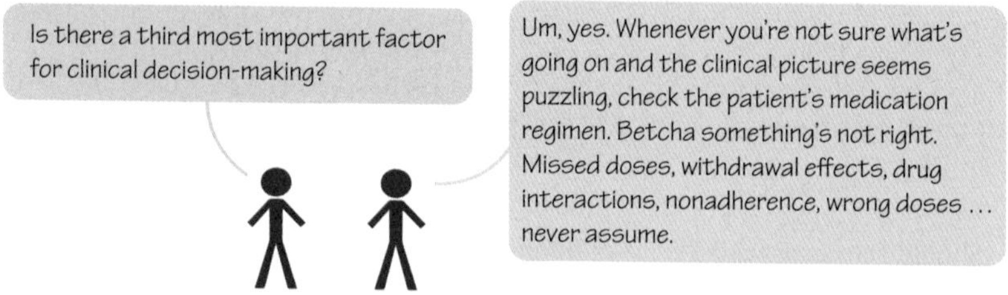

D USING THE RIGHT TOOL FOR THE RIGHT JOB

The above discussion brings us to a broader consideration around clinical decision-making regarding differential therapeutics, including pharmacotherapies. Our focus in this book has not been to review the relative evidence bases that exist to support the use of one potential pharmacotherapy relative to another, based on patient-specific characteristics – a topic for which we refer the reader to our earlier volume, *Practical Psychopharmacology* (Goldberg and Stahl, 2021). However, we would here touch on recognizing the basic appropriateness versus inappropriateness of distinct pharmacotherapy choices, appreciating whether or not class effects are evident across drugs that share certain mechanisms of action, and recognizing factors that point toward (or away from) one pharmacotherapy versus another when constructing a decision tree for a given patient.

This vast topic involves, among other things, recognizing when randomized trials have demonstrated where a drug is indisputably effective (e.g., lamotrigine for prevention of depression relapse in bipolar I disorder (Bowden et al., 2003; Calabrese et al., 2003)), demonstrably ineffective (e.g., topiramate for adult bipolar mania (Kushner et al., 2006)), or simply rationale-based but under-studied for efficacy (e.g., atomoxetine, based on its mechanism of action, for major depression). Related questions involve how clinicians make nuanced distinctions between two or more drugs that share similar-enough degrees of efficacy (e.g., deciding from among SSRIs to treat a first episode of major depression or generalized anxiety disorder – where comparative tolerability or data in special populations (e.g., pregnancy, children, or adolescents) may guide decision-making). There are also what should be obvious instances in which the intended use of a particular medication is inconsistent with the database to support that use, as illustrated by several representative examples in Boxes 10.2 and 10.3. Tables 10.1 and 10.2 summarize the existing evidence base for second-generation antipsychotic medications as monotherapies or adjuncts in the treatment of mood disorders, as does Table 10.3 for drugs commonly referred to as mood stabilizers.

Box 10.2

Examples of non-evidence-based pharmacotherapies in mood disorders

- **Gabapentin for mood disorders**: randomized trials in mania show no difference from placebo (Pande et al., 2000); there are no placebo-controlled studies in bipolar depression; one small (n = 25) randomized maintenance trial found a significant effect using the Clinical Global Impressions scale but, curiously, no differences from placebo in any specific mood rating or anxiety scale scores (Vieta et al., 2006)
- **Lamotrigine in acute mania**: there are nonpublished negative randomized trials in mania, and no database to suggest efficacy in this setting; relapse prevention data also demonstrate efficacy to prevent impending depressive but not manic episodes in bipolar disorder (Bowden et al., 2003; Calabrese et al., 2003)
- **Lamotrigine in major depressive disorder**: only negative published clinical trial data exist (Barbosa et al., 2003) – though admittedly the lack of an extensive database may reflect more the evidence of absence rather than the absence of evidence
- **Paroxetine for bipolar depression**: if one is going to choose a monoaminergic antidepressant medication to treat bipolar depression, it is better to pick one that does not have only multiple negative randomized trials (Nemeroff et al., 2001; Sachs et al., 2007; McElroy et al., 2010) and no positive trials

Box 10.3

Examples of non-evidence-based pharmacotherapies in anxiety disorders

- **Bupropion for the treatment of generalized anxiety disorder or panic disorder**: while there remains debate as to whether or not bupropion may be an "activating" and potentially anxiogenic agent for some patients, there is no body of evidence to support its use as a primary therapeutic agent to treat anxiety disorders, particularly in the absence of depression
- **Amphetamine salts or methylphenidate for anxiety symptoms**: tricky here is the question of whether an individual with ADHD or similar attentional complaints attributes subjective anxiety symptoms to problems with attentional processing; conceivably, "anxiolysis" could occur as a downstream consequence of improved attentional or executive functioning brought about by a psychostimulant
- **Escalating doses of long-term benzodiazepines for chronic anxiety in the setting of pharmacodynamic tolerance**: while the safety and efficacy of long-term benzodiazepines in anxiety disorders remains a subject of debate (Shinfuku et al., 2019), the development of tolerance (in which increasingly higher doses may be needed to recapture a lost response) is widely regarded as a slippery slope for which continued dosage escalations are not considered an advisable mitigation strategy

Table 10.1 Efficacy across mood states with second-generation antipsychotic partial agonists

	Mood state			
Agent	**Mania**	**Bipolar depression**	**Bipolar maintenance**	**Major depressive disorder**
Aripiprazole	>2 positive RCTS [1,2]	2 negative RCTs [3]	Prevents mania but not depression [4,5]	≥2 positive adjunctive RCTs [6]
Brexpiprazole	2 negative RCTs [7]	No data	No data	≥2 positive adjunctive RCTs [8]
Cariprazine	2 positive RCTs [9]	>2 positive RCTs [10-12]	No data	≥2 positive adjunctive RCTs [13,14]

Abbreviations: RCT, randomized controlled trial. References: [1] Keck et al., 2009; [2] Keck et al., 2003; [3] Thase et al., 2008a; [4] Keck et al., 2008; [5] Calabrese et al., 2017b; [6] Thase et al., 2008b; [7] Vieta et al., 2021; [8] Thase et al., 2019; [9] Earley et al., 2017; [10] Earley et al., 2019; [11] Earley et al., 2020; [12] Durgam et al., 2016a; [13] Durgam et al., 2016b; [14] Sachs et al., 2023.

Table 10.2 Efficacy across mood states with second-generation antipsychotic full antagonists

	Mood state			
Agent	**Mania**	**Bipolar depression**	**Bipolar maintenance**	**Major depressive disorder**
Asenapine	>2 positive RCTs [1-3]	No data	2 positive RCTs [4]	No data
Lumateperone	No data	2 positive RCTs [5]	No data	No data
Lurasidone	No data	2 positive RCTs [6,7]	1 negative RCT [8]	No data
Olanzapine	>2 positive RCTs [9]	2 positive RCTs [10]	Prevents both mania and depression [11, 12]	5 positive RCTs with OFC in treatment-resistant depression [13]
Paliperidone	>2 positive RCTs [14, 15]	No data	Prevents mania but not depression [16]	No data
Quetiapine	4 positive RCTs [17]	>2 positive RCTs [18]	Prevents both mania and depression (adjunctive) [19]	3 positive adjunctive RCTs [20]
Risperidone	6 positive RCTs [21]	No data	Prevents mania but not depression (LAI) [22, 23]	4 positive adjunctive RCTs [24]
Ziprasidone	>2 positive RCTs [25]	No data	(Adjunctive) prevents mania but not depression [26]	1 positive adjunctive RCT with escitalopram [27]

Abbreviations: LAI, long-acting injectable; OFC, olanzapine–fluoxetine combination; RCT, randomized clinical trial. Note, no large published RCTs in mood disorders exist with either clozapine or iloperidone. References: [1] McIntyre et al., 2009; [2] McIntyre et al., 2010; [3] Landbloom et al., 2016; [4] Szegedi et al., 2018; [5] Calabrese et al., 2021; [6] Loebel et al., 2014a; [7] Loebel et al., 2014b; [8] Calabrese et al., 2017a; [9] Chengappa et al., 2003; [10] Tohen et al., 2013; [11] Tohen et al., 2005; [12] Tohen et al., 2006; [13] Tohen et al., 2010; [14] Vieta et al., 2010; [15] Berwaerts et al., 2012a; [16] Berwaerts et al., 2012b; [17] Vieta et al., 2007; [18] Kishi et al., 2019; [19] Suppes et al., 2013; [20] Maneeton et al., 2012; [21] Rendell et al., 2006; [22] Quiroz et al., 2010; [23] Vieta et al., 2012; [24] Owenby et al., 2011; [25] Lombardo et al., 2012; [26] Bowden et al., 2010; [27] Papakostas et al., 2015.

Table 10.3 Choosing from among mood-stabilizing agents in bipolar disorder

Agent	Optimal clinical profile
Lithium	Few lifetime episodes (Gelenberg et al., 1989)
	Pure "euphoric" (rather than dysphoric) manias; absence of mixed features (Swann et al., 1997)
	Predominance of manic rather than depressive episodes (so-called "polarity proneness") (Scott et al., 2020)
	Absence of more than four episodes per year (i.e., rapid cycling) (Dunner and Fieve, 1974)
	Absence of psychosis (Scott et al., 2020)
	Absence of comorbid alcohol or substance use disorders (Scott et al., 2020)
	Family history of lithium-responsive bipolar disorder (Grof et al., 2002)
Divalproex	Equally responsive in multi-episode presentations (Swann et al., 1999)
	Equally responsive in pure or mixed/dysphoric presentations (Swann et al., 1997)
	Potentially more effective than lithium in reducing alcohol use patterns (Salloum et al., 2005)
Lamotrigine	Prevents depressive episodes much more than manic/hypomanic episodes (Bowden et al., 2003; Calabrese et al., 2003)
	For acute depression, may synergize with lithium (van der Loos et al., 2009) or quetiapine (Geddes et al., 2016)
	May have some greater anxiolytic properties than placebo but less than olanzapine (Maina et al., 2008)

To the above summary we would add several more nuanced points regarding possible pharmacodynamic distinctions among second-generation antipsychotic medications, as noted in Box 10.4.

Box 10.4

Additional considerations regarding second-generation antipsychotic medication choices in mood disorders

- **Asenapine**: has demonstrated efficacy in bipolar depression with mixed features (along with lumateperone (McIntyre et al., 2023) and lurasidone (McIntyre et al., 2015)); magnitude of antimanic response and remission is less than seen with olanzapine (McIntyre et al., 2010)
- **Cariprazine**: potent dopamine D_3 binding may suggest theoretical value in reward-based features such as anhedonia; anxiolytic properties demonstrated at low (i.e., 1–5 mg/day) but not high (i.e., 3 mg/day) doses (Earley et al., 2019, 2020)

Box 10.4 (cont.)

- **Lumateperone**: perhaps the most weight-neutral of second-generation antipsychotic medications; markedly greater serotonin 5-HT_{2A} than D_2 binding suggests particular value in patients who may be especially sensitive to extrapyramidal side effects
- **Lurasidone**: may have particular value to address cognitive symptoms in bipolar disorder (Yatham et al., 2017)
- **Olanzapine**: comparable antimanic efficacy to haloperidol but significantly less likely to lead to a depressive episode following mania (Tohen et al., 2003); while most clinicians are likely aware that olanzapine–fluoxetine combination is an established and on-label treatment for both bipolar depression and treatment-resistant depression, two olanzapine monotherapy randomized controlled trials have established its (off-label) use as a monotherapy for bipolar depression (Tohen et al., 2013)
- **Quetiapine**: has an extensive (off-label) database in targeting anxiety symptoms (Maneeton et al., 2016) as well as PTSD (Villarreal et al., 2016)

E A WORD ON THE IMPACT OF THIRD-PARTY CONSTRAINTS IN THE DECISION-MAKING PROCESS

It would be disingenuous to ignore the reality posed by third-party payers for mental health treatment as a factor in decision-making processes. For most patients, third-party payers absorb costs related to medications, hospitalizations, outpatient visits, intermediate levels of care, and even the extent and scope of appointments (e.g., can a reimbursable family therapy appointment occur on the same day as an individual psychotherapy appointment, or an appointment focused mainly on pharmacotherapy?). Tiered levels of approval for iterative treatments are often determined not by patient-specific symptoms and past nonresponses, but by raw cost, linked with assumptions that drugs within a broad class are sufficiently equivalent in their range of pharmacodynamic properties. Generic risperidone, aripiprazole, or ziprasidone each may be less costly than a branded antipsychotic medication to treat bipolar depression, but there are no data to support efficacy for those agents for that use (see Table 10.2). Even within a single institution, formulary restrictions or policies about access to levels of care may drive decision-making in ways that may not necessarily converge with evidence-based practices.

If there exists a solution to such healthcare policy dilemmas, it probably starts with the astute clinician maintaining a dual focus of thinking. One focus involves recognizing the evidence base and patient-specific characteristics that are likely to yield the best clinical outcomes, while avoiding options that are either irrelevant or otherwise counterproductive. The second focus involves an awareness of the limited resources available for a given patient in a given situation. And then brokering the best compromise possible, without sacrificing basic principles or yielding to inappropriate treatment injunctions. Perhaps a superbly trained surgeon can operate with primitive tools on a desert island and improvise to the best of their ingenuity, following as best they can their knowledge of core principles (aseptic technique; an excellent knowledge of anatomy) that limits interference by outside elements as much as possible. They also would not confuse the imposition of limited resources with best care practices. Mental health practitioners can adopt the same stance and not sacrifice knowledge of excellent decision-making even when circumstances limit their ability to implement best decisions.

F DIFFERENTIATING ON- OR OFF-LABEL VERSUS EVIDENCE-BASED PHARMACOTHERAPIES

From the larger clinical trials evidence base, clinicians should be aware of when a potential pharmacotherapy has or has not been studied for a particular purpose, whether the database behind that purposeful use is robust, preliminary, or contradictory, and whether there is a clear rationale behind the use of any proposed pharmacotherapy and the target symptoms of interest. One limitation in this area involves the commercial interests of proprietary drug (or device) manufacturers. Pharmaceutical manufacturers undertake studies of treatments for conditions that are likely to lead to US Food and Drug Administration approvals and commercial licensure to advertise the use of a medication for a specific purpose. However, the resultant database does not necessarily reflect a comprehensive assessment of the entire pharmacopoeia so much as the presence of a commercially viable marketplace to justify a return on the investment of costs associated with product development. Drugs with waning or expired patent lives are unlikely to see the expansion of new commercial uses, even if they may be clinically or scientifically compelling, when there is no prospect of a return on the investment of sponsor resources.

G AIN'T BROKE DON'T FIX

The temptation to alter a stable pharmacotherapy regimen likely afflicts all stakeholders (patients, caregivers, prescribers, and nonprescribing therapists) at one time or another. Sometimes the decision to alter a stable regimen is thoughtful, judicious, and auspicious – a sufficient period of time has elapsed since symptoms were last present that the idea of simplifying a regimen may arise organically; or it may arise through planning and anticipation, following some basic ground rules (such as, a period of relative calm in someone's life with no major life transitions or stresses on the immediate or foreseeable horizon). Sometimes, as illustrated in Clinical Vignette 10.8, requests to tamper with a treatment regimen soon after an apparent successful outcome is attained can result in disaster.

Clinical Vignette 10.8

Cheryl was a 42-year-old married woman with chronic major depression with comorbid borderline personality disorder. She had emotionally volatile relationships and several brief affairs, which her dynamically informed therapist called "acting out her anger" toward emotionally unavailable early caregivers. She tended to see the people in her life as being all good or all bad and was prone to suspect anyone who came close to her as having exploitative intentions. It was hard to tell how much her anger and distrust of others drove her depression or vice-versa. She acknowledged low self-worth and often felt hopeless and passively suicidal. Her overall condition markedly stabilized on a regimen of semi-weekly intranasal esketamine plus olanzapine–samidorphan 5 mg–10 mg/day, as well as lithium carbonate 600 mg/day, lamotrigine 300 mg/day, and gabapentin used for anxiolysis at 300–600 mg nightly; she appeared euthymic for the first time in many years and, soon thereafter, the question was raised as to whether her pharmacology regimen could become more streamlined. When queried about side effects, she expressed more awareness of a sense of sedation, particularly after well-intended family members told her it was better for her to be on the fewest medicines possible. Her psychiatrist described the perils of pharmacological Jenga® (Chapter 9, Section O) and expressed concern that premature tinkering with her regimen could jeopardize her relatively nascent remission of symptoms. Nevertheless, sheer curiosity and external pressures ultimately gave way to caution and she insisted on stopping olanzapine–samidorphan. Within 2 weeks she was bedbound, hopeless, passively suicidal, and convinced that her marriage was the source of her unhappiness and she needed to leave it as soon as possible.

Important to the experiment that was Cheryl's olanzapine–samidorphan discontinuation is the role of a controlled observation paradigm. Decisions about when to time a discontinuation experiment are particularly important if they are proposed soon after improvement because premature drug cessation can obscure a possible transient placebo response. Additionally, changing only one variable at a time is essential to concluding whether the consequences of discontinuing this one component of her regimen likely takes either full credit or full blame for whatever the result may be. Were it the case that the outgoing drug had a longer half-life than olanzapine–samidorphan, the time frame for judging pharmacodynamic consequences would be longer than the 2 weeks observed in Cheryl's case. It can also be helpful to formulate a kind of advanced psychiatric directive with a patient such as Cheryl in making clear her wishes in the event that the experimental results lead to relapse, as seemingly occurred here. The assumption is that restarting the discontinued medication should restore euthymia, although sheer disruption to a stable equilibrium state might in itself lead to ongoing repercussions and a bumpier course than otherwise expected to regain lost strides. These would count as known risks in the informed consent process for engaging Cheryl's request to conduct a drug discontinuation experiment.

At the other end of the spectrum lies empirical testing to determine if a component of a medication regimen is indeed relevant –a question that is often best answered by purposefully stopping it under controlled conditions and observing for clinical worsening. A brief example is illustrated in Clinical Vignette 10.9.

Clinical Vignette 10.9

Casey was a 28-year-old woman with difficult-to-treat OCD that involved germ phobias, noting only partial improvement in her Yale-Brown Obsessive-Compulsive Scale scores despite optimized trials of various serotonergic antidepressant medications with second-generation antipsychotic augmentations as well as adjunctive trials of N-acetylcysteine and memantine. Diligently changing only one variable at a time, she reported feeling "spacey and fuzzy," with no diminished intensity of obsessive thoughts around contamination, since starting memantine initially at 10 mg/day with a subsequent increase to 20 mg/day. The mutual decision was made to stop the memantine to determine its culpability as well as apparent lack of efficacy 5 weeks after its initiation.

And finally, consider the potential sanctity of a longstanding equilibrium state, and the risks involved in imposing any disruption – even when there may be a sense that a treatment regimen could be improved upon. There are instances in which patients present with ongoing symptoms (or, at least, complaints about how they feel) paired with a medication regimen that may seem antiquated, suboptimal, or even inappropriate. But before unsheathing any weaponry, wait – how longstanding is the regimen? Like a tumor wrapped around an extensive tangle of nerves and blood vessels, chopping away at an entrenched regimen could fundamentally disrupt a longstanding homeostasis and bring about disaster if done without delicacy and caution.

H HOLD THAT POSE

Altering a stable regimen is often unwise before a clear signal of sustained wellness has been established. Some experts advocate a period of not less than 6 months following the occurrence of a stable remission before even contemplating the alteration of any components of an apparently successful treatment regimen, short of substantial adverse effects. Why 6 months? For one reason, that is the time frame conventionally adopted for defining recovery in a consensus statement from the American College of Neuropsychopharmacology (Rush et al., 2006) and by the MacArthur Foundation (Frank et al., 1991). It is also the time frame in which the greatest likelihood exists for observing a return of symptoms from the index episode, across most disorders.

I ON-OFF-ON DESIGNS

Note as a corollary to the hypothesis-testing scenario illustrated in Casey's situation, in Clinical Vignette 10.9, is the on–off–on experimental design – readily implemented in an individual patient as an *n*-of-1 trial. Here, when a causal effect (either good or bad) from a particular intervention is ambiguous, one might propose stopping the agent and then restarting it as a way to test the likelihood of a true drug effect. Clinician-observers must take into consideration the terminal elimination half-life of the drug in question (agents with particularly long half-lives, such as fluoxetine, aripiprazole, or cariprazine, may take longer to judge the effects of discontinuation; and agents with especially short half-lives (such as risperidone or ziprasidone, and many SSRIs) may trigger rebound effects of abrupt cessation rather than being gradually stopped).

Closely following decisions about matching the right level of care with the gravity, severity, and nature of an individual clinical presentation is the *choice of treatment modalities*. Many of the pertinent decisions here echo themes discussed throughout Chapter 5; sometimes, decision-making can have an honest degree of arbitrariness. As we saw in Chapter 5, the decision to treat mild-to-moderate forms of depression with psychotherapy versus pharmacology versus both may hinge more on patient preference than on an evidence base favoring the efficacy of one approach over another. In other instances, seasoned clinicians often bring to bear some wisdom and experience for gauging the likelihood that pharmacology would be more helpful than futile; or that symptoms arising within a compelling psychosocial context are perhaps more deserving of psychotherapeutic interventions as a more contextually specific than arbitrary treatment modality. Consider the "fit" of the psychotherapy modality in Clinical Vignette 10.10.

Clinical Vignette 10.10

Charles was a 23-year-old man treated for major depression, who recently completed college, was searching diligently for employment, and lived with his parents. They felt that he invoked the idea of "being" depressed as a "crutch" to explain away his failure to procure work, and criticized his efforts toward achieving independence by highlighting his perceived failures and discounting small inroads such as arranging a job interview. His parents also were philosophically opposed to the idea of seeking mental health treatment and belittled his efforts to find a therapist or take medications. They micromanaged his decision-making and hovered extensively over his activities and interactions with others. His self-esteem suffered. Charles eventually found a self-identified "supportive" therapist who was untrained in family systems theory. She validated his feelings but made no comments on the impact of expressed emotion and verbal criticism as exacerbating his mood or posing obstacles toward his problem-solving efforts to improve his circumstances.

It is certainly possible that Charles might make some therapeutic inroads by working with the therapist he found, but there is an important psychosocial architecture that contextualizes his self- and world-views, which a nondirective supportive therapy is unlikely to bring to the forefront of his attention, or prompt changes in his point of view or sense of social competence. Perhaps a family-focused or even cognitively oriented psychotherapy would be a more precise tool for the job he is trying to tackle.

J WHEN AND HOW TO SUMMON YOUR INNER STATISTICIAN

Statisticians construct models to explain the variability of a phenomenon based on how well a set of variables governs that phenomenon. We would propose that clinicians might find it useful to adopt the mindset of a statistician when trying to understand or reason through the various factors that might account for the phenomenological presentation of a given patient. If the patient were one big regression model, the clinician's inner statistician would apportion different degrees of importance to the plethora of candidate factors that might account for what they see.

> **Tip**
> Linear regression is a statistical approach in which one examines how well a number of variables can independently and collectively explain the amount of variability in a parameter of interest (say, overall symptom severity).

How *much* does family history contribute to the observable phenomenology? How about interpersonal style and personality structure? Does a trauma history account for the magnitude of symptom severity, medication resistance, or emotional distress with which a given patient presents? What about past substance abuse? Is a history of head injury a small or large contributor to the overall clinical picture? Statisticians are thrilled when they capture enough relevant variables that explain a high proportion of the variance, as elaborated further in Box 10.5.

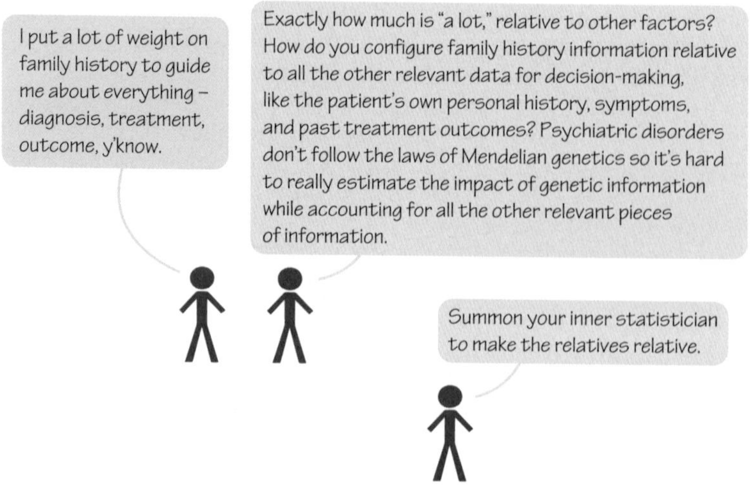

Box 10.5

Proportion of explained variance

In statistics - specifically, linear regression - the **proportion of explained variance** is a quantity expressed as R^2. It is essentially yet another way of describing an effect size. A large R^2 means that the collection of variables one has assembled accounts for a substantial amount of the variability one sees in the phenomenon being studied. A model with an R^2 of 100% would be stupendous, and rather impossible - every last morsel of relevant information has been accounted for. In real-world statistics, an R^2 of just 9% is considered to be a medium effect, and an R^2 of 25% is considered a large effect.

"Variance" is statistical parlance for how much the value of something is spread out from its mean value. Take intelligence quotient (IQ) as an example. If the mean IQ of a population is 100, and one wanted to identify factors that could account for meaningfully higher or lower values than 100, one might explore relevant explanatory variables (such as education level, socioeconomic status, and inherent motivation). Now take someone's Hamilton Anxiety Scale (HAM-A) score as the (dependent) variable of interest. We could hypothesize for a given individual that their duration of symptoms, comorbid depression, sleep quality, and level of social supports might explain much of the variance in their current symptom severity. We can test that hypothesis by targeting these variables in a treatment plan; if improved depression, sleep quality, and social supports lessens their HAM-A score (we cannot really leverage chronicity), our hypothesis would seem to be correct.

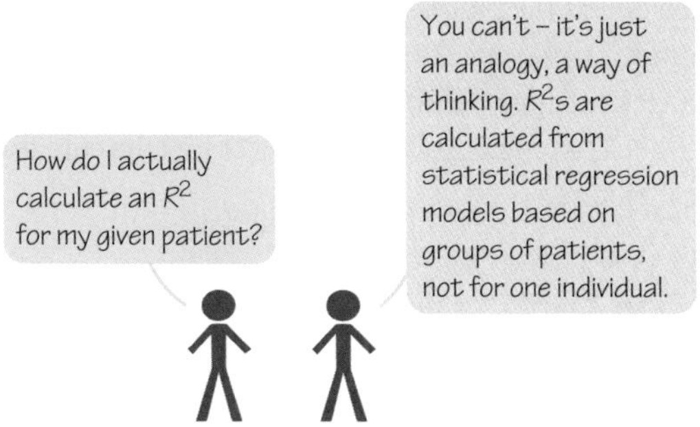

Now let us apply the same reasoning process of constructing an explanatory model to assemble the elements of a coherent and relevant treatment plan. Strong statistical models are said to have high explanatory power, meaning they have ruled in variables that are most relevant and ruled out those that are extraneous for a given patient. Box 10.6 provides some examples of potentially relevant "candidate parameters" one might want to account for when creating a mental "regression model" to explain the variance in a given patient's presentation.

Box 10.6

Examples of clinical factors that can influence variance in observed psychiatric symptoms

• Age	• Distress tolerance
• Mood	• Attentional processing
• Energy	• Cognitive flexibility
• Thought processes	• Chronicity
• Personality structure	• Past treatment response/nonresponse
• Impulse control	• Intact reality-testing

When clinical decision-makers have identified a reasonable and appropriate panel of factors that likely account sufficiently for explaining the variance in a clinical phenomenon, a treatment plan can then be developed which appropriately and relevantly targets the fundamental elements of the model. This means that extraneous factors get rejected because they may be tangential or otherwise not so relevant to the variables that explain the phenomenon. Throwing lithium into the mix of an eating disorder regimen is out of place because it fails to address the processes that underlie eating disorders. So does amphetamine for panic attacks or buspirone for negative symptoms in schizophrenia. A treatment model should be based on rationales and evidence that is targeted to (i.e., has high explanatory power for) the core features driving the overall clinical picture.

J.1 Goodness of Fit

How well the proposed interventions conform to the model brings us to the statistical concept of **goodness of fit**. As the term implies, goodness of fit refers to how well empirical observations align with the theory, or hypotheses, being tested to explain or account for the clinical phenomena being treated.

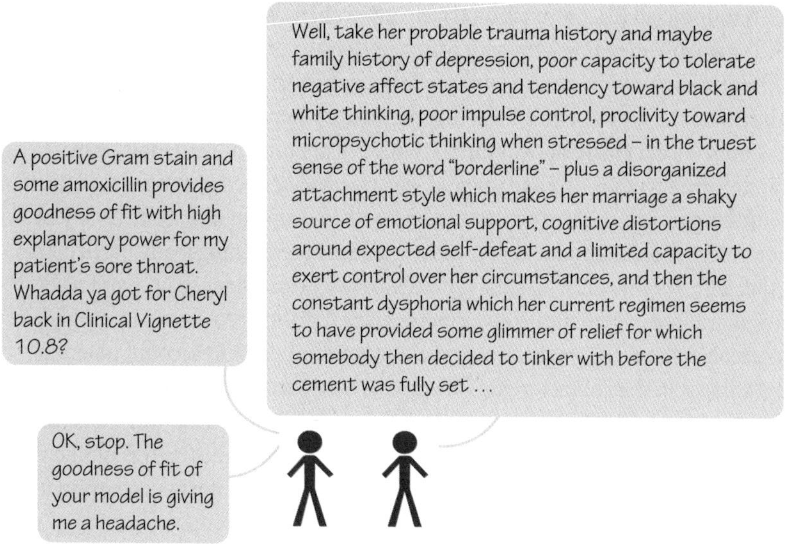

J.2 Interaction Effects

An interaction effect means that two or more variables exert some influence on each other, which in turn produces a unique effect on the phenomenon being studied. Examples of interaction effects might include the interaction between age and antidepressant medication exposure influencing the risk of suicidal behavior when taking antidepressants, age and declining metabolic clearance, and pharmacokinetic effects when one drug inhibits the metabolism of another.

K TREATMENT ENDPOINTS REVISITED

Perhaps one of the most underappreciated deficiencies in both psychopharmacology teaching and the evidence-based literature is knowing when to stop a treatment after it has produced a benefit. We previously touched briefly on this issue in Chapter 5, Section N. Arbitrariness, or happenstance, often ends up dictating such decisions by default; a patient runs out of a medication after a period of wellness and decides to see what happens if they remain off. Someone pauses a treatment due to a medical illness or a perceived side effect, which then abates, and they then similarly decide to continue off the medication to determine if it was really so necessary. Or a third-party payer or manufacturer may sometimes dictate a pharmacological endpoint when a drug either is no longer available or no longer financially feasible to continue. Planned discontinuations on clinical grounds, and parameters to guide or inform such decisions, are seldom articulated.

Randomized discontinuation trials, rather than observational studies, are the only truly meaningful way in which to draw scientific inferences about the optimal duration of drug efficacy for purposes of relapse prevention, or to anticipate the kinds of problems that may arise when a long-term medication is stopped for a particular condition. A logistical problem with long-term randomized trials is dropout; over a 1-year period, it is common for two-thirds to three-quarters of an intent-to-treat sample to drop out of a study (often not at random; healthier patients may lose interest in remaining study participants, especially as other activities may increasingly take precedence in their lives). Resultant loss of statistical power then makes it difficult to draw meaningful inferences about the medication effects without taking into account potential differences in the characteristics of patients who leave early or stay for the duration of a trial. Moreover, given that the vast majority of clinical trials research worldwide is conducted by the private pharmaceutical industry, it is unlikely that the field will ever see a dedicated study designed to inform consumers about when they should no longer purchase a manufacturer's product.

Even in the case of psychotherapy, treatment endpoints are not well described in the literature, apart from brief psychotherapies that are deliberately time-limited and have a prespecified number of sessions. (And, in reality, "booster" follow-up sessions after completion of a brief therapy "module" are often acknowledged as having value on an as-needed basis.) Let us also not consider psychotherapy "endpoints" that are arbitrarily determined by third-party insurers who impose reimbursement limits on the number of "allowed" appointments over a period of time. Curiously, we are aware of no formal guidelines issued by any professional society that articulate criteria for planning and implementing the termination of a psychotherapy unless the modality is prespecified as "brief therapy." Some authors on the topic of psychotherapy termination point out that treatment should end when its goals have been achieved, that is, when symptoms and functioning are improved (Joyce et al., 2007), perhaps with less focus on lifelong conditions whose symptoms may wax and wane indefinitely. Defining "goal achievement" in psychotherapy becomes more tangible when the outcome is a depression rating scale score than when the substrate for psychotherapy involves trying to modify engrained maladaptive personality traits (such as, entitlement, lack of empathy, interpersonal exploitativeness, or tendencies toward self-sabotage).

Psychotherapy ideally, and as much as pharmacotherapy, instills a preventative action plan to manage relapses and provide skills for managing recurrent or chronic symptoms or stresses that may be incidental to a psychiatric diagnosis. Observational studies have shown that patients who carry the diagnosis of a "major mental illness" are more likely to be viewed as candidates for indefinite psychotherapy in some form or other, with no notion of a prespecified intended endpoint (Friedlander et al., 2014). In such instances, one might wonder if psychotherapy as a formal intervention may risk becoming conflated with the concept of "case management" for a potentially lifelong chronic condition (or, said differently, indefinite psychosocial assessments may be an integral component of a disease management, rather than disease-modifying, mode of intervention).

One would imagine that "endpoint" criteria for psychotherapy termination would entail achieving the goals and objectives that were initially identified at the start of treatment. However, to the extent that psychotherapy often explicitly focuses more on making strides in quality of life, rather than achieving syndromal remission in a traditional disease-state model, one might argue that the idea of such an endpoint is necessarily subjective, or at least more a matter of relative degree (of life satisfaction) than a binary construct (such as, "recovered, yes or no?").

L THE PALLIATIVE MODEL WHEN FACING PHARMACOLOGICAL FUTILITY

At many points along the way in this book we have touched on the importance of recognizing when the probability of successive therapeutic interventions with the same modality (say, monoaminergic antidepressant medications for treatment-resistant depression) incurs diminishing returns. And that there likely comes a point that few clinicians (or patients) ever wish to acknowledge in which the probability of achieving greater strides after multiple failed treatment efforts greatly diminishes. Ethical dilemmas arise for the clinician. On the one hand, they may assume that the only way to instill and preserve hope is never to yield to the notion of defeat and continue prescribing medications ad infinitum rather than declare pharmacological futility. On the other hand lies the alternative honest reframing of a problem for which there may be no curative or even meaningfully beneficial intervention to offer. The focus then shifts from disease modification to disease management with greater emphasis placed on coping and acceptance under a chronic illness model.

Here is where the concept of managing a chronic illness comes into critical focus, and borrows heavily from the acceptance and commitment model described in Chapter 5. Pharmacological futility is not synonymous with untreatability or divestment of hope for any improvement, but it does mean adopting a realistic in-the-moment approach (it is unlikely that persistent, treatment-resistant symptoms will be going away any time soon). Some key principles that borrow from models of palliative care and chronic disease management are summarized in Box 10.7.

Box 10.7

Principles for a chronic medical management model in psychiatry

- Offer an honest appraisal that after many appropriate and adequate treatments have failed to yield a clear benefit, the probability is low that a new intervention will create a substantial improvement in symptoms, based on existing technology

Box 10.7 (cont.)

- Assure that diagnoses are accurate, to the best of one's ability, and that no psychiatric, medical, or substance use disorder comorbidities have been missed
- Assure that nonadherence or pharmacokinetic interactions have not caused pseudo-treatment resistance
- Deprescribe medications of no obvious benefit, changing only one variable at a time whenever possible
- Differentiate when residual symptoms or medication side effects are uncomfortable but manageable versus intolerable or hazardous
- Encourage second opinions or additional consultations with caution, if they run the risk of fostering unrealistic appraisals or magical thinking about disease modification
- Spare patients burdensome, overzealous, costly, or potentially exploitative interventions that have a low likely yield of benefit
- Revise the goals of treatment; this may include managing (rather than trying to eliminate) chronic suicidality, depressed mood, or persistent anxiety; attempt to make inroads in select target symptoms if feasible (such as chronic insomnia)
- Focus on strategies that can foster hope and a future orientation through resilience, coping, and identifying meaningful life goals within the framework of an acceptance and commitment therapy model

TAKE-HOME POINTS

- Recognize which clinical decisions take priority over others, including treatment setting, level of care, and appropriate fit between interventions and clinical presentations
- Pharmacological, psychotherapeutic, or other interventions should enter into a decision tree with a rationale and purpose, which includes patient preference and the evidence base to support a given modality for a unique patient's clinical presentation
- Favor decisions to stop a treatment in a nonarbitrary manner after the elapse of sufficient time to judge a sustained period of wellness, while considering the risk for decompensation if removing a treatment component proves that it had been integral to sustained wellness
- Do not confuse pharmacological futility with having nothing more to offer patients; ultra-treatment-resistant conditions often require a reorientation from disease-modification to disease-management approaches, with attention redirected toward living with and managing a chronic condition, revising the goals of treatment, focusing on quality of life, and minimizing adverse treatment effects

References

American Psychiatric Association. Diagnostic and Statistical Manual of Mental Disorders, 4th edition, text revision (DSM-IV-TR). Washington, DC: American Psychiatric Association, 2000

Barbosa L, Berk M, Voster M. A double-blind, randomized, placebo-controlled trial of augmentation with lamotrigine or placebo in patients concomitantly treated with fluoxetine for resistant major depressive episodes. J Clin Psychiatry 2003; 64: 403–407

Berwaerts J, Xu H, Nuamah I, et al. Evaluation of the efficacy and safety of paliperidone extended-release in the treatment of acute mania: A randomized, double-blind, dose-response study. J Affect Disord 2012a; 136 (1–2): e51–e60

Berwaerts J, Melkote R, Nuamah I, et al. A randomized, placebo- and active-controlled study of paliperidone extended-release as maintenance treatment in patients with bipolar I disorder after an acute manic or mixed episode. J Affect Disord 2012b; 138: 247–258

Bowden CL, Calabrese JR, Sachs G, et al. A placebo-controlled 18-month trial of lamotrigine and lithium maintenance treatment in recently manic or hypomanic patients with bipolar I disorder. Arch Gen Psychiatry 2003; 60: 392–400

Bowden CL, Vieta E, Ice KS, et al. Ziprasidone plus a mood stabilizer in subjects with bipolar I disorder: A 6-month, randomized, placebo-controlled, double-blind trial. J Clin Psychiatry 2010; 71: 130–137

Calabrese JR, Bowden CL, Sachs G, et al. A placebo-controlled 18-month trial of lamotrigine and lithium maintenance treatment in recently depressed patients with bipolar I disorder. J Clin Psychiatry 2003; 64: 1013–1024

Calabrese JR, Pikalov A, Streicher C, et al. Lurasidone in combination with lithium or valproate for the maintenance treatment of bipolar I disorder. Eur Neuropsychopharmacol 2017a; 27: 865–876

Calabrese JR, Sanchez R, Jin N, et al. Efficacy and safety of aripiprazole once-monthly in the maintenance treatment of bipolar I disorder: A double-blind, placebo-controlled, 52-week randomized withdrawal study. J Clin Psychiatry 2017b; 78: 324–331

Calabrese JR, Durgam S, Satlin A, et al. Efficacy and safety of lumateperone for major depressive episodes associated with bipolar I or bipolar II disorder: a phase 3 randomized placebo- controlled trial. Am J Psychiatry 2021; 178: 1098–1106

Chengappa KNR, Baker RW, Shao L, et al. Rates of response, euthymia and remission in two placebo-controlled olanzapine trials for bipolar mania. Bipolar Disord 2003; 5: 1–5

Dunner DL, Fieve RR. Clinical factors in lithium carbonate prophylaxis failure. Arch Gen Psychiatry 1974; 30: 229–233

Durgam S, Earley W, Lipschitz A, et al. An 8-week randomized, double-blind, placebo-controlled evaluation of the safety and efficacy of cariprazine in patients with bipolar I depression. Am J Psychiatry 2016a; 173: 271–281

Durgam S, Earley W, Guo H, et al. Efficacy and safety of adjunctive cariprazine in inadequate responders to antidepressants: A randomized, double-blind, placebo-controlled study in adult patients with major depressive disorder. J Clin Psychiatry 2016b; 77: 371–378

Earley W, Durgam S, Lu K, et al. Tolerability of cariprazine in the treatment of acute bipolar I mania: A pooled post hoc analysis of 3 phase II/III studies. J Affect Disord 2017; 215: 205–212

Earley W, Burgess MV, Rekeda L, et al. Cariprazine treatment of bipolar depression: A randomized double-blind placebo-controlled phase 3 study. Am J Psychiatry 2019; 176: 439–448

Earley WR, Burgess MV, Khan B, et al. Efficacy and safety of cariprazine in bipolar I depression: A double-blind, placebo-controlled phase 3 study. Bipolar Disord 2020; 22: 372–384

Frank E, Prien RF, Jarrett RB, et al. Conceptualization and rationale for consensus definitions of terms in major depressive disorder. Remission, recovery, relapse, and recurrence. Arch Gen Psychiatry 1991; 48: 851–855

Friedlander ML, Austin CL, Cabrera P. When psychotherapy is indefinite and there is no final outcome: Case study of a community mental health clinic. Psychotherapy (Chic) 2014; 51: 580–594

Geddes JR, Gardiner A, Rendell J, et al. Lurasidone versus treatment as usual for cognitive impairment in euthymic patients with bipolar I disorder: A randomised, open-label, pilot study. Lancet Psychiatry 2016; 3: 31–39

Gelenberg AJ, Kane JM, Keller MB, et al. Comparison of standard and low serum levels of lithium for maintenance treatment of bipolar disorder. N Engl J Med 1989; 321: 1489–1493

Goldberg JF, Stahl SM. Practical Psychopharmacology: Translating Findings from Evidence-Based Trials into Real-World Clinical Practice. Cambridge: Cambridge University Press, 2021

Grof P, Duffy A, Cavazzoni P, et al. Is response to prophylactic lithium a familial trait? J Clin Psychiatry 2002; 62: 942–947

Høglend P, Sørbye Ø, Sørlie T, et al. Selection criteria for brief dynamic psychotherapy: Reliability, factor structure and long-term predictive value. Psychother Psychosom 1992; 57: 67–74

Joyce AS, Piper WE, Ogrodniczuk JS, et al. Termination in Psychotherapy: A Psychodynamic Model of Processes and Outcomes. Washington, DC: American Psychological Association, 2007

Kayser A, Robinson DS, Nies A, et al. Response to phenelzine among depressed patients with features of hysteroid dysphoria. Am J Psychiatry 1985; 142: 486–488

Keck PE Jr., Marcus R, Tourkodimitris S, et al. A placebo-controlled, double-blind study of the efficacy and safety of aripiprazole in patients with acute bipolar mania. Am J Psychiatry 2003; 160: 1651–1658

Keck PE Jr., Calabrese JR, McIntyre RS, et al. Aripiprazole monotherapy for maintenance therapy in bipolar I disorder: A 100-week, double-blind study versus placebo. J Clin Psychiatry 2008; 68: 1480–1491

Keck PE Jr., Orsulak PJ, Cutler AJ, et al. Aripiprazole monotherapy in the treatment of acute bipolar I mania: A randomized, double-blind, placebo- and lithium-controlled study. J Affect Disord 2009; 112 (1–3): 36–49

Kishi T, Ikuta T, Sakuma K, et al. Comparison of quetiapine immediate- and extended-release formulations for bipolar depression: A systematic review and network meta-analysis of double-blind, randomized placebo-controlled trials. J Psychiatr Res 2019; 115: 121–128

Klein DF, Liebowitz MR. Hysteroid dysphoria. Am J Psychiatry 1982; 139: 1520–1521

Kushner SF, Khan A, Lane R, et al. Topiramate monotherapy in the management of acute mania: Results of four double-blind placebo-controlled trials. Bipolar Disord 2006; 8: 15–27

Landbloom RL, Mackle M, Wu X, et al. Asenapine: efficacy and safety of 5 and 10mg bid in a 3-week, randomized, double-blind, placebo-controlled trial in adults with a manic or mixed episode associated with bipolar I disorder. J Affect Disord 2016; 190: 103–110

Loebel A, Cucchiaro J, Silva R, et al. Lurasidone monotherapy in the treatment of bipolar I depression: A randomized, double-blind, placebo-controlled study. Am J Psychiatry 2014a; 171: 160–168

Loebel A, Cucchiaro J, Silva R, et al. Lurasidone as adjunctive therapy with lithium or valproate for the treatment of bipolar I depression: A randomized, double-blind, placebo-controlled study. Am J Psychiatry 2014b; 171: 169–177

Lombardo I, Sachs G, Kolluri S, et al. Two 6-week, randomized, double-blind, placebo-controlled studies of ziprasidone in outpatients with bipolar I depression: Did baseline characteristics impact trial outcome? J Clin Psychopharmacol 2012; 32: 470–478

Maas Genannt Bermpohl F, Hülsmann L, Martin A. Efficacy of mindfulness- and acceptance-based cognitive–behavioral therapies for bodily distress in adults: A meta-analysis. Front Psychiatry 2023; 14: 1160908

Maina G, Albert U, Rosso G, et al. Olanzapine or lamotrigine addition to lithium in remitted bipolar disorder patients with anxiety disorder comorbidity: A randomized, single-blind, pilot study. J Clin Psychiatry 2008; 69: 609–616

Maneeton N, Maneeton B, Srisurapanont M, et al. Quetiapine monotherapy in acute phase for major depressive disorder: A meta-analysis of randomized, placebo-controlled trials. BMC Psychiatry 2012; 12: 160

Maneeton N, Maneeton B, Woottiluk P, et al. Quetiapine monotherapy in acute treatment of generalized anxiety disorder: A systematic review and meta-analysis of randomized controlled trials. Drug Des Devel Ther 2016; 10: 259–276

McElroy SL, Weisler RH, Chang W, et al. A double-blind, placebo-controlled study of quetiapine and paroxetine as monotherapy in adults with bipolar I depression (EMBOLDEN II). J Clin Psychiatry 2010; 71: 163–174

McIntyre RS, Cohen M, Zhao J, et al. A 3-week, randomized, placebo-controlled trial of asenapine in the treatment of acute mania in bipolar mania and mixed states. Bipolar Disord 2009; 11: 673–686

McIntyre RS, Cohen M, Zhao J, et al. Asenapine in the treatment of acute mania in bipolar I disorder: A randomized, double-blind, placebo-controlled trial. J Affect Disord 2010; 122 (1–2): 27–38

McIntyre RS, Cucchiaro J, Pikalov A, et al. Lurasidone in the treatment of bipolar depression with mixed (subsyndromal hypomanic) features: Post hoc analysis of a randomized placebo-controlled trial. J Clin Psychiatry 2015; 76: 398–205

McIntyre RS, Durgam S, Huo J, et al. The efficacy of lumateperone in patients with bipolar depression with mixed features. J Clin Psychiatry 2023; 84(3): 22m14739

Nemeroff CB, Evans DL, Gyulai L, et al. Double-blind, placebo-controlled comparison of imipramine and paroxetine in the treatment of bipolar depression. Am J Psychiatry 2001; 158: 906–912

Owenby RK, Brown LT, Brown JN. Use of risperidone as augmentation treatment for major depressive disorder. Ann Pharmacother 2011; 45: 95–100

Pande AC, Crockatt JG, Janney CA, et al. Gabapentin in bipolar disorder: A placebo-controlled trial of adjunctive therapy. Gabapentin Bipolar Disorder Study Group. Bipolar Disord 2000; 2: 249–255

Papakostas GI, Fava M, Baer L, et al. Ziprasidone augmentation of escitalopram for major depressive disorder: Efficacy results from a randomized, double-blind, placebo-controlled study. Am J Psychiatry 2015; 172: 1251–1258

Quiroz JA, Yatham LN, Palumbo JM, et al. Risperidone long-acting injectable monotherapy in the maintenance treatment of bipolar I disorder. Biol Psychiatry 2010; 68: 156–162

Rendell JM, Gijsman HS, Bauer MS, et al. Risperidone alone or in combination for acute mania. Cochrane Database Syst Rev 2006; 1: CD004043

Roth A, Fonagy P. What Works for Whom?, 2nd edition. New York: Guilford Press, 2005

Rush AJ, Kraemer H, Sackeim HA, et al. Report by the ACNP task force on response and remission in major depressive disorder. Neuropsychopharmacology 2006; 31: 1841–1853

Sachs GS, Nierenberg AA, Calabrese JR, et al. Effectiveness of adjunctive antidepressant treatment for bipolar depression. N Engl J Med 2007; 356: 1711–1722

Sachs GS, Yeung PP, Rekeda L, et al. Adjunctive cariprazine for the treatment of patients with major depressive disorder: A randomized, double-blind, placebo-controlled phase 3 study. Am J Psychiatry 2023; 180: 241–251

Salloum IM, Cornelius JR, Daley DC, et al. Efficacy of valproate maintenance in patients with bipolar disorder and alcoholism: A double-blind placebo-controlled study. Arch Gen Psychiatry 2005; 62: 37–45

Scott J, Bellivier F, Manchia M, et al. Can network analysis shed light on predictors of lithium response in bipolar I disorder? Acta Psychiatr Scand 2020; 141: 522–533

Shinfuku M, Kishimoto T, Uchida H, et al. Effectiveness and safety of long-term benzodiazepine use in anxiety disorders: A systematic review and meta-analysis. Int Clin Psychopharmacol 2019; 34: 211–221

Sifneos P. Short-term Dynamic Psychotherapy. New York: Plenum, 1979

Suppes T, Vieta E, Gustafsson U, et al. Maintenance treatment with quetiapine when combined with either lithium or divalproex in bipolar I disorder: Analysis of two large randomized, placebo-controlled trials. Depress Anxiety 2013; 30: 1089–1098

Swann AC, Bowden CL, Morris D, et al. Depression during mania. Treatment response to lithium or divalproex. Arch Gen Psychiatry 1997; 54: 37–42

Swann AC, Bowden CL, Calabrese JR, et al. Differential effect of number of previous episodes of affective disorder on response to lithium or divalproex in acute mania. Am J Psychiatry 1999; 156: 1264-1266

Szegedi A, Durgam S, Mackle M, et al. Randomized, double-blind, placebo-controlled trial of asenapine maintenance therapy in adults with an acute manic or mixed episode associated with bipolar I disorder. Am J Psychiatry 2018; 175: 71–79

Thase ME, Jonas A, Khan A, et al. Aripiprazole monotherapy in nonpsychotic bipolar I depression: Results of 2 randomized, placebo-controlled studies. J Clin Psychopharmacol 2008a; 28: 13–20

Thase ME, Trivedi MH, Nelson JC, et al. Examining the efficacy of adjunctive aripiprazole in major depressive disorder: A pooled analysis of 2 studies. Prim Care Compan J Clin Psychiatry 2008b; 10: 440–447

Thase ME, Zhang P, Weiss C, et al. Efficacy and safety of brexpiprazole as adjunctive treatment in major depressive disorder: Overview of four short-term studies. Expert Opin Pharmacother 2019; 20: 1907–1916

Tohen M, Goldberg JF, Gonzalez-Pinto Arrillaga AM, et al. A 12-week, double blind comparison of olanzapine vs. haloperidol in the treatment of acute mania. Arch Gen Psychiatry 2003; 60: 1218-1226

Tohen M, Greil W, Calabrese JR, et al. Olanzapine versus lithium in the maintenance treatment of bipolar disorder: A 12-month, randomized, double-blind, controlled clinical trial. Am J Psychiatry 2005; 162: 1281–1290

Tohen M, Calabrese JR, Sachs GS, et al. Randomized, placebo-controlled trial of olanzapine as maintenance therapy in patients with bipolar I disorder responding to acute treatment with olanzapine. Am J Psychiatry 2006; 163: 247–256

Tohen M, Case M, Trivedi MH, et al. Olanzapine/fluoxetine combination in patients with treatment-resistant depression: Rapid onset of therapeutic response and its predictive value for subsequent overall response in a pooled analysis of 5 studies. J Clin Psychiatry 2010; 71: 451–462

Tohen M, Katagiri H, Fujikoshi S, et al. Efficacy of olanzapine monotherapy in acute bipolar depression: A pooled analysis of controlled studies. J Affect Disord 2013; 149 (1-3): 196–201

van der Loos ML, Mulder PG, Hartong EG, et al. Efficacy and safety of lamotrigine as add-on treatment to lithium in bipolar depression: A multicenter, double-blind, placebo-controlled trial. J Clin Psychiatry 2009; 70: 223-231

Vieta E, Goikolea JM, Martínez-Arán A, et al. A double-blind, randomized, placebo-controlled, prophylaxis study of adjunctive gabapentin for bipolar disorder. J Clin Psychiatry 2006; 67: 473–477

Vieta E, Goldberg JF, Mullen J, et al. Quetiapine in the treatment of acute mania: Target dose for efficacious treatment. J Affect Disord 2007; 100 (suppl 1): S23–S31

Vieta E, Nuamah IF, Lim P, et al. A randomized, placebo- and active-controlled study of paliperidone extended release for the treatment of acute manic and mixed episodes of bipolar I disorder. Bipolar Disord 2010; 12: 230–243

Vieta E, Montgomery S, Sulaiman AH, et al. A randomized, double-blind, placebo-controlled trial to assess prevention of mood episodes with risperidone long-acting injectable in patients with bipolar I disorder. Eur Neuropsychopharmacol 2012; 22: 825–835

Vieta E, Sachs G, Chang D, et al. Two randomized, double-blind, placebo-controlled trials and one open-label, long-term trial of brexpiprazole for the acute treatment of bipolar mania. J Psychopharmacol 2021; 35: 971–982

Villarreal G, Hamner MB, Cañive JM, et al. Efficacy of quetiapine monotherapy in posttraumatic stress disorder: A randomized, placebo-controlled trial. Am J Psychiatry 2016; 173: 1205–1212

Yatham LN, Mackala S, Basivireddy J, et al. Lurasidone versus treatment as usual for cognitive impairment in euthymic patients with bipolar I disorder: A randomised, open-label, pilot study. Lancet Psychiatry 2017; 4: 208–217

Index